MW00844756

Social Aspects of HIV

Volume 5

Series Editors

Peter Aggleton, Centre for Social Research in Health, UNSW Sydney, Kensington, Sydney, NSW, Australia

Seth Kalichman, Psychology, University of Connecticut, Storrs, CT, USA

Susan Kippax, Social Policy Research Center, UNSW Sydney, Kensington, Sydney, NSW, Australia

Richard Parker, Mailman School of Public Health, Columbia University, New York, NY, USA

John de Wit, Interdisciplinary Social Science, Utrecht University, Utrecht, The Netherlands

Since the start of the epidemic, HIV and AIDS have fired the imaginations of social as well as medical and public health scientists. This innovative series of books offers a setting in which to publish the very best of social scientific thinking and research. The Social Aspects of HIV series offers readers authoritative introductions and overviews, together with summaries of enduring and cutting edge concerns. The series is international and multidisciplinary in focus, including contributions from psychology, sociology, anthropology, education, economic, political and social theory, and international development. Individual volumes offer scholarly overviews of key topics and concerns but also address 'big issues' relevant to HIV prevention, treatment and care. Sexual and drug-related practices; adherence; disclosure; and stigma and discrimination are among topics focused upon, alongside broader cultural, political and social responses to the epidemic, including globalisation and internationalisation. The political economy of AIDS, links to broader questions of sexual health and rights, and the progressive biomedicalisation of the response, will also be among key issues examined. The series will appeal to those working in public health, health psychology, medical sociology, medical anthropology, health promotion, social work and international development. Individual volumes are relevant to students, teachers, researchers and practitioners within each of these disciplines as well as program developers and managers working across a variety of contexts.

More information about this series at http://www.springer.com/series/11922

Sarah Bernays • Adam Bourne • Susan Kippax •
Peter Aggleton • Richard Parker
Editors

Remaking HIV Prevention in the 21st Century

The Promise of TasP, U=U and PrEP

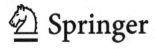 Springer

Editors
Sarah Bernays
School of Public Health
University of Sydney
Sydney, New South Wales, Australia

Adam Bourne
Australian Research Centre in Sex, Health and
Society
La Trobe University
Melbourne, Victoria, Australia

Susan Kippax
Social Policy Research Centre
UNSW Sydney
Kensington, New South Wales, Australia

Peter Aggleton
Centre for Social Research in Health
UNSW Sydney
Kensington, New South Wales, Australia

Richard Parker
Department of Sociomedical Sciences,
Mailman School of Public Health
Columbia University
New York, USA

ISSN 2509-6559   ISSN 2509-6567   (electronic)
Social Aspects of HIV
ISBN 978-3-030-69818-8   ISBN 978-3-030-69819-5   (eBook)
https://doi.org/10.1007/978-3-030-69819-5

© Springer Nature Switzerland AG 2021
Chapters "Anticipating Policy, Orienting Services, Celebrating Provision: Reflecting on Scotland's PrEP Journey", "How the Science of HIV Treatment-as-Prevention Restructured PEPFAR's Strategy: The Case for Scaling up ART in 'Epidemic Control' Countries", "Stigma and Confidentiality Indiscretions: Intersecting Obstacles to the Delivery of Pre-Exposure Prophylaxis to Adolescent Girls and Young Women in East Zimbabwe" and "The Drive to Take an HIV Test in Rural Uganda: A Risk to Prevention for Young People?" are licensed under the terms of the Creative Commons Attribution 4.0 International License (http://creativecommons.org/licenses/by/4.0/). For further details see license information in the chapters.
This work is subject to copyright. All rights are reserved by the Publisher, whether the whole or part of the material is concerned, specifically the rights of translation, reprinting, reuse of illustrations, recitation, broadcasting, reproduction on microfilms or in any other physical way, and transmission or information storage and retrieval, electronic adaptation, computer software, or by similar or dissimilar methodology now known or hereafter developed.
The use of general descriptive names, registered names, trademarks, service marks, etc. in this publication does not imply, even in the absence of a specific statement, that such names are exempt from the relevant protective laws and regulations and therefore free for general use.
The publisher, the authors, and the editors are safe to assume that the advice and information in this book are believed to be true and accurate at the date of publication. Neither the publisher nor the authors or the editors give a warranty, expressed or implied, with respect to the material contained herein or for any errors or omissions that may have been made. The publisher remains neutral with regard to jurisdictional claims in published maps and institutional affiliations.

This Springer imprint is published by the registered company Springer Nature Switzerland AG.
The registered company address is: Gewerbestrasse 11, 6330 Cham, Switzerland

Acknowledgements

We thank Tom, June, Jacob, Kit, Preecha and Vagner for their understanding and support while preparing this book.

Thanks also go to Sarah Hoile for her editorial support throughout the process of preparing the manuscript for publication.

Contents

1 Remaking HIV Prevention: The Promise of TasP, U=U
   and PrEP.. 1
   Sarah Bernays, Adam Bourne, Susan Kippax, Peter Aggleton,
   and Richard Parker

Part I Efficacy and Effectiveness: Shaping Policy and Informing
        Interventions

2 'PrEP Is a Programme': What Does this Mean for Policy........ 21
   Hakan Seckinelgin

3 Making the Ideal Real: Biomedical HIV Prevention as Social
   Public Health..................................... 35
   Mark Davis

4 PrEP, HIV, and the Importance of Health Communication....... 47
   Josh Grimm and Joseph Schwartz

5 Anticipating Policy, Orienting Services, Celebrating Provision:
   Reflecting on Scotland's PrEP Journey..................... 59
   Ingrid Young

6 Fighting for PrEP: The Politics of Recognition and Redistribution
   to Access AIDS Medicines in Brazil....................... 73
   Felipe de Carvalho Borges da Fonseca, Pedro Villardi,
   and Veriano Terto Jr

Part II Pleasure, Agency and Desire

7 The Beatification of the Clinic: Biomedical Prevention
   'From Below'...................................... 91
   Kane Race

8   New Potentials for Old Pleasures: The Role of PrEP in Facilitating
    Sexual Well-being among Gay and Bisexual Men   105
    Bryan A. Kutner, Adam Bourne, and Will Nutland

9   New Hierarchies of Desirability and Old Forms of Deviance
    Related to PrEP: Insights from the Canadian Experience   117
    Adrian Guta, Peter A. Newman, and Ashley Lacombe-Duncan

10 Agency, Pleasure and Justice: A Public Health Ethics Perspective
    on the Use of PrEP by Gay and Other Homosexually-Active Men . . .   131
    Julien Brisson, Vardit Ravitsky, and Bryn Williams-Jones

Part III   Provision Politics and New Forms of Governmentality

11 The Political Life of PrEP in England: An Ethnographic
    Account   145
    Sara Paparini

12 Implementation Science or 'Show' Trial? England's PrEP Impact
    Study   159
    Catherine Dodds

13 The Stigma Struggles of Biomedical Progress: Understanding
    Community Engagement with PrEP by People Who Use Drugs . . .   173
    Andy Guise

14 How the Science of HIV Treatment-as-Prevention Restructured
    PEPFAR's Strategy: The Case for Scaling up ART in 'Epidemic
    Control' Countries   187
    Ryan Whitacre

15 Getting Real on U=U: Human Rights and Gender as Critical
    Frameworks for Action   201
    Laura Ferguson, William Jardell, and Sofia Gruskin

16 Falling Short of 90-90-90: How Missed Targets Govern Disease
    Elimination   219
    Kari Lancaster and Tim Rhodes

Part IV   Anticipating and Understanding the Consequences
          of Biomedicine

17 Stigma and Confidentiality Indiscretions: Intersecting Obstacles
    to the Delivery of Pre-Exposure Prophylaxis to Adolescent Girls
    and Young Women in East Zimbabwe   237
    Morten Skovdal, Phyllis Magoge-Mandizvidza,
    Rufurwokuda Maswera, Melinda Moyo, Constance Nyamukapa,
    Ranjeeta Thomas, and Simon Gregson

**18   Imagined Futures and Unintended Consequences in the Making
        of PrEP: An Evidence-Making Intervention Perspective**   249
        Martin Holt

**19   The Drive to Take an HIV Test in Rural Uganda: A Risk to
        Prevention for Young People?**   265
        Sarah Bernays, Allen Asiimwe, Edward Tumwesige, and Janet Seeley

20   Entangled Bodies in a PrEP Demonstration Project   277
        Lisa Lazarus, Robert Lorway, and Sushena Reza-Paul

**21   An Unfinished History: A Story of Ongoing Events and Mutating
        HIV Problems**   289
        Marsha Rosengarten

Editors and Contributors

About the Editors

Sarah Bernays is a senior lecturer in global health at the University of Sydney and an associate professor at the London School of Hygiene and Tropical Medicine. An anthropologist by training, she specialises in co-designing and evaluating interventions to support communities to engage in infectious disease control and treatment. She has developed long-term partnerships with national research institutions and leading sexual and mental health programmes working with young people in South Africa, Uganda and Zimbabwe as part of a collaborative effort to invest in capacity building and translating knowledge into policy and practice. Her work also extends to South East Asia, Europe and Australia. She has recently worked with the WHO to inform their global guidelines for adolescents living with HIV.

Adam Bourne is an associate professor of public health and Deputy Director of the Australian Research Centre in Sex, Health and Society at La Trobe University in Melbourne, as well as a senior visiting fellow at the Kirby Institute, UNSW Sydney. A health psychologist by training, he has led numerous studies examining the perception and management of HIV-related risk among gay, bisexual men and other men who have sex with men in the context of new prevention technologies, as well as the treatment and care experiences of those living with diagnosed HIV. His work extends across Europe, Eastern and Southern Africa, South East Asia and Australia and incorporates HIV-related research among people who use drugs (particularly in sexual contexts) as well as female sex workers. Adam is an associate editor of the journal *Sexually Transmitted Infections*, is a member of the Victorian Whole of Government LGBTIQ Taskforce and, between 2016 and 2018, was a member Global Advocacy Platform to Fast-Track the HIV and Human Rights Response for Men who have Sex with Men, hosted by the MSM Global Forum and UNAIDS.

Susan Kippax has a PhD in Social Psychology and is a Fellow of the Academy of the Social Sciences of Australia. In 2019, she was awarded an Order of Australia (AO). She is an emeritus professor in the Social Policy Research Centre, UNSW Sydney, having retired from the position of Director of the National Centre in HIV Social Research (1995–2007). Professor Kippax has an extensive research track record in the areas of sexuality and health and has published a number of books and research papers. She played a central role in framing Australia's response to HIV and AIDS and has served on many international and national advisory panels and committees. She was joint editor-in-chief of the *Journal of the International AIDS Society* (2009–2019) and a founding editor of *Culture, Health and Sexuality*.

Peter Aggleton holds professorial positions in the Centre for Gender and Global Health at UCL in London, in the Centre for Social Research in Health at UNSW Sydney, in the School of Sociology at the Australian National University, and in the Australian Research Centre for Sex, Health and Society at La Trobe University, Melbourne. He has published extensively on the social and educational aspects of HIV and sexual health, and is editor-in-chief of three international journals *Culture, Health and Sexuality*, *Sex Education* and the *Health Education Journal*. In addition to his academic work, Peter has served as a senior adviser to UNAIDS, UNESCO, UNFPA and WHO. He lives in Bath and has worked extensively in Africa, Asia and Latin America.

Richard Parker is senior visiting professor in the Institute for the Study of Collective Health at the Federal University of Rio de Janeiro as well as Professor Emeritus of Sociomedical Sciences and Anthropology and a member of the Committee on Global Thought (http://cgt.columbia.edu/) at Columbia University in New York City. He is President of the Brazilian Interdisciplinary AIDS Association (ABIA), one of the leading non-governmental AIDS advocacy, research and service organisations in Brazil (http://www.abiaids.org.br); founder and Co-Chair of Sexuality Policy Watch, a global coalition of researchers, policymakers and activists from a wide range of countries and regions with secretariat offices in Rio de Janeiro and New York City (http://www.sxpolitics.org); editor-in-chief of the journal, *Global Public Health* (http://www.tandfonline.com/loi/rgph20#.UiemgryE71s); and a founding editor of the journal *Culture, Health and Sexuality*.

Contributors

Allen Asiimwe Social Science Department, MRC/UVRU & LSHTM Uganda Research Unit, London School of Hygiene and Tropical Medicine, Entebbe, Uganda

Sarah Bernays School of Public Health, University of Sydney, Sydney, Australia

Adam Bourne Australian Research Centre in Sex, Health and Society, La Trobe University, Melbourne, Victoria, Australia

Julien Brisson Bioethics Program, Department of Social & Preventive Medicine, School of Public Health, University of Montreal, Montreal, Canada

Felipe de Carvalho Borges da Fonseca Brazilian Interdisciplinary AIDS Association, Rio de Janeiro, Brazil

Mark Davis School of Social Sciences, Monash University, Melbourne, Australia

Catherine Dodds School for Policy Studies, University of Bristol, Bristol, UK

Laura Ferguson USC Institute on Inequalities in Global Health, University of Southern California, Los Angeles, California, USA

Simon Gregson Manicaland Centre for Public Health Research, Biomedical Research and Training Institute, Harare, Zimbabwe
Department of Infectious Disease Epidemiology, Imperial College London, London, UK

Josh Grimm Manship School of Mass Communication, Lousiana State University, Baton Rouge, USA

Sofia Gruskin USC Institute on Inequalities in Global Health, University of Southern California, Los Angeles, California, USA

Andy Guise Faculty of Life Sciences & Medicine, King's College, London, UK

Adrian Guta School of Social Work, University of Windsor, Windsor, Canada

Martin Holt Centre for Social Research in Health, UNSW Sydney, Sydney, Australia

William Jardell USC Institute on Inequalities in Global Health, University of Southern California, Los Angeles, California, USA

Bryan A. Kutner HIV Center for Clinical and Behavioral Studies, New York State Psychiatric Institute and Colombia University, New York, NY, USA

Ashley Lacombe-Duncan School of Social Work, University of Michigan, Michigan, USA

Kari Lancaster Centre for Social Research in Health, UNSW Sydney, NSW, Australia

Lisa Lazarus Institute for Global Public Health, Rady Faculty of Health Sciences, University of Manitoba, Winnipeg, Canada

Robert Lorway Institute for Global Public Health, Rady Faculty of Health Sciences, University of Manitoba, Winnipeg, Canada

Phyllis Magoge-Mandizvidza Manicaland Centre for Public Health Research, Biomedical Research and Training Institute, Harare, Zimbabwe

Rufurwokuda Maswera Manicaland Centre for Public Health Research, Biomedical Research and Training Institute, Harare, Zimbabwe

Melinda Moyo Manicaland Centre for Public Health Research, Biomedical Research and Training Institute, Harare, Zimbabwe

Peter A. Newman Factor-Inwentash Faculty of Social Work, University of Toronto, Toronto, Canada

Will Nutland Department of Public Health, Environments and Society, London School of Hygiene and Tropical Medicine, London, UK

Constance Nyamukapa Manicaland Centre for Public Health Research, Biomedical Research and Training Institute, Harare, Zimbabwe
Department of Infectious Disease Epidemiology, Imperial College London, London, UK

Sara Paparini Nuffield Department of Primary Care Health Sciences, University of Oxford, Oxford, UK

Kane Race Department of Gender and Cultural Studies, University of Sydney, Sydney, Australia

Vardit Ravitsky Bioethics Program, Department of Social & Preventive Medicine, School of Public Health, University of Montreal, Montreal, Canada

Sushena Reza-Paul Institute for Global Public Health, Rady Faculty of Health Sciences, University of Manitoba, Winnipeg, Canada
Ashodaya Samithi, Mysore, India

Tim Rhodes University of New South Wales, Sydney, NSW, Australia
London School of Hygiene and Tropical Medicine, London, UK

Marsha Rosengarten Goldsmiths, University of London, London, UK

Joseph Schwartz College of Arts, Media and Design, Northeastern University, Boston, USA

Hakan Seckinelgin Department of Social Policy, LSE, London, UK

Janet Seeley Department of Global Health and Development, London School of Hygiene and Tropical Medicine, London, UK

Social Science Department, MRC/UVRU & LSHTM Uganda Research Unit, London School of Hygiene and Tropical Medicine, Entebbe, Uganda
African Health Research Institute, Durban, South Africa

Morten Skovdal Department of Public Health, University of Copenhagen, Copenhagen, Denmark

Veriano Terto Jr Brazilian Interdisciplinary AIDS Association, Rio de Janeiro, Brazil

Ranjeeta Thomas Department of Health Policy, London School of Economics and Political Science, London, UK

Edward Tumwesige Social Science Department, MRC/UVRU & LSHTM Uganda Research Unit, London School of Hygiene and Tropical Medicine, Entebbe, Uganda

Pedro Villardi Brazilian Interdisciplinary AIDS Association, Rio de Janeiro, Brazil

Ryan Whitacre Anthropology and Global Health, Graduate Institute of International and Development Studies, Geneva, Switzerland

Bryn Williams-Jones Bioethics Program, Department of Social & Preventive Medicine, School of Public Health, University of Montreal, Montreal, Canada

Ingrid Young Centre for Biomedicine, Self and Society, Usher Institute, University of Edinburgh, Edinburgh, UK

Chapter 1
Remaking HIV Prevention: The Promise of TasP, U=U and PrEP

Sarah Bernays, Adam Bourne, Susan Kippax, Peter Aggleton, and Richard Parker

1.1 Why this Book?

HIV has always been, and continues to be, as much a social phenomenon and challenge as it is a clinical one. Controlling transmission and containing the virus relies on engaging with and adjusting the social contours of behaviours and practices. Efforts to prevent acquisition and enable 'protection' against HIV continue to illuminate the complexity, multiplicity and dynamism of relationships in context,

S. Bernays (✉)
School of Public Health, Faculty of Medicine and Health, University of Sydney, Sydney, Australia

Department of Global Health and Development, London School of Hygiene and Tropical Medicine, London, UK
e-mail: sarah.bernays@sydney.edu.au

A. Bourne
Australian Research Centre in Sex, Health and Society, La Trobe University, Melbourne, Australia

Kirby Institute, UNSW Sydney, Sydney, Australia

S. Kippax
Social Policy Research Centre, UNSW Sydney, Sydney, Australia

P. Aggleton
Centre for Social Research in Health, UNSW Sydney, Sydney, Australia

Centre for Gender and Global Health, UCL, London, UK

R. Parker
Institute for the Study of Collective Health, Federal University of Rio de Janeiro, Rio de Janeiro, Brazil

Sociomedical Sciences and Anthropology, Colombia University, New York, USA

Brazilian Interdisciplinary AIDS Association (ABIA), Rio de Janeiro, Brazil

© Springer Nature Switzerland AG 2021
S. Bernays et al. (eds.), *Remaking HIV Prevention in the 21st Century*, Social Aspects of HIV 5, https://doi.org/10.1007/978-3-030-69819-5_1

from the micro level of person to person interaction extending up to the global stage of political economies. Despite major biomedical breakthroughs over the course of the HIV epidemic, the influence of the social has not diminished. What risks being diluted through the optimism evoked by the biomedical promise though is how immediately visible and relevant the role of the social remains in efforts to prevent, control and perhaps 'eliminate' HIV.

The current 'biomedical' response to the HIV epidemic has been framed as a shift from an understanding of prevention as dependent on changes in social norms and practices and political responses to one predominately associated with pill-taking and injectables by individuals. This biomedical turn within HIV prevention has been interpreted by some, falsely we believe, as indicative of the failure of the earlier social programmes and associated behavioural interventions. Furthermore, such a framing serves only to create or maintain a false separation, as biomedical responses always depend on social processes in order to be put into practice (Hankins and de Zalduondo 2010). Treatment as Prevention (TasP), through consistently adhering to anti-retroviral treatment (ART), or negotiating Pre-Exposure Prophylaxis (PrEP) use, rely on behavioural responses as much as interventions explicitly referred to in behavioural terms, such as condom use or serosorting. The effectiveness of biomedical methods is shaped by, and indeed dependent upon, social processes, which are indivisible from their prescribing, delivery and consumption contexts.

Since the early days of the HIV epidemic, social scientists have understood that behavioural responses are essentially social. The same is true in relation to the responses of people to the HIV-related biomedical programmes and interventions we see around us now. These have, in many respects, been brought into being by global advocacy and social movements. They have been made accessible (in some contexts) by activism, by politics and by sustained civil society engagement. They have been made acceptable (to some) by community organising, peer-based communication and other creative ways of facilitating awareness, interest and uptake. It is also social and cultural forces that have restricted access for some, and that have denied the possibilities afforded by the biomedical to some groups, particularly those most stigmatised or criminalised. The success or failure of prevention interventions in achieving an end to the epidemic, and in ensuring health equity, will rest heavily on the ability, willingness or determination of societies and cultures to drive change. This was integral to the emphasis of combination prevention, which reflected a concerted effort, especially in resource-stretched settings, to ensure that the learning about the value of structural interventions and attending to the intersection of social practices across a range of distinct but complementary prevention options was not lost in the rush to embrace biomedical prevention (UNAIDS 2009; Hankins and de Zalduondo 2010; Kurth et al. 2011). Despite this approach losing political favour in some places, such as Brazil, in recent years (Montenegro et al. 2020), there remains much to be learned from how biomedical approaches can be incorporated into existing approaches and programmes, rather than framed as substituting them (Brown et al. 2015; Cáceres et al. 2015; Mahase 2020; O'Reilly et al. 2020; Tolley et al. 2020).

Much of the optimism generated through the expectation that biomedical prevention will accelerate progress towards HIV elimination, and in doing so will redress
the 'failings' of earlier behavioural interventions, has been derived from efficacy
data generated under controlled trial conditions. Producing similar levels of effectiveness within the messy contexts of everyday life has proved more challenging
(Cohen et al. 2011; Kippax 2003). This illustrates not only the entanglement
between biomedical interventions and behaviours, but also the interconnected social,
economic and political spheres which constitute the conditions in which HIV
prevention must operate. How these interventions have come to be framed, shaped
and experienced through this nexus of social conditions and across various contexts
is the focus of this book.

In this edited collection, we consider the effects of the increasing forms of
biomedical prevention through developments such as Treatment as Prevention
(TasP), Undetectable equals Untransmittable (U=U) and Pre-Exposure Prophylaxis
(PrEP) on continually reframing policy, practice and research. Although these
approaches are commonly described under the collective banner of biomedical
prevention, it is constructive to delineate how they differ in form and effect. PrEP
is a medication taken in the form of a pill or injection to prevent acquiring HIV. TasP
exists both as a treatment policy and as a powerful slogan to inspire engagement in
this treatment policy because it also prevents transmission: U=U. Although intan-
gible, the value of TasP and U=U as slogans reflects the ongoing powerful influence
of community advocacy in shaping the aspirational course of global HIV policy in
the pursuit of the 'elimination' of AIDS. The subsequent appeal of these slogans
rests in part in their capacity to produce powerful possibilities about how HIV risk
can be managed and controlled. Although predicated on universal opportunity, the
extent to which they are feasible under current conditions across communities is
much more fractured.

For many people and communities, these developments have increased hope for
the future, even if the attainment of this promise has been unevenly experienced so
far. These new forms of prevention raise a number of political, social, cultural and
ethical issues that thus far have received insufficient attention. As with all behaviours
or practices, there is a need to acknowledge the central role of these concerns in
influencing the delivery, consumption and effects of biomedical prevention, which
in turn is influencing the success or failure of current HIV prevention efforts.

Thus, while accepting that TasP, U=U and PrEP hold great promise, this book
takes a broad social science stance and examines the social and political impacts of
the recent and ongoing move to biomedical prevention and the variable attention
paid to combined prevention. This is vital to illuminate the influence of the social on
the effects, mechanisms and outcomes of interventions, which are now predominantly framed as being biomedical. We argue that a social lens, one that illuminates
affected communities' active and creative appropriation of biomedical information
and technologies, including those whose participation may be indirectly impeded, is
essential to distinguish more or less effective developments in prevention. Attending
to what becomes visible through this lens is necessary to ensure that we are
responding to the opportunities to maximise the success of biomedical and other

'new' technologies and are able to adapt programmes to meet the varying needs of all those at risk of acquiring HIV. We intend that the analyses of a range of political, economic and cultural concerns, which coalesce to create the 'social', across the chapters of this book should offer a clear call for biomedical and social scientists to ensure together that the realities of everyday life are understood as central to the success of all forms of HIV prevention and to avoid the pitfalls of unintended and unwanted outcomes.

1.2   Situating Biomedical Prevention

1.2.1   Treatment as Prevention (TasP) and Undetectable=Untransmittable

The term Treatment as Prevention (TasP) refers to the range of biomedical prevention methods and programmes that use antiretroviral treatment (ART) to decrease the risk of HIV transmission. There is increasingly clear evidence that when people adhere consistently to ART, on a treatment regimen to which they are not resistant, the HIV viral load in their blood or other bodily fluids (semen, vaginal fluid and rectal fluid) can be reduced to such a low level that blood tests cannot detect it (Cohen et al. 2011; Rodger et al. 2019). This is described as viral suppression or an 'undetectable' viral load. In such circumstances, not only is a person's health not affected by HIV but also, they cannot transmit HIV to others. This advance has given rise to the 'undetectable equals untransmittable' (U=U) campaign to enhance awareness that if a person has an undetectable viral load and takes their ART medications as prescribed, they will not transmit HIV to their sexual partners (Eisinger et al. 2019).

The concept of expanded access to ART to curb the epidemic through a 'treat-all' strategy was initially proposed by UNAIDS and then formally recognised by the World Health Organization (WHO) in 2015, which recommended that all those diagnosed with HIV should be started on ART immediately, regardless of HIV viral load. It is anticipated that this approach will decrease community viral load (the average viral load across a certain group) and thereby reduce the rate of new infections. This underpins the WHO's 95-95-95 strategy (95% of people living with HIV knowing their HIV status; 95% of people who know their HIV status on treatment; and 95% of people on treatment with suppressed viral loads) and is an essential component of the modelling studies that have predicted that TasP could lead to HIV transmission being dramatically reduced if not eliminated. Despite consensus to work towards these goals, the powerful rhetoric encapsulated within these slogans can serve to overstate the progress being made on the ground, given the existing limitations in treatment access and coverage, rendering the gaps between aspirational policy and reality less visible. We argue that in spite of these positive developments, the approaches and models that provide the foundation for current global AIDS policies and programmes face major challenges when rolled out in the real world: a world characterised by limited resources, variable political will, continued HIV-related stigma and discrimination, and social and economic inequality.

1.2.2   Pre-Exposure Prophylaxis

Pre-exposure prophylaxis (PrEP) is a course of anti-retroviral treatment taken by HIV-negative people to protect them against HIV infection. Truvada, which was first approved in the USA for use as PrEP in 2012 and has since been approved in dozens of countries, is a single pill combining two anti-retroviral treatments, tenofovir and emtricitabine. In some settings, generic alternatives have also been approved for use as PrEP (Mameletzis et al. 2018; Hodges-Mameletzis et al. 2019). Injectables and other long-acting options have also been developed and may serve to further increase the appeal and scalability of PrEP coverage globally. A number of large, high profile clinical trials have shown the efficacy of PrEP in preventing HIV, if taken correctly. It is evident that under controlled conditions, the harms associated with particular sexual practices and with illicit injection drug use have been dramatically reduced by the presence of PrEP. Mathematical modelling studies have predicted that among populations of gay, bisexual and other men who have sex with men; a large and early effect on HIV incidence can be achieved if PrEP is implemented with high coverage of those at risk. This has changed the face of HIV prevention, especially for gay and other men who have sex with men in the high-income countries of the world.

Ongoing research continues to investigate levels of knowledge about and attitudes towards PrEP, to measure levels of uptake and adherence, and, more generally, to evaluate the impact of PrEP on a number of different populations over time, that is, to investigate effectiveness. As alternative formulations become available, such long-acting injectables, the appeal, scalability and impact of PrEP for a wider range of populations groups, in particular heterosexual men and women, is likely to change too (Mahase 2020; Tolley et al. 2020). Addressing contested questions such as for whom PrEP is for and how to ensure greater equity in its availability and accessibility, as well as exploring its varied appeal and ability to meet the needs (and risks) of potential users, particularly women and those in resource-constrained settings, have been shown to be much more complicated.

1.3   HIV Prevention for all?

Learning from HIV prevention spans almost four decades and has consistently shown that there is no one approach that will work for everyone all of the time. Indeed, prior to the advent of biomedical approaches, combination prevention—involving a range of safer sex and safer drug use options—was often advocated as the strategy to adopt, in recognition of people's and communities different (and often changing) circumstances and needs.

Importantly, the opportunities afforded by biomedical interventions do not negate the need for a continued emphasis on combination approach, which are tailored to population groups, attentive to social marginalisation and adapted to be delivered at scale. There is no intrinsic tension in this approach. However, there is a risk that in the pursuit of biomedical interventions there may be a neglect of the pertinence of social structures and contexts in shaping effectiveness as interventions are rolled out at scale. In so doing, the narrative which blames the intended user for not adequately engaging with the intervention may gain traction, reproducing or creating new forms of inequity, detracting attention from how biomedical methods need to be adjusted to improve equity and to better meet the prevention needs of individuals and groups.

In recognition of this, we pay particular attention to the political and economic motivations behind the roll-out of recent innovations in HIV prevention. Policymaking with regards to TasP, U=U and PrEP varies significantly internationally and highlights not only continued inequities between the global North and global South, but also in-country divisions between those who are economically and socially marginalised, and those who are not.

The active embrace of TasP, and its ensuing success in reducing new infection, has been concentrated in resource-rich countries, primarily in the global North. It is within such contexts that not only are good quality second and third-line treatment regimens with low level side effects available, but also civil society organising and activism has, to date, been most effectively focused towards the needs of ethnically and economically dominant groups. While numerous high-income countries have observed declines in HIV incidence associated with TasP among white, middle class, native-born gay and bisexual men, such success has not often been achieved among those from minority ethnic backgrounds, Indigenous communities or among migrants. In the context of low- and middle-income countries, primarily in the global South, where supply chain management may be weaker (especially in the absence of donor support), older treatment regimens with significant side effects (and related challenges for the levels of adherence necessary to avoid viral resistance) are often the only options that are available. This has created a tier of relatively affordable but 'second class' accessible treatments in many resource-constrained settings. Despite improving rates of global treatment coverage, which is celebrated within annual reports, the limited effectiveness and tolerability of available ART regimens impede the chances of the success of TasP and widespread viral suppression. In addition, across contexts the communication of the U=U message has not always been coherent and/or straightforward, being influenced by and framed by political and social complexities and tensions. The heterogeneity in progress, including the time that it will take to attain the global targets (if ever), are commonly obscured within the buoyancy of these slogans and global reports. We aim to draw attention to the uneven topography by attending to the variation across contexts in achieving viral suppression and thus realising the promise of TasP and U=U.

Similar inequities exist with regard to PrEP. Whereas most of the research related to use by gay, bisexual and other men who have sex with men has occurred in North

America, Europe and Australia, with the notable exceptions of intense research activity on PrEP in Peru (Perez-Brumer 2019), most of the sex worker related research has taken place in Africa (Eakle et al. 2018; Busza et al. 2020), where there is also an emerging focus on transgender women (Poteat et al. 2020). Furthermore, access to PrEP for use in public health prevention programmes continues to be disproportionately available principally in high-income economies and for certain population groups. The uneven effect of PrEP, even within countries which have demonstrated successes (Laborde et al. 2019), indicates that its positive impact currently remains more posited than proven (Rosengarten and Murphy 2019) and reflects the power invested in promises to leverage funding and to guide global HIV policy. Promising 'the end of AIDS' in resource rich countries thus goes hand in hand with the politics of outsourcing clinical trials for biomedical prevention methods to low- and middle-income countries (as well as those in unsympathetic political regimes), while in many middle- and low-income countries access to PrEP is all but impossible and/or limited to those enrolled in 'demonstration' trials (Patton and Kim 2012; Kenworthy et al. 2018).

The positive impact of PrEP has not yet been broadly realised in many low-income settings. Although there are some notable exceptions to this trend in Latin America (Galea et al. 2018; Luz et al. 2019), again we must be cautious to avoid assuming that positive outcomes are uniform across different populations and subgroups (Torres-Cruz and Suárez-Díaz 2020). Retention in PrEP trials and demonstration projects by key populations in numerous countries in Sub Saharan Africa (e.g. Kenya) has been very low (Wahome et al. 2020). Similarly, adherence to PrEP in South Africa, Uganda and other contexts has not met expectations (Mayer et al. 2019; Kinuthia et al. 2020; Pillay et al. 2020), which suggests there is much still to understand about the cultural context within which this new intervention is perceived, understood and actioned. Decades of research relating to HIV testing and treatments has taught us the value of local wisdom in facilitating uptake and adherence and this remains true for newer forms of biomedicine (Cowan et al. 2016). It has always been, and will continue to be, inappropriate and ineffective to transfer interventions conceived and developed in one context into another without examining and attending to the diverse, nuanced and creative situated reality (Syversten 2019; Well and Ledin 2019).

These disparities are compounded by inequalities in the ways in which science operates globally. While scientific decision-making and authority, as well as most major funding is concentrated in the hands of scientists from the global North, the implementation of trials has taken place primarily in the global South, sub-contracted to local institutions and more junior co-investigators. Such inequities reflect the power of Big Pharma and existing trade regulations, which, when combined with how science gets done, places low- and middle-income countries at a significant disadvantage. Existing intellectual property rights and commercial trade regulations create significant barriers to access for new biomedical approaches in low- and middle-income countries, and pharmaceutical companies in the global North have consistently fought against the approval of generic versions of PrEP in countries across the global South.

The move to biomedical prevention reflects a shift from the community to the clinic, which has been associated with the individualising and privatisation of prevention. The physician's office and clinic offer very different contexts from the settings in which most of the early successful epidemic responses took place. As a result of social solidarity and collective action among gay, bisexual and other men who have sex with men, injection drug users and sex workers, social norms were developed over time, which protected community members from HIV transmission. HIV prevention, whether it involved condom use, serosorting, the education of clients by sex workers, or the use of sterile needles and syringes was intimately tied to the sexual or injection act and depended on communication between social actors. The development and strength of social and community norms, which are themselves so central to the take up of new technologies, depend on such conversation and talk. HIV prevention remains a deeply social practice and, in order for biomedical prevention to be effective, it too must be understood as a social practice and interventions be developed through participatory dialogue.

One example of the dynamic and divergent social practices, which emerge from engaging with biomedical prevention, is pill-taking. If pill-taking can be done privately, then this can have distinct advantages for those who wish to avoid the stigma associated with being known as gay or a person who injects drugs or a sex worker, as it reduces the likelihood of talk and communication between community members, but this absence of talk may undermine needed communication. Furthermore, the experience of PrEP use itself may produce stigma and discrimination. On the one hand, PrEP has been associated with promiscuity and pleasure and those using PrEP in the gay community have been subject to 'slut-shaming' discourse, while, on the other hand, gay, bisexual and other men who have sex with men choosing not to use PrEP may find themselves subject to social censure and questions about 'good gay' citizenship.

Stigma may also be produced among young women. For example, the advocacy in some southern African countries to place all young women on PrEP because they are 'vulnerable' to infection, is likely to position (once again) women as 'vessels of disease' responsible for HIV transmission. For some, such interventions may have a liberating influence: for others, without due attention to how meanings are produced and intersect with existing disadvantage, the unintended effects of biomedical prevention may further solidify inequity.

1.4   Blind Spots

While the emphasis on biomedical prevention can detract from and blur the visibility of social influences that moderate their effectiveness, it is also vital to illuminate the blind spots that exist within this book. The chapters follow the trajectory of the development of biomedical HIV prevention within HIV policy, tracking the implementation of interventions within and beyond trials into programmes. As such, this is a collection of insights and reflections which maps the social effects of what *is* being implemented rather than what is not. Being predominately empirically informed, in each chapter the authors broadly focus their analytical attention on the presence of biomedical interventions, rather than its absence. The resulting limitations in coverage both reflects and reproduces the centripetal force which guides empirical research attention and funding. In pursuit of the operation of biomedical prevention, the chapters reveal the hierarchy of concerns which are driven by profit margins and systemic opportunities in which some population groups are prioritised over others.

Within this collection there is only limited attention to people who use drugs or transgender people. This does, however, reflect the fact that, comparatively speaking, far less research has been conducted with and for these populations, which itself reflects a lack of political attention or will (and thus funding) to engage with populations that are doubly disadvantaged, highly stigmatised and whose experiences and needs have often been placed on the periphery of the HIV response. Although the chapters deliberately highlight who or what may be explicitly or indirectly left out of existing scientific and programmatic classifications and mechanisms, our focus on all population groups is partial at best, and broadly incomplete.

A pertinent example of this are the debates which coalesce around PrEP, which have predominately considered gay, bisexual and other men who have sex with men. There is much to be learnt from the groups that continue to be framed as absent from the discussion, as well as the reasons why they are indirectly excluded. The blind spots around how biomedical prevention can engage with the needs of specific and marginalised population groups, such as trans women or trans men, as well as extensive, but also at times invisible, populations such as women living in poverty and men and women in migration, demand more empirical and analytical attention.

Having outlined the purpose of this book, as well as identifying its limitations, we turn next to explaining how the book is structured and the chapters organised thematically.

1.5   Efficacy and Effectiveness: Shaping Policy and Informing Interventions

As we navigate an era of new HIV biomedical technologies, social scientists across the world have sought to examine how the promise such interventions offer within tightly controlled trial settings can be—or has been—realised in real world settings.

Chapters in this first part—which focuses largely on the opportunities and difficulties associated with PrEP—pose important questions about how biomedical science is understood and acknowledged in policy, programming and health promotion, as well as how effectiveness is advanced through social action. By so doing, this part raises important questions about the growing emphasis on biomedical interventions in an epidemic that is intensely social in character, including the need to acknowledge the interwoven relationships between the biomedical, social and political.

In the first chapter, Hakan Seckinelgin invites readers to consider the idea of PrEP as a programme rather than just a pill. By reconsidering what exactly PrEP trials have demonstrated in terms of efficacy and what efficacy might mean for policy in non-trial contexts, the chapter raises critical questions about the relationship between biomedical interventions and the contexts in which they are applied. Related ideas are explored in Mark Davis' chapter which follows. This interrogates how dominant assumptions about biomedical HIV prevention view social factors as largely secondary to effectiveness, either as barriers to the rollout and uptake of interventions or as conduits for the same processes. Such an approach marginalises the reflexivity of those who are the subjects of HIV prevention, ignoring the unanticipated effects this may have on social and sexual lives. The chapter encourages a rethinking of biomedical HIV prevention as an assemblage of biomedical, social and political forces and effects, each of which is necessary for the approach to be effective. The next chapter, by Josh Grimm and Joseph Schwartz, focuses on PrEP, HIV and health communication. Engaging with the idea that messages and messaging matters, it argues that communication in general and mass media, interpersonal communication and app-based communication, in particular, are valuable tools to increase awareness and adoption of biomedical HIV prevention such as PrEP. When employed strategically, mass media can encourage discussion—helping build relationships and support the adoption of PrEP. Dating and hookup apps such as Grindr and Scruff provide additional ways of reaching gay, bisexual and other men who have sex with men providing hyper-local information about PrEP, HIV and sexual health resources.

Building on some of these ideas the final two chapters in this part, focusing on two different contexts—Scotland and Brazil respectively—shift the focus to examine the effects of PrEP and related forms of biomedical HIV prevention on the everyday experiences of those who use them, as well as for the communities of which they are a part. Ingrid Young's chapter signals how the arrival of PrEP in Scotland came with expectation and celebration. As the first country in the UK to offer PrEP through the national health service, Scotland was heralded as a leader in HIV prevention. The chapter asks how anticipation of PrEP and its focus on specific risk practices affected not only awareness, access and use, but also wider narratives about prevention, inequality and 'progress'. The chapter signals how PrEP roll-out contributes to an orientation towards certain (gendered) PrEP users and PrEP use. It considers how the anticipation of PrEP as a biotechnology for particular risk practices, bodies and communities shaped promissory HIV prevention futures and determined what success and 'celebration' could be like. The struggle for PrEP access figures strongly in Felipe de Carvalho Borges da Fonseca, Pedro Villardi and Veriano Terto Jr's chapter that follows. This chapter addresses, through a historical perspective, the role of organised civil society in the struggle for access to HIV medicines in Brazil. Through concepts of recognition and redistribution, the text shows how recognition of the rights of people living with HIV and the participation of the AIDS social movement in policymaking were decisive in the establishment and sustainability of universal access to HIV treatment in Brazil. Over the course of the past decade, activism around new HIV prevention methods such as PrEP has shown that expanded access to these technologies depends on the fight against both moral and market barriers. The future is far from certain, as recent setbacks to democracy both in Brazil and elsewhere mean less recognition of civil rights and threats to universal access to medicines and HIV prevention tools.

1.6   Pleasure, Agency and Desire

Part II of this book moves beyond effects, efficacy and effectiveness to consider questions of agency, pleasure and desire. PrEP, TasP and the opportunities provided by U=U afford HIV affected populations the opportunity to have sex without condoms—with both regular and other partners—in ways that reduce or eliminate the chances of acquiring or transmitting HIV. After more than 30 years of 'use a condom every time' messaging, this represents a fundamental change in how people understand and operationalise constructions of sexual safety in negotiation or combination with forms of sexual pleasure. The new biomedical and technological affordances have been acknowledged and embraced by actors in some settings who have sought to promote PrEP. However, while they may facilitate new forms of sexual satisfaction, they also intensify opportunities for the policing of groups and their practices (both internally within communities and externally by others), especially when considered in isolation from the assemblages that shape or foster desire. In other contexts, notions of pleasure have been ignored and reproduced the denial of sexual agency and the right to pleasure that has permeated much of the HIV epidemic response to date.

These and other issues are examined in Kane Race's chapter on biomedical prevention 'from below'. With the introduction of biomedical prevention, gay community-based agencies have sought to optimise biomedical prevention by establishing non-judgemental, anonymous community-based clinics offering rapid HIV and STI testing in shopfronts, mobile clinics and gay neighbourhoods. To maximise accessibility these services have framed sex as a valid form of pleasure and experimentation rather than an object of moral correction. While these modes of implementing biomedical prevention represent a case of intensified biomedicalisation, they are continuous with a history of collective experimentation with bodies, pleasures and care practices that has long distinguished gay community responses to HIV. Bryan A. Kutner, Adam Bourne and Will Nutland's chapter develops similar ideas to show how by decoupling fear about HIV from the sex lives of gay, bisexual and other men who have sex with men, PrEP presents an opportunity to broaden programmes and interventions beyond HIV prevention to embrace sexual wellbeing more generally. Case studies from organisations and advocacy groups that have worked to acknowledge and promote pleasure are explored together with the cultural and structural forces that seek to deny pleasure as a healthy feature of the sex lives of gay, bisexual and other men who have sex with men in many parts of the world.

The following chapter by Adrian Guta, Peter A. Newman and Ashley Lacombe-Duncan shifts the focus slightly to consider new hierarchies of desirability in the context of PrEP availability. Through a new materialist-informed reading of qualitative data collected from PrEP users and non-users in Toronto, Canada and health promotion campaigns, they explore how PrEP-mediated desirability is produced and deployed within a neoliberal context. For some gay, bisexual and other men who have sex with men, PrEP is experienced as empowering and offers anxiety-free condomless sexual exploration. For others, PrEP remains aspirational, and a condition of their desirability. Between, there is considerable ambiguity, flexibility and movement. Their analysis considers emerging hierarchies of desirability within an assemblage of bodies, relations, affects, pills, evidence, technologies, discourses and material conditions, which expands theorising about PrEP beyond it being a repressive biomedical prevention technology. Developing issues of empowerment further, Julien Brisson, Vardit Ravitsky and Bryn Williams-Jones's chapter on agency, pleasure and justice offers a public health ethics perspective on the use of PrEP by gay and other homosexually active men. It argues that such men should be understood as agentic in their use of PrEP as opposed to being the passive victims of biomedicalisation. Applying a reproductive justice framework, the chapter argues that the worldwide inaccessibility of PrEP constitutes a more serious ethical issue than the medicalisation of gay men's sexuality.

1.7 Provision Politics and New Forms of Governmentality

Like all actions in response to HIV, TasP, PrEP and U=U are intensely political. Structurally, they have raised significant questions regarding access, the division of resources and the role of targets in shaping epidemic responses, which have produced new or altered forms of governmentality for the individual and for heavily affected communities. As has been evident at so many points in the history of the HIV epidemic, community activism has once again been central to ensuring access and facilitating uptake, often coming into conflict with political forces that have sought to pit one community or population against another in the struggle for attention and resources. The four chapters included in this part, in their different ways engage with the politics at work here and the forms of governmentality they imply.

Sara Paparini's chapter on the political life of PrEP in England offers an ethnographic account of these developments. It took six years from the first release of the results of the PROUD PREP trial for NHS England to begin to provide PrEP as a routine service to people considered at high risk of acquiring HIV. These years have been marked by significant controversy, activism, a court case and heated media debate. The chapter tells the story of the emergence of PrEP in England through the accounts of key stakeholders showing how new HIV prevention technologies intensifying the relationship between pharmaceutical private interest and public health have a political life animated by moral, legal and material antagonisms.

Such antagonisms leverage clinical evidence and activist alliances to extend the history of HIV politics into new realms. In a complementary account to that offered above, Catherine Dodds traces the policy events that gave rise to the Impact trial in England, which followed several years after PROUD and provided a means of accessing PrEP for some gay and bisexual men while ostensibly examining real-world integration within relevant health systems. Interviews with key stakeholders demonstrate that rather than achieving its aims as a practical implementation trial that might have enabled and shared learning on the best ways to roll out PrEP, the Impact trial was designed as a 'show trial' to help manage a policy and financial impasse. But because the trial's power dynamics were rooted in traditional hierarchies concerning the production of evidence, this undermined its potential as anything other than a stop-gap measure. Ultimately, rather than enabling the identification of lessons for those planning England's future PrEP services, the trial's legacy will largely be about the divisions and inequalities that it exacerbated.

Community responses to PrEP diverge. For some communities PrEP has offered a 'revolution' in HIV prevention; for others—including people who use drugs—PrEP access and use is complicated by on-going struggles for health and rights. Andy Guise's chapter explores diverging responses of revolution and struggle to PrEP with a particular focus on people who use drugs. Building on an analysis of community engagement in the early HIV epidemic response as well as recent stigma scholarship, the chapter explains how PrEP is bound up in long-running processes of resistance to stigma. The character of these 'stigma struggles' shapes the potential for PrEP to be experienced as either revolution or struggle, while the norms of biomedical science exacerbate and complicate these struggles, through their symbolic power to erase history from analysis. The chapter concludes by reflecting on how an analysis of stigma struggles and their role in biomedical progress can inform relevant and tailored HIV prevention strategies.

The following two chapters progress the widening of focus that has occurred throughout this volume. In his chapter, Ryan Whitacre considers how the advent of TasP restructured the strategy adopted by the US President's Emergency Plan for AIDS Relief (PEPFAR). It demonstrates how TasP, conceptualised as an 'evidence-based' solution for effectively treating and preventing HIV, came progressively to inform the organisation's use of metrics for evaluating performance, and decisions for allocating funds to specific programmes and countries. Whereas under previous efforts to 'lead the global response' to the epidemic, PEPFAR supported a wide variety of programme areas, including strengthening health systems, following the advent of TasP, PEPFAR came to prioritise treatment programmes over and above all others. Emphasising the clinical logic of TasP, PEPFAR justified spending on a limited number of programmes in a small set of countries that could produce what it defined as the right kinds of outcomes. This ultimately laid the groundwork for the retreat of US foreign aid.

In their chapter entitled 'Getting Real on U=U: Human rights and gender as critical frameworks for action', Laura Ferguson, William Jardell and Sofia Gruskin push this analysis further by pointing to the selective way in which international non-governmental organisations and UN system bodies selectively engaged with the opportunities and constraints which Undetectable equals Untransmittable (U=U) offered, subsequent to the roll-out of TasP by PEPFAR and other agencies. Reminding us of the importance of gender and human rights to any understanding of justice and equality in HIV prevention, their analysis highlights the challenges posed by the complex institutional landscape and the sometimes inconsistent policies and contested politics of the different agencies and systems that have grown rapidly as a result of the global scale-up of the HIV response, signalling the key role of international non-governmental organisations and civil society movements in seeking to monitor and advocate for more effective policies internationally.

In the chapter which brings to close this third part of the book, Kari Lancaster and Tim Rhodes consider how all too often global health targets are not met. Writing in the context of the COVID-19 pandemic, and as the anticipated future of 2020 imagined in the UNAIDS targets becomes the past, their chapter considers how missed targets such as these come to govern disease elimination. Drawing on studies of numbering practices in science and technology studies, their chapter explores how global health targets continue to govern even when they fail to be achieved. Enumerating prevention (and other health) targets—and progress towards them—does its work through progression and not completion, constructing disease elimination as but a vague predicate. Success or failure in HIV prevention (by biomedical means or otherwise) thereby has a latitude which makes ongoing governance and imagined futures possible. Within the context of HIV, 90-90-90 targets afford the possibility of virtual elimination—even as they fall short. Taking this reality seriously requires us to think differently about the timescapes of disease elimination and what the outcome of global targets such as these might be.

1.8 Anticipating and Understanding the Consequences of Biomedicine

Like all actions that take place in the social world, the introduction of PrEP, TasP and U=U has not been without its consequences. Some of these may be intended, embraced or celebrated as evidence of efficacy or impact, others perhaps not. This final part of the book focuses on a range of anticipated and unanticipated issues, including those related to broader health benefits and dis-benefits; human rights and social justice; intended and unanticipated community and political responses; the status and engagement (or otherwise) of particular populations such as sex workers and young people; and other issues. In doing so, authors of the chapters connect the current phase of an increasingly biomedicalised response to the epidemic with challenges pervasive throughout its history, particularly in respect of gender equity, HIV stigma and discrimination.

Morten Skovdal, Phyllis Magoge-Mandizvidza, Rufurwokuda Maswera, Melinda Moyo, Constance Nyamukapa, Ranjeeta Thomas and Simon Gregson commence this work with a chapter focusing on obstacles to the delivery of

Pre-Exposure Prophylaxis to adolescent girls and young women in east Zimbabwe. Despite efforts to scale-up biomedical HIV prevention such as PrEP, many countries and regions are off–track in reaching HIV prevention targets. Uptake of, and adherence to, PrEP amongst adolescent girls and young women in sub-Saharan Africa is particularly challenging. Drawing on qualitative individual interviews and focus group discussions with thirty participants in east Zimbabwe, as well as interviews with healthcare providers, this chapter looks at the root causes of this challenge. Stigma and the worry that privacy and confidentiality cannot be maintained in health clinics and by local healthcare providers, presents a major barrier to young women's uptake of PrEP. Action is needed to tackle the socio-cultural norms and practices that interact to make engagement with PrEP an (im)-possible and (un)desirable thing to do for many adolescent girls and young women.

The next chapter by Martin Holt considers the way in which pre-exposure prophylaxis (PrEP) was imagined before it was widely used, the evidence generated as it has been trialled and implemented, and how knowledge-making practices have been incorporated into the making of PrEP as an HIV prevention strategy. The analysis attends to the ways in which unintended consequences (such as difficulties with adherence, high rates of discontinuation, reduced condom use and sexually transmitted infections) have been conceptualised and responded to as PrEP has been trialled and implemented. A tension is identified between considering PrEP as a discrete and stable intervention that can traverse contexts unchanged, and as an emergent process or assemblage that is enmeshed within local conditions and enacted in practice. Responses to unintended consequences suggest that it is not possible to separate PrEP from existing practices like condom use, or longstanding arguments about appropriate forms of sexual conduct and responsibility. To make PrEP work effectively, we should recognise the dense networks of relations on which it relies, and the positive and disruptive effects it can simultaneously provoke.

A key component of current global HIV prevention efforts is widespread HIV testing. This strategy in part reflects the focus on the broader global targets to eliminate AIDS by achieving high rates of viral suppression. Sarah Bernays, Allen Asiimwe, Edward Tumwesige and Janet Seeley's chapter examines young people's engagement with HIV prevention options in South-West Uganda. A qualitative approach is used to examine how young people aged 16–24 years old navigate risks and opportunities within their daily lives. These risks include HIV, but also economic precarity. Within a context in which using HIV prevention methods, such as condoms or abstinence, is severely compromised by contextual realities, some young people report relying on irregular HIV testing as their primary method of prevention. One unintended consequence of the 'push' for HIV testing may be that it overrides other behavioural prevention strategies. Findings illustrate the impact such biomedical interventions may have if implemented in isolation from the structural drivers of vulnerability and the social context of young people's lives.

This theme of unintended consequences is extended in Lisa Lazarus, Robert Lorway and Sushena Reza-Paul's ethnographic study of a PrEP demonstration project in South India among female sex workers. The authors analyse a set of narratives in which participants claim PrEP as a 'cure all' for a range of physical ailments. What becomes clear is how participation in the demonstration project has intensified a relationship with their bodies, leading women to reflect on and track various changes pertaining to bodily wellness. 'The body' thereby becomes a highly reactive site that entangles global HIV science, sex workers' engagements with health promotion, and regimes of self-care. Engaging with these local biologies holds important insights for the design and implementation of future biomedical interventions.

Marsha Rosengarten's chapter ends our book by pointing to an unfinished history of constantly changing HIV problems. It takes as its focus the thinking that has come to prevail with regard to women and HIV and, by so doing, working backwards through the genealogy of the development of PrEP. Without disputing the affordances of PrEP, in either pill or long-term form, it is suggested that WHO/UNAIDS 90-90-90 goals and optimism for a future end to the epidemic are founded on a misplaced conception of what is at stake. Drawing on process philosophy and 'event-thinking', it argues that if biomedicine is to be responsive to the what is most relevant to those affected by HIV, a more open conception of what is assumed by international health authorities as the 'dynamics of the epidemic' may be warranted. This is especially pertinent to the situation of women in heavily affected communities whose reluctance to participate in the community trials of PrEP documented in the chapter should be understood as a profoundly ethical stance raising questions about for whom, and in what ways, biomedical advance proves beneficial. What is at stake here is that through their discourse, international agencies and national authorities, as well as most in biomedicine and public health, have positioned and continue to position women as both vulnerable and yet responsible for the heterosexual transmission of sexually transmissible infection.

Throughout this book, authors attempt to draw attention to the social dimension to what is often construed as 'biomedical' HIV prevention. We invited them to do so because ultimately biomedicine is as much a social enterprise as it is a biological and medical undertaking. The programmes and interventions developed, the priorities they respond to, and the aims and ambitions of scientists and clinicians are as much cultural enterprises as they are scientific ones. They are driven by the passions and interests of individuals and communities—of scientists as well as advocates, activists and people living with HIV—which in turn reflect broader (and sometimes narrower) social priorities and concerns. To deny this, or to pretend otherwise, is not only blinkered but dishonest. Too often, initiatives such as TasP, PrEP and U=U have been promoted as 'good things' simply because they represent what is thought to be the latest advance in HIV prevention. To do this, however, is to present them shorn of their genealogy, significance and placement alongside other elements of the social assemblage that comprises HIV prevention today. Our call here is for an opening up of discourse and dialogue about these 'goods' in the hope that this may lead to a more critical appreciation of their strengths and limitations for some people, in some contexts, some of the time. We hope you feel inspired to contribute to this work.

References

Brown, G., Reeders, D., Dowsett, G. W., Ellard, J., Carman, M., Hendry, N., et al. (2015). Investigating combination HIV prevention: Isolated interventions or complex system. *Journal of the International AIDS Society, 18*(1), 20499.

Busza, J., Phillips, A. N., Mushati, P., Chiyaka, T., Magutshwa, S., Musemburi, S., et al. (2020). Understanding early uptake of PrEP by female sex workers in Zimbabwe. *AIDS Care.* https://doi.org/10.1080/09540121.2020.1832192.

Cáceres, C. F., Koechlin, F., Goicochea, P., Sow, P. S., O'Reilly, K. R., Mayer, K. H., et al. (2015). The promises and challenges of pre-exposure prophylaxis as part of the emerging paradigm of combination HIV prevention. *Journal of the International AIDS Society, 18*, 19949.

Cohen, M. S., Chen, Y. Q., McCauley, M., Gamble, T., Hosseinipour, M. C., Kumarasamy, N., et al. (2011). Prevention of HIV-1 infection with early antiretroviral therapy. *New England Journal of Medicine, 365*(6), 493–505.

Cowan, F. M., Delany-Moretlwe, S., Sanders, E. J., Mugo, N. R., Guedou, F. A., Alary, M., et al. (2016). PrEP implementation research in Africa: What is new? *Journal of the International AIDS Society, 19*, 21101.

Eakle, R., Bourne, A., Mbogua, J., Mutanha, N., & Rees, H. (2018). Exploring acceptability of oral PrEP prior to implementation among female sex workers in South Africa. *Journal of the International AIDS Society, 21*(2), e25081.

Eisinger, R. W., Dieffenbach, C. W., & Fauci, A. S. (2019). HIV viral load and transmissibility of HIV infection: Undetectable equals Untransmittable. *JAMA, 321*(5), 451–452.

Galea, J. T., Baruch, R., & Brown, B. (2018). ¡ PrEP Ya! Latin America wants PrEP, and Brazil leads the way. *The Lancet HIV, 5*(3), e110–e1e2.

Hankins, C. A., & de Zalduondo, B. O. (2010). Combination prevention: A deeper understanding of effective HIV prevention. *AIDS, 24*, S70–S80.

Hodges-Mameletzis, I., Fonner, V. A., Dalal, S., Mugo, N., Msimanga-Radebe, B., & Baggaley, R. (2019). Pre-exposure prophylaxis for HIV prevention in women: Current status and future directions. *Drugs, 79*(12), 1263–1276.

Kenworthy, N., Thomann, M., & Parker, R. (2018). From a global crisis to the 'end of AIDS': New epidemics of signification. *Global Public Health, 13*(8), 960–971.

Kinuthia, J., Pintye, J., Abuna, F., Mugwanya, K. K., Lagat, H., Onyango, D., et al. (2020). Pre-exposure prophylaxis uptake and early continuation among pregnant and post-partum women within maternal and child health clinics in Kenya: Results from an implementation programme. *The Lancet HIV, 7*(1), e38–e48.

Kippax, S. (2003). Sexual health interventions are unsuitable for experimental evaluation. In J. M. Stephenson, J. Imrie, & C. Bonell (Eds.), *Effective sexual health interventions* (pp. 17–48). Oxford: Oxford University Press.

Kurth, A. E., Celum, C., Baeten, J. M., Vermund, S. H., & Wasserheit, J. N. (2011). Combination HIV prevention: Significance, challenges, and opportunities. *Current HIV/AIDS Reports, 8*(1), 62–72.

Laborde, N. D., Spinello, M., & Whitacre, R. (2019, June 17). *"Zero infections. Zero deaths. Zero stigma."* Somatosphere. Retrieved November 26, 2020, from http://somatosphere.net/2019/zero-infections-zero-deaths-zero-stigma.html/.

Luz, P. M., Veloso, V. G., & Grinsztejn, B. (2019). The HIV epidemic in Latin America: Accomplishments and challenges on treatment and prevention. *Current Opinion in HIV and AIDS, 14*(5), 366.

Mahase, E. (2020). HIV prevention injection is more effective than daily pill, trials show. *British Medical Journal, 371*, m4433.

Mameletzis, I., Dalal, S., Msimanga-Radebe, B., & Rodolph, M. (2018). Going global: The adoption of the World Health Organization's enabling recommendation on oral pre-exposure prophylaxis for HIV. *Sexual Health, 15*(6), 489.

Mayer, C. M., Owaraganise, A., Kabami, J., Kwarisiima, D., Koss, C. A., Charlebois, E. D., et al. (2019). Distance to clinic is a barrier to Pr EP uptake and visit attendance in a community in rural Uganda. *Journal of the International AIDS Society, 22*(4), e25276.

Montenegro, L., Velasque, L., LeGrand, S., Whetten, K., Rafael, R. D. M. R., & Malta, M. (2020). Public health, HIV care and prevention, human rights and democracy at a crossroad in Brazil. *AIDS and Behavior, 224*(1), 1–4.

O'Reilly, K. R., Fonner, V. A., Kennedy, C. E., Yeh, P. T., & Sweat, M. D. (2020). The paradox of HIV prevention: Did biomedical prevention trials show how effective behavioral prevention can be? *AIDS, 34*(14), 2007–2011.

Patton, C., & Kim, H. J. (2012). The cost of science: Knowledge and ethics in the HIV pre-exposure trials. *Journal of Bioethical Inquiry, 9*, 295–310.

Perez-Brumer, A. (2019). *HIV biomedical prevention science and the business of gender and sexual diversity*. Doctoral thesis. Columbia University, New York.

Pillay, D., Stankevitz, K., Lanham, M., Ridgeway, K., Murire, M., Briedenhann, E., et al. (2020). Factors influencing uptake, continuation, and discontinuation of oral PrEP among clients at sex worker and MSM facilities in South Africa. *PLoS One, 15*(4), e0228620.

Poteat, T., Malik, M., van der Merwe, L. L. A., Cloete, A., Adams, D., Nonyane, B. A., et al. (2020). PrEP awareness and engagement among transgender women in South Africa: A cross-sectional, mixed methods study. *The Lancet HIV, 7*(12), e825–e834. https://doi.org/10.1016/S2352-3018(20)30119-3.

Rodger, A. J., Cambiano, V., Bruun, T., Vernazza, P., Collins, S., Degen, O., et al. (2019). Risk of HIV transmission through condomless sex in serodifferent gay couples with the HIV-positive PARTNER taking suppressive antiretroviral therapy (PARTNER): Final results of a multicentre, prospective, observational study. *Lancet, 393*(10189), 2428–2438.

Rosengarten, M., & Murphy, M. (2019). 'A wager on the future': A practical response to HIV pre-exposure prophylaxis (PrEP) and the stubborn fact of process. *Social Theory and Health, 18*(1), 1–15.

Syversten, J. L. (2019, August 12). *The social life of PrEP in Kenya*. Somatosphere. Retrieved November 26, 2020, from http://somatosphere.net/2019/the-social-life-of-prep-in-kenya.html/

Tolley, E. E., Zangeneh, S. Z., Chau, G., Eron, J., Grinsztejn, B., Humphries, H., et al. (2020). Acceptability of long-acting injectable Cabotegravir (CAB LA) in HIV-uninfected individuals: HPTN 077. *AIDS and Behavior, 24*(9), 2520–2531.

Torres-Cruz, C., & Suárez-Díaz, E. (2020). The stratified biomedicalization of HIV prevention in Mexico City. *Global Public Health, 14*(4), 598–610.

UNAIDS. (2009). Combination prevention: Strategic HIV prevention programmes founded on good practice. In *A background paper for the UNAIDS prevention reference group meeting, 3–5 December 2009*. Geneva: UNAIDS.

Wahome, E. W., Graham, S. M., Thiong'o, A. N., Mohamed, K., Oduor, T., Gichuru, E., et al. (2020). PrEP uptake and adherence in relation to HIV-1 incidence among Kenyan men who have sex with men. *EClinicalMedicine, 26*, 100541.

Well, B., & Ledin, C. (2019, November 4). *PrEP at the after/party: The 'post-AIDS' politics of Frank Ocean's "PrEP+"*. Somatosphere. Retrieved November 26, 2020, from http://somatosphere.net/2019/prep-at-the-after-party.html/.

Part I
Efficacy and Effectiveness: Shaping Policy and Informing Interventions

Chapter 2
'PrEP Is a Programme': What Does this Mean for Policy

Hakan Seckinelgin

2.1 Introduction

The purpose of this chapter is to reconsider the idea of *PrEP is a programme rather than simply a pill*. My analysis makes a distinction between what is meant by programme, that is indicating considerations of clinical support mechanisms to deal with the PrEP implementation issues and programme as including the context within which PrEP outcomes are produced. The latter, unlike the former, considers how assumptions about efficacy are already embedded in the contexts of Randomised Control Trials (RCTs) and other demonstration projects. This distinction then allows a coherent way to think about PrEP policy in different contexts. In the rest of this chapter I explore this way of thinking about the meaning of *PrEP is a programme*. I do this by reconsidering what exactly PrEP trials demonstrate in terms of efficacy and what that efficacy means for getting that result to work as policy in non-trial contexts. By policy, PrEP-based prevention policy, I mean a set of coherent interrelated activities involving knowledge of behaviour, medicine availability, access, and the clinical and social conditions for sustainable use of PrEP. These are necessary for creating an outcome both for those who are using it (that they are not infected) and for the public (gradual reduction of transmission). In the next section I provide general background on the emergence of both PrEP as a prevention tool and the idea of *PrEP is a Programme*.

This project has received funding from the European Research Council (ERC) under the European Union's Horizon 2020 research and innovation programme (grant agreement no 667526). The views expressed here reflect only the author's view and that the Agency is not responsible for any use that may be made of the information it contains.

H. Seckinelgin (✉)
Department of Social Policy, LSE, London, UK
e-mail: M.H.Seckinelgin@lse.ac.uk

© Springer Nature Switzerland AG 2021
S. Bernays et al. (eds.), *Remaking HIV Prevention in the 21st Century*, Social Aspects of HIV 5, https://doi.org/10.1007/978-3-030-69819-5_2

2.2   Background and Emergence of PrEP

Since 2010, a series of clinical trials have demonstrated that daily, or on-demand, use of specific antiretrovirals before sex, has significantly reduced the risk of HIV transmission among the vast majority of groups considered to be at risk (Grant et al. 2010; Baeten et al. 2012; Choopanya et al. 2013; Cremin et al. 2015; McCormack et al. 2016; Molina et al. 2015). While there were trials showing no efficacy in some groups, the successful demonstrations of efficacy have made *pre-exposure prophylaxis* (PrEP) an important tool for HIV prevention. The PrEP approach combines a pharmaceutical tool, a pill (tenofovir disoproxil fumarate-TDF, alone or in combination with emtricitabine-FTC) with a specific behaviour—adherence—to produce health outcomes for individuals who are HIV negative. International guidelines have been developed to set procedures for PrEP provision for HIV-infection in high-risk groups (WHO 2015, 2017). PrEP and its scaling up are also considered to be one of the critical prevention policies to reach 2020 targets to reduce infections. PrEP is presented as having the potential to stop HIV transmission if used correctly.

However, Robert Grant, the leading medical scientist in PrEP research, argues that 'the premise of PrEP remains unfulfilled' (2019). This observation reflects several parallel processes that followed the announcement of research results. While the policy world focused on the trial results to develop prevention strategies and policy guidelines for interventions, within the scientific community a number of critical challenges emerged with reference to PrEP use. Simultaneously, the long-awaited positive results of these trials created a new treatment activism. Many activists, who as members of the target communities had participated in these trials, made demands from authorities that PrEP be made available immediately to those who would like to use it.

2.2.1   Science, Policy and Activism Entangled

Despite the euphoria in medical and HIV policy circles, the policy uptake has been slow and challenging. There are various reasons for this. It is possible to divide these reasons into two groups: (a) cost considerations of a possible PrEP-based prevention policy in middle and low-income settings and (b) questions about the implications of PrEP use on sexual behaviour and implications of this in turn on HIV (Abbas et al. 2013). According to some, the cost of providing PrEP is a concern for many governments across the world (Venter et al. 2015; Hodges-Mameletzis et al. 2018). This concern relates to the sustainability of access in context, from gaps in existing public health infrastructure: 'making PrEP easily accessible where people live requires that local medical providers are aware of and comfortable with pre-scribing PrEP. Indeed, most clinicians around the world are not prepared to deliver this service yet' (Zablotska et al. 2018, p. 482; also see Di Ciaccio et al. 2018, p. 42) and that lack of data is impacting designing policies 'to offer PrEP' (Coleman 2018, p. 486). These concerns do not question the PrEP efficacy claims. Instead, they point to resource allocation challenges arising from these new medical developments given the existing capacities.

The second group of concerns which has contributed to the reluctance on PrEP implementation relate to the efficacy of PrEP in everyday contexts. There are several issues here: one concern is about adherence (van der Elst et al. 2013): with low adherence HIV prevention is compromised (see below). Another concern is about risk compensation and whether PrEP-use would increase risky sexual behaviour leading to a possible increase in sexually transmitted diseases in general (Marcus et al. 2013; Rojas Castro et al. 2019). Research on this question is ongoing with some studies demonstrating no risk compensation while others are highlighting challenges to the consistent adherence to PrEP (Sagaon-Teyssier et al. 2016; Lal et al. 2017). Another issue focuses on the 'long term side effects of using PrEP' and their potential for 'HIV resistance to emerge if breakthrough infections occur[red]' (Gafos et al. 2019).

Both sets of concerns illustrate the difficulty of moving from efficacy demonstrated by clinical trials to PrEP-use as a prevention policy in different *real world* contexts. As Catherine Hankins, Ruth Macklin and Mitchell Warren put it 'the extraordinary feat of proving PrEP's efficacy may turn out to have been easier than ensuring it is used well' (2015, p. 75). Put simply, the translation of trial results into policy that needs to work in the contexts of implementation is not straightforward. These critical concerns and observations about PrEP caution against the establishment of a direct link that expects the efficacy of PrEP observed in trial settings to be straightforwardly replicated in everyday contexts.

These critical and cautionary concerns on PrEP policy have been countered by treatment activists. *We want PrEP and we want it now* has become a widely used slogan (see https://www.iwantprepnow.co.uk/; Hildebrandt 2018). For activists the efficacy demonstrated in the trials warrants that PrEP be made available for all those who would like to use it, independent of the emerging concerns discussed above. In their demand to have access to PrEP, activists have developed a direct answer to challenges in order that availability and PrEP access not be hampered. When views on PrEP as a pill are expressed, the activists respond forcefully that 'PrEP is not a pill. It is a programme'. This statement has become a refrain deployed by PrEP activists such as *Prepsters* to counter the criticism that the PrEP is a pill (Prepsters 2020). They point out that while availability and access are central, PrEP should be considered as a programme with its required routine clinical tests to support those who use the medicine. Under this view of *PrEP as a programme*, both policy guidelines and the activist positions suggest that the efficacy of the antiretroviral medicine in protecting people without HIV from acquiring HIV should be the main basis for thinking about policy directions. The activists' urgency was also taken up by international policy makers.

The World Health Organization (WHO) published the first PrEP guidelines in 2012, targeting specific risk groups such as MSM and sex-workers. These were then expanded by WHO in 2015 (WHO 2012). The new recommendation states that 'Oral

PrEP containing TDF [tenofovir disoproxil fumarate] should be offered as an additional prevention choice for people at substantial risk of HIV infection as part of combination HIV prevention approaches' (WHO 2015, p. 42). The document states that the recommendation is based on the analysis of 'twelve trials of the effectiveness of oral PrEP' and that 'adherence is considered to be a central moderator for the positive outcome of PrEP use' in all of these trials (WHO 2015, p. 42). In its analysis of *Equity and Acceptability* the document points out that access to PrEP facilitates access to other relevant health systems for those who are at risk with limited 'opportunities to have access to health services' (WHO 2015, p. 45). These guidelines show that the WHO is also taking a view on PrEP as a programme, a programme of standard medical interventions, despite its admission in its 2017 guidelines that 'there has been limited experience with providing PrEP outside research and demonstration projects in low- and middle-income countries' (WHO 2017, p. 2; see Hodges-Mameletzis et al. 2018, p. 496).

These guidelines strengthened treatment activism to put pressure on policymakers for PrEP access. In activists' language, there is often a move from the position described as *we want PrEP and we want it now,* about the activists themselves who are in the resource rich settings (such as Australia, France, the UK, the USA), to the position that *we want PrEP for everyone/everywhere.* This move prioritises making PrEP as a pill available in resource poor settings including many contexts in Sub-Saharan Africa. The move is evidenced by a number of demonstration projects/trials to assess the acceptability and feasibility of providing PrEP in different contexts (Kibengo et al. 2013; O'Malley et al. 2019). These projects/trials generally accept that PrEP works and want to assess whether a target population in those contexts, a risk group such as gay men, MSM, Transwomen, sex workers, and others, will use it to assess the feasibility of providing PrEP in different contexts. In this process there is a further move from the idea of *PrEP is a programme* to *let's just provide the pill* as the most important and urgent part for the prevention. In this the importance of clinical support is not ignored, but assumed to be either available or something that needs to be provided once access to the pill is possible and demand has been created. It is an understandable move and aspiration within a general treatment activism underpinned by a sense of solidarity.[1]

---

[1]Observations, findings, that are discussed here are based on analysing the PrEP debate since 2010 and following the emergence of new research findings and policy directions. I followed the interactions between various actors at the 2018 22nd International AIDS Conference in Amsterdam (https://www.aids2018.org/) and other meetings around it: conference organised by the Association for the Social Sciences and Humanities in HIV (ASSHH) -*Intensifying the social in the biomedical era* and a workshop by M-pact Global Action on 22 July 2018 *Out with it – Community Solutions for the Sexual Health and Rights of Young Gay and Bisexual Men* (https://mpactglobal.org/wp-content/uploads/2018/07/Out-With-It-2018-Program-Book.pdf)

2.2.2 What Is the Problem?

While the tensions mentioned earlier are observable in many discussions on PrEP, critical questions about PrEP policy are often responded to with findings showing the acceptability of PrEP among risks groups, including in resource poor settings, on the basis of specific trials/projects (see Hoagland et al. 2017). These findings are used as justifications for further PrEP roll-out. But they are implicitly limited in their scope being tied to a generic category of risk group. There is often limited understanding of what it will mean for people to request PrEP in their everyday contexts. These considerations may or may not fit the assumptions made about how people targeted under these risk categories will behave. Didier Eribon's (2004) critical observation that revealing one's HIV status is more than just a medical statement because it reveals details of one's life is highly relevant here: seeking PrEP reveals much more than being health conscious. In different contexts what is revealed is a desire to have sex, or to have sex in a certain way, which will have direct and wide-ranging implications for those seeking PrEP. These raise challenging questions for any PrEP guideline or policy. When questioned on this basis, some researchers and activists tend to argue, drawing on the words of a number of activists that: 'PrEP is a programme and not a pill' and that it is about 'delivering on people's right to health' and that 'all other concerns can be gradually addressed once people have access to PrEP'. Arguably, the core demand in these claims is still about having access to the pill. The language of *a programme* acts as an important public statement, a good advocacy tool, to counter critical questions about PrEP policy. This is done by implying that *programme* means 'using PrEP will involve routine clinical monitoring, users will be monitored for all possible problems around STIs. Therefore, PrEP might be more cost-effective as a prevention tool'. However, the focus of most discussions and policy drives—particularly in relation to resource-poor settings, where routine clinical support is not readily available—seems to be on the medicine and its availability.

2.3 Rethinking PrEP Policy as a Programme

In this section I use an analytical lens to re-think the statement that *PrEP is a programme*. The aim is to decentre the idea of PrEP as a pill that informs the idea of PrEP is a programme and the many policy initiatives and assessments that rely on it. In many of these assessments what is assessed is if it is feasible for the target group to use PrEP and if there is a demand for PrEP in this group or if it is absent whether it can be created (see Mugo et al. 2016; Heffron et al. 2018; Hoagland et al. 2017; Dunbar et al. 2018; Schwartz et al. 2018; AVAC 2019). The point is to establish how we should understand PrEP as a programme if there is going to be a PrEP-based prevention policy, implemented to help people in their everyday lives beyond making pills available. I argue that if we unpack what is meant by *PrEP is a programme,* we see a number of components: a biomedical tool- the pill, biomedical clinical monitoring, health infrastructure, human resources and conditions that facilitate the choices of those who want to use PrEP. The latter is fundamental for any PrEP policy outcome given adherence is central to producing efficacy. The projected outcome, benefits, of PrEP as prevention policy, are produced by factors that interact. The policy outcomes are underpinned by these behavioural interactions that support use of a biomedical tool. It is on these interactions that I want to focus on to explore what *PrEP as a programme* needs to inform policy directions.

2.3.1   Conceptual Considerations

Here I consider the idea of *PrEP is a programme* as an 'installation' (Lahlou 2017). This is useful for considering how PrEP is supposed to work, how human activity is supposed to be 'constructed and channelled' through PrEP policy (Lahlou 2017, p. 94). From this perspective, PrEP policy becomes a way of constructing and channelling individuals' behaviour, both in relation to sexual activity and HIV prevention. The central point of this approach is to consider 'the situations where individual needs, desires and will combine with the reality of the context to produce a behavioural outcome' (Lahlou 2017, p. 94). For PrEP, 'situation' would cover the introduction of new policy that needs to be implemented within target groups' everyday lives. As a part of this, people are expected to 'learn and relearn how to behave' from the perspective of the policy as it relates to their everyday lives. According to Saadi Lahlou each such situation is composed of three layers: 'individuals and their embodied competencies, the material environment and social regulation' (Lahlou 2017, pp. 94–95). These three layers come together 'locally to produce activity' or in our case to make possible individuals in target groups engage with PrEP in such ways to produce the expected policy outcomes. Therefore, considering PrEP as an installation allows one to think about PrEP as a programme in terms of the intersections of personal capacities, material environment and social regulation.

There are various competencies individuals need to develop for PrEP policies: an ability and desire to use the pill within their everyday sexual practices and; the capacity to engage with the clinical support systems within a set of norms and rules that exist in various contexts. These competencies don't exist or function in abstract. They are facilitated, developed or constrained by the existing social regulations that formally or informally sanction certain behaviours. In practice, the above defined competencies will develop and be exercised within material environments where material is not limited to 'single policy objects' such as the pill but also include other elements that are 'as-a-whole relevant for action' such as clinics and hospitals as well as new ways of thinking about sexual behaviour. For PrEP policy the material environment combines, among other aspects, the availability of pills (this involves political decisions and considerations of opportunity costs), clinical services, training of clinical professionals (not only on PrEP but also on particular target groups that will need to have access to these services) to be able to engage with PrEP policy and how these environments function, and function interactively, to allow the channelling of individual behaviours to produce expected outcomes. These material and social capacities of the systems to engage with the target groups are significant (see Mack et al. 2015). The possibility of exercising individual capacity to act, to use PrEP as a pill, is also conditioned by social perceptions of what it means to be a PrEP user and to be in legal contexts where revealing oneself as MSM will have consequences (see Haire 2015). According to Lahlou, installation theory brings together these three components to 'create a functional system that produces projected outcomes' (2017, p. 95). The issue here is the relationship between objects and the actions that they 'inform, support and constrain' (Lahlou 2017, p. 97). Applying this, PrEP as a programme is then not only about a pill or about specific support services, but it is about how, in a policy process, these act together to guide behaviour or action of people deliberately 'to elicit or support specific behaviour'. As a result, people's abilities to act also become part of the programme.

One critical component of this thinking is the idea of *affordances* that are about what an environment, an installation, allows individuals or objects to do. According to J. J. Gibson, 'the affordances of things are what they furnish, for good or ill, that is what they afford the observer...they are ecological, in the sense that they are properties of the environment ... Affordances do not cause behaviour but constrain or control it' (Gibson in Lahlou 2017, p. 46; also see Gibson 1977). Affordances account for how subjects perceive the pragmatic potential of their environment 'or opportunities for action, such as graspability' (Good 2007, p. 270). The idea can simply be described as 'subjects perceive directly the behavioural possibilities that the environment affords them' (Gibson in Lahlou 2017, p. 45; see also Gibson 1977). I argue that the idea of *PrEP is a programme* describes an installation that attempts to create affordances for individuals to achieve expected policy outcomes, namely to prevent individuals from catching HIV. In this the label, *programme*, is important because it indicates an attempt to create an environment that guides individuals to achieve these particular outcomes. The affordance that is embedded in a PrEP programme is produced on the basis that 'the production of action depends both on the agency of the objects present in the context, and of the position of the subject' (Lahlou 2017, p. 55). So, it is clear that PrEP as a pill contributes to affordance, but this takes place within PrEP as a programme. The latter is assumed to create affordances by also positioning and enabling those subjects who are supposed to utilise the pill. Thus, the approach presents an interactive mechanism that provides coherence to the idea of a programme. It leads policy thinking to consider how PrEP programme as a mechanism might function, thus creating affordances for PrEP policy in different contexts.

Summarising, treating a PrEP policy as an installation that creates affordances to produce expected outcomes allows a re-analysis of the research findings that have guided the policy thinking. In what follows, I argue that to better understand the policy relevance of the research guiding PrEP policy, we need to re-consider the research underlying it, particularly from RCTs and other field experiments, as installations that create environments with affordances that lead to the research results. This approach allows the understanding of the conditions that have created specific affordances that ultimately ground the possibility of the results reported in those trials.

2.3.2   PrEP Trials as Installations

Looking at the medical science journals that report on PrEP trial results can provide good insights about why thinking about these as installations matter. The Preexposure Prophylaxis Initiative's (iPrEx) reporting is a typical example (see Thigpen et al. 2012; Choopanya et al. 2013; Molina et al. 2015; McCormack et al. 2016). In December 2010 the iPrEx team reported the results of research conducted in six countries in the New England Journal of Medicine. The trial team led by Robert M. Grant, reported that their work demonstrated the significant preventative efficacy of using antiretrovirals for HIV negative people who are at risk: 'Oral FTC-TDF provided protection against the acquisition of HIV among the subjects. Detectable blood levels strongly corelated with the prophylactic effect' (Grant et al. 2010, p. 2587). As per usual, the reporting included a methodology section to explain how the trial was structured and how the randomisation was done, how the recruitment of subjects was conducted and what procedures were followed throughout the trial. They reported under three headings *Study Visits, Standard Preventing Interventions* and *Laboratory Testing* the sets of procedures that were used in the trial to keep subjects engaged. Looking at these sections reveals a very close engagement between research/trial staff and the subjects participating in research through the various steps of the trial. It is worthwhile here to use extended quotations to highlight the structure of the trial.

Once subjects were selected from targeted risk groups through the inclusion criteria, participants expected to follow a process:

> Every 4 weeks after enrolment, each 4-week visit included drug dispensation, pill count, adherence counselling, rapid testing for HIV antibodies and taking medical history. Chemical and haematological analyses were performed at weeks 4, 8, 12, 16 and 24 and every 12 weeks thereafter. During screening, a computer-assisted structured interview collected information about education level, self-identified sex, and alcohol use, along with subjects' perceived study-group assignment at week 12. High-risk behaviour was assessed by interview every 12 weeks, and physical examinations and evaluations for sexually transmitted infections were performed at least every 12 weeks (Grant et al. 2010, p. 2588).

So, in this mapping of the process we observe clearly the creation of a community around the intervention. The process not only repeatedly engages subjects through the provision of pills but creates a social regulation through its monitoring. The monitoring procedure aims to maintain participation of the subjects through the process. Moreover, the monitoring also creates social measures of evaluation of right and wrong behaviours in relation to the trial aims.

Participants were also given set of standard prevention tools:

[A]t every scheduled visit, subjects received a comprehensive package of prevention services, including HIV testing, risk-reduction counselling, condoms, and diagnosis and treatment of symptomatic sexually transmitted infections, including gonorrhoea and chlamydia urethritis, syphilis and herpes simplex virus type 2 (HSV-2)... All subjects were instructed to protect themselves from HIV with conventional methods, since they were unaware of their study-group assignment. Subjects who reported a recent unprotected exposure to an HIV-infected partner were referred for postexposure prophylaxis (at sites where such therapy was available)...Vaccination against hepatitis B virus (HBV) was offered to all susceptible subjects (Grant et al. 2010, p. 2589).

The nature of clinical support provided was comprehensive and significant given the intervals at which subjects were seen. The monitoring of sexual health of subjects was conducted by biological tests '[T]esting for HIV antibody was performed on whole blood with use of two different tests at every scheduled visit, and reactive rapid tests were tested with the use of Western blot analysis of serum'...Testing for drug resistance genotyping was performed with use of clinically validated assays' (Grant et al. 2010, p. 2589). These tests were routine during the trial, additional to tests conducted to enrol subjects to the trial. The measures discussed in this manner were created to monitor and motivate adherence.

Amico et al., analysing adherence procedures in number of these trials, point out that in the iPrEx RCT '[A]n adherence working group (AWG) was formed to investigate the potential discrepancy between the measurement of study product use and its actual use, and to offer potential recommendations' (2013, p. 2149). Given the importance of adherence to daily use for the outcomes of the RCT in the trial's diverse sites, this group suggested a number of strategies ''[C]onversations about product-use stressed the need for taking the daily dose at a specific time, and prescribed strategies to achieve this regularity. Tools were also provided to promote daily product use, including pill cases, where available, and key fobs or dose-carrying tools' (Amico et al. 2013, pp. 2149–2150).

Furthermore, they developed a specific counselling strategy 'Next Step Counselling (NSC) to support product use and Neutral Assessment' (Amico et al. 2013, pp. 2149–2150). This counselling approach is based on communication between subjects and the staff in the trial to facilitate self-reporting on product and sexual behaviour. According to Amico et al. '[T]he approach is designed with flexible content to be culturally adaptive and responsive to individual needs. The NSC approach recommends a general flow for product-use discussions and a climate to establish open conversation, while specific wording and guidance that the counsellors use are entirely individualized and make use of locally available resources' (2013, p. 2150).

While these aspects are presented in brief, and mostly as a background information to show how they maintained the integrity of the trial process, I argue that all of these aspects of the iPrEx trial together constitute a programme. With this programme, the trial informs participants' sexual and health behaviour during the trial. Subjects are gradually, at each visit, conditioned and taught how to be within the procedures of the trial. These aspects of the trial do not just attempt to reduce the chances of people dropping out of the trial, jeopardising its integrity. They are measures central for producing the efficacy results that were presented. These measures create an environment that aims to control and influence subjects' adherence to the procedures for the pill use and change sexual practices during the trial (see Grant et al. 2010, p. 2590). The affordances of the trial setting in this way are part of the efficacy demonstrated for the PrEP in this and other similar trials (including demonstration studies see van der Elst et al. 2013; Hoagland et al. 2017). What matters, therefore, is not only the proof of efficacy of a pill or a particular regimen in which the pill is used but also how it was possible to use that pill in that particular way over time: what enabled participants to go through this process in the right ways to produce efficacy.

2.3.3   From Trial to Policy What Do we Need to Know?

If trials are also environments that allow affordances, with specific social regulations, to maintain the integrity of research, we then need to think how such affordances are, or could be, related to everyday environments, that have different affordances, for people expected to engage with PrEP policy outside of trials. PrEP trials, as installations, bring together the above-mentioned three components: 'individuals and their embodied competencies, the material environment and social regulation' (Lahlou 2017, pp. 94–95). In the iPrEx trial I observed how the installation works by bringing together these components: (a) the trial brought together resources to enable participants to understand and use the medical regimen. The trial was an attempt to develop individuals' competencies. Part of this was the support mechanism used at each visit to motivate participants to adhere to the required regimen of behaviour and medicine within their everyday sexual lives; (b) the material environment that was created by the trial was extensive. It included clinical support mechanisms that provided extensive material capacity, including trained clinical support staff who were able to engage at multiple levels from laboratory testing to counselling; and (c) all of these were located within a system of norms and rules that framed the trial to create the adherence needed for positive research results. For instance, participants were encouraged, indeed required, to talk about their sexual behaviours and experiences. Furthermore, participants were made clearly aware that testing as HIV positive would end their participation in the trial and the access to the resources provided by the trial, strengthening their incentives to adhere.

The trial as an installation created its own social and behavioural environment. I argue that the iPrEx, and other PrEP related trials, are not just about demonstrating the efficaciousness of a pharmaceutical product or about showing that adherence matters. They are also about how the conditions for adherence can be created to motivate and support a group of people to engage with a pharmaceutical product given a context. The specific aspects of this process, as described above, come together in the context of the trial to produce a positive outcome. It is this coming together, being an installation, that needs to be considered as policy relevant. So, PrEP becomes a programme through the trial that worked for a group of people with specific characteristics. The question for PrEP becoming a programme for wider policy then becomes about how to translate the trial as installation into relevant policies for different contexts (see Hellström and Jacob 2017).

2.4 Conclusions

By way of conclusion, I argue that PrEP policy is indeed a programme that needs to guide and support different people in different places through their sexual lives. The chapter highlighted that PrEP research shows how an installation is needed to produce certain affordances to guide participants to achieve results. PrEP policy needs to work as a programme for the pharmaceutical product to work for prevention.

Considering how trials guide behaviour, the role of specific affordances becomes central for considering a PrEP policy as a programme. But a caution is required. A programme developed through a trial is unlikely to be replicable to produce similar results when its affordances are taken to be policy relevant as a general policy for different contexts. The affordances in trials are created for specific participant groups and according to their needs in each trial. So, the point here is that PrEP as a programme in different contexts needs to consider different and relevant affordances for people in those contexts. The idea of a programme needs to understand people, their needs and their behaviour within their specific contexts as underpinned by their contextual norms, values and social expectations, rather than thinking using limited generic risk categories such as gay, MSM or sex worker or heterosexual. The engagement with PrEP as a prevention tool is likely to be perceived differently by different groups in different contexts. While it is important to look at the successful research to understand how the given success was created there, what are the mechanisms that support such success, the components of required affordances in relation to specific groups need to be considered in each context for PrEP policy as a programme. PrEP policy as a programme needs to think about affordances that are directly relevant for everyday lives where for instance same-sex relations or sex-work might be criminalised and/or stigmatised. To work PrEP is a programme should not just be about a generic programme but rather a *contextualised programme* for the particular target groups and their needs in those contexts.

References

Abbas, U. L., Glaubius, R., Mubayi, A., Hood, G., & Mellors, J. W. (2013). Antiretroviral therapy and pre-exposure prophylaxis: Combined impact on HIV transmission and drug resistance in South Africa. *Journal of Infectious Diseases, 208*(2), 224–234.

Amico, K. R., Mansoor, L. E., Corneli, A., Torjesent, K., & van der Straten, A. (2013). Adherence support approaches in biomedical prevention trials: Experiences, insights and future directions from four multisite prevention trials. *AIDS Behaviour, 17*, 2143–2155.

AVAC. (2019). *On going and planned PrEP open label demonstration and implementation projects*. Retrieved March 25, 2020, from https://www.avac.org/sites/default/files/resource-files/ongoing_planned_oralPrEP_studies_april2019.pdf

Baeten, J. M., Donnell, D., Ndase, P., Mugo, N. R., Campbell, J. D., Wangisi, J., et al. (2012). Antiretroviral prophylaxis for HIV prevention in heterosexual men and women. *New England Journal of Medicine, 367*(5), 399–410.

Choopanya, K., Martin, M., Suntharasamai, P., Sangkum, U., Mock, P. A., Leethochawalit, M., et al. (2013). Antiretroviral prophylaxis for HIV infection in injecting drug users in Bangkok, Thailand (the Bangkok Tenofovir study): A randomised, doubleblind, placebo-controlled phase 3 trial. *Lancet, 381*(9883), 2083–2090.

Coleman, R. (2018). Setting the scene, setting the targets. Joint United Nations Programme on HIV/AIDS prevention targets of 2016 and estimated global pre-exposure prophylaxis targets. *Sexual Health, 15*, 485–488.

Cremin, I., Morales, F., Jewell, B. L., O'Reilly, K. R., & Hallett, T. B. (2015). Seasonal PrEP for partners of migrant miners in southern Mozambique: A highly focused PrEP intervention. *Journal of Intentional AIDS Society, 18*(4 Suppl 3), 19946.

Di Ciaccio, M., Protiere, C., Castro, D. R., Suzan-Monti, M., Chas, J., Cotte, L., et al. (2018). The ANRS-Ipergay trial, an opportunity to use qualitative research to understand the perception of the "participant"-physician relationship. *AIDS Care, 30*(Suppl. 2), 41–47.

Dunbar, M., Kripke, K., Haberer, J., Castor, D., Dalal, S., Mukoma, W., et al. (2018). Understanding and measuring uptake and coverage of oral pre-exposure prophylaxis delivery among adolescent girls and young women in sub-Saharan Africa. *Sexual Health, 15*(6), 513–521.

Eribon, D. (2004). *Insult and the making of the gay self*. (M. Lucey, Trans.). Durham and London: Duke University Press.

Gafos, M., Horne, R., Nutland, W., Bell, G., Rae, C., Wayal, S., et al. (2019). The context of sexual risk behaviour among men who have sex with men seeking PrEP, and the impact of PrEP on sexual behaviour. *AIDS and Behaviour, 23*(7), 1708–1720.

Gibson, J. J. (1977). Theory of affordance, chapter 3. In R. Shaw & J. Bransford (Eds.), *Perceiving, acting and knowing: Toward an ecological psychology* (pp. 67–87). Hillsdale, NJ: Lawrence Erlbaum Ass.

Good, J. J. M. (2007). The affordances for social psychology of the ecological approach to social knowing. *Theory & Psychology, 17*(2), 265–295.

Grant, R. M. (2019). *Testimony of Robert M Grant – Hearing on 'HIV prevention drug: Billions in corporate profits after millions in taxpayer investment'*. U.S. House of Representatives House Committee on Oversight and Reform. Retrieved November 27, 2019, from https://docs.house.gov/Committee/Calendar/ByEvent.aspx?EventID=109486.

Grant, R. M., Lama, J. R., Anderson, P. L., McMahan, V., Liu, A. Y., Vargas, L., et al. (2010). Preexposure chemoprophylaxis for HIV prevention in men who have sex with men. *New England Journal of Medicine, 363*(27), 2587–2599.

Haire, B. G. (2015). Preexposure prophylaxis-related stigma: Strategies to improve uptake and adherence-a narrative review. *HIV/AIDS Research and Palliative Care, 7*, 241–249.

Hankins, C., Macklin, R., & Warren, M. (2015). Translating PrEP effectiveness into public health impact: Key considerations for decision-makers on cost-effectiveness, price, regulatory issues, distributive justice and advocacy for access. *Journal of International AIDS Society, 18*(Suppl. 3), 19973.

Heffron, R., Ngure, K., Odoyo, J., Bulya, N., Tindimwebwa, E., Hong, T., et al. (2018). Pre-exposure prophylaxis for HIV-negative persons with partners living with HIV: Uptake, use, and effectiveness in an open-label demonstration project in East Africa. *Gates Open Research, 1*, 3.

Hellström, T., & Jacob, M. (2017). Policy instrument affordances: A framework for analysis. *Policy Studies, 38*(6), 604–621.

Hildebrandt, T. (2018, September 27). No more excuses: The NHS must fund the drug that stops people getting HIV. *The Guardian.* https://www.theguardian.com/commentisfree/2018/sep/27/nhs-fund-anti-hiv-drugs-prep.

Hoagland, B., Moreira, R. I., De Boni, R. B., Kallas, E. G., Madruga, J. V., Vasconcelos, R., et al. (2017). High pre-exposure prophylaxis uptake and early adherence among men who have sex with men and transgender women at risk for HIV infection: The PrEP Brasil demonstration project. *Journal of the International AIDS Society, 20*(1), 21472.

Hodges-Mameletzis, I., Dalal, S., Msimanga-Radebe, B., Rodolph, M., & Baggaley, R. (2018). Going global: The adoption of the World Health Organization's enabling recommendations on oral pre-exposure prophylaxis for HIV. *Sexual Health, 15*, 489–500.

Kibengo, F. M., Ruzagira, E., Katende, D., Bwanika, A. N., Bahemuka, U., Haberer, J. E., et al. (2013). Safety, adherence and acceptability of intermittent tenofovir/emtricitabine as HIV pre-exposure prophylaxis (PrEP) among HIV-uninfected Ugandan volunteers living in HIV-serodiscordant relationships: A randomized, clinical trial. *PLoS One, 8*(9), e74314.

Lahlou, S. (2017). *Installation theory: The societal construction and regulation of behaviour.* Cambridge: CUP.

Lal, L., Audsley, J., Murphy, D. A., Fairley, C. K., Stoove, M., Roth, N., et al. (2017). Medication adherence, condom use and sexually transmitted infections in Australian preexposure prophylaxis users. *AIDS, 31*(12), 1709–1714.

Mack, N., Wong, C., McKenna, K., Lemons, A., Odhiambo, J., & Agot, K. (2015). Human resource challenges to integrating HIV pre-exposure prophylaxis (PrEP) into the public health system in Kenya: A qualitative study. *African Journal of Reproductive Health, 19*, 54–62.

Marcus, J. L., Glidden, D. V., Mayer, K. H., Liu, A. Y., Buchbinder, S. P., Amico, K. R., et al. (2013). No evidence of sexual risk compensation in the iPrEx trial of daily oral HIV preexposure prophylaxis. *PLoS One, 8*(12), e81997.

McCormack, S., Dunn, D. T., Desai, M., et al. (2016). Pre-exposure prophylaxis to prevent the acquisition of HIV-1 infection (PROUD): Effectiveness results from the pilot phase of a pragmatic open-label randomised trial. *The Lancet, 387*, 53–60.

Molina, J. M., Capitant, C., Spire, B., Pialoux, G., Cotte, L., Charreau, I., et al. (2015). On-demand Preexposure prophylaxis in men at high risk for HIV-1 infection. *New England Journal of Medicine, 373*(23), 2237–2246.

Mugo, N. R., Ngure, K., Kiragu, M., Irungu, E., & Kilonzo, N. (2016). The preexposure prophylaxis revolution; from clinical trials to programmatic implementation. *Current Opinion in HIV and AIDS, 11*(1), 80–86.

O'Malley, G., Barnabee, G., & Mugwanya, K. (2019). Scaling-up PrEP delivery in sub-Saharan Africa: What can we learn from the scale-up of ART? *Current HIV/AIDS Reports, 16*(2), 141–150.

Prepsters. (2020). *Questions and answers on PrEP.* Retrieved November 25, 2019, from https://prepster.info/prep-faqs/

Rojas Castro, D., Delabre, R. M., & Molina, J. M. (2019). Give PrEP a chance: Moving on from the "risk compensation" concept. *Journal of International AIDS Society, 22*(Suppl6), e25351.

Sagaon-Teyssier, L., Suzan-Monti, M., Demoulin, B., Capitant, C., Lorente, N., Preau, M., et al. (2016). Uptake of PrEP and condom and sexual risk behavior among MSM during the ANRS IPERGAY trial. *AIDS Care - Psychological and Socio-Medical Aspects of AIDS/HIV, 28*, 48–55.

Schwartz, K., Ferrigno, B., Vining, S., Gomez, A., Briedenhann, E., Gardiner, E., et al. (2018). PrEP communications accelerator: A digital demand creation tool for sub-Saharan Africa. *Sexual Health, 15*, 570–577.

Thigpen, M. C., Kebaabetswe, P. M., Paxton, L. A., Smith, D. K., Rose, C. E., Segolodi, T. M., et al. (2012). Antiretroviral preexposure prophylaxis for heterosexual HIV transmission in Botswana. *The New England Journal of Medicine, 367*(5), 423–434.

van der Elst, E. M., Mbogua, J., Operario, D., Mutua, G., Kuo, C., Mugo, P., et al. (2013). High acceptability of HIV pre-exposure prophylaxis but challenges in adherence and use: Qualitative insights from a phase I trial of intermittent and daily PrEP in at-risk populations in Kenya. *AIDS Behaviour, 17*(6), 2162–2172.

Venter, W. D. F., Cowan, F., Black, V., Rebe, K., & Bekker, L. G. (2015). Pre-exposure prophylaxis in southern Africa: Feasible or not? *Journal of International AIDS Society, 18* (suppl 3), 35–41.

WHO. (2012). *Guidance on pre-exposure Oral prophylaxis (PrEP) for serodiscordant couples, men and transgender women who have sex with men at high risk of HIV: Recommendations for use in the context of demonstration projects?* Geneva: WHO.

WHO. (2015). *Guideline on when to start antiretroviral therapy and on pre-exposure prophylaxis for HIV*. Geneva: WHO.

WHO. (2017). *WHO implementation tool for pre-exposure prophylaxis (PrEP) for HIV infection (module 1 clinical)*. Geneva: WHO.

Zablotska, I. B., Beaten, J. M., Panuphak, N., McCormack, S., & Ong, J. (2018). Getting pre-exposure prophylaxis (PrEP) to the people: Opportunities, challenges and examples of successful health service models of PrEP implementation. *Sexual Health, 15*, 481–484.

Chapter 3
Making the Ideal Real: Biomedical HIV Prevention as Social Public Health

Mark Davis

3.1 Introduction

As previous chapters in this volume have shown, a variety of experts have speculated that the 'end of AIDS' is now possible due to the use of antiretroviral treatments to reduce the transmission of HIV (sometimes called treatment as prevention, TasP). In support of such a claim, a 2019 article in the online version of *The Guardian* carried the following headline: 'End to AIDS in sight as huge study finds drugs stop HIV transmission' (Boseley and Devlin 2019). As news media often do, the item reported on the publication of an article in *The Lancet* summarising findings from the PARTNER study in Europe (Rodger et al. 2019), which showed that TasP considerably reduces the risk of HIV transmission to the regular partners of gay men with HIV. The lead researcher of the PARTNER study reportedly said that:

> Our findings provide conclusive evidence for gay men that the risk of HIV transmission with suppressive ART [antiretroviral therapy] is zero. Our findings support the message of the international U=U campaign that an undetectable viral load makes HIV untransmittable. This powerful message can help end the HIV pandemic by preventing HIV transmission, and tackling the stigma and discrimination that many people with HIV face (Boseley and Devlin 2019).

These findings, as welcome as they are, are particular since they pertain to gay men in ongoing regular partnerships. This important proviso with respect to the apparently universal notion of U=U will be considered in what is to follow. *The Guardian* article also cites a commentary on the PARTNER study by Myron Cohen, who says:

> It has taken considerable time and massive effort to prove that antiretroviral drugs can prevent HIV through treatment or as PrEP. During the course of these studies, antiretroviral

M. Davis (✉)
School of Social Sciences, Monash University, Melbourne, Australia
e-mail: mark.davis@monash.edu

© Springer Nature Switzerland AG 2021
S. Bernays et al. (eds.), *Remaking HIV Prevention in the 21st Century*, Social Aspects of HIV 5, https://doi.org/10.1007/978-3-030-69819-5_3

drugs have become more effective, reliable, durable, easier to take, well tolerated, and much less expensive. The results of the PARTNER2 study provide yet one more catalyst for a universal test-and-treat strategy to provide the full benefits of antiretroviral drugs. This and other strategies continue to push us toward the end of AIDS (Cohen 2019, p. 2367).

Cohen admits, however, that achieving this goal may not be easy,

Yet maximising the benefits of ART has proven daunting, especially for MSM. It is not always easy for people to get tested for HIV or find access to care; in addition, fear, stigma, homophobia, and other adverse social forces continue to compromise HIV treatment. Furthermore, diagnosis of HIV infection is difficult in the early stages of infection when transmission is very efficient, and this limitation also compromises the treatment as prevention strategy (2019, pp. 2366–2367).

Such a way of talking about the pandemic—as welcome as the end of AIDS would be—gives the impression that it is only now, through the use of diagnostic and pharmaceutical measures, that the end of AIDS is imaginable and possible. This approach has been criticised for its incipient erasure of the social knowledge and political action that first made the prevention of HIV possible (Nguyen et al. 2011; Kippax and Stephenson 2016). It also glosses over the currents and eddies produced by biotechnology's contribution to HIV prevention, for example, 'treatment optimism' and its influence on the risk practices of people with HIV (Elford et al. 2002). It also identifies psychosocial dynamics—fear, stigma, prejudice, homophobia—as the principal barrier to TasP, as if the eradication of these factors would allow TasP to operate without impediment. Casting society as the problematic other exposes the axiomatic, reductive rationality of biomedicalising HIV prevention. Another effect of this perspective is to do disservice to the many people who have been affected by the pandemic across the decades and throughout the world, and who have laboured to prevent the infection and moderate its effects. Affected individuals and communities have strived under often pressing conditions to work towards the end of AIDS using whatever tools and techniques came to hand, often by adapting biomedical methods of prevention to address the social conditions of their existence. HIV prevention has always been framed by an imaginary of how the end of AIDS might be possible.

It is not difficult to find examples of HIV prevention activity that attest to the complexities somewhat obscured by reductive talk of the end of AIDS. In 1986, as a volunteer for the lesbian and gay switchboard in Brisbane, Queensland, Australia, I helped to facilitate a number of Stop AIDS workshops in community settings. Stop AIDS was developed in the United States by gay communities in response to HIV and employed small group-based experiential learning activities (Robert and Rosser 1990). The workshops brought together small groups of gay and bisexual men who wanted to find out more about HIV and how infection could be prevented through the use of condoms for anal sex. These workshops were important moments for these men because they happened at a time when biomedicine and its institutional frameworks were able to provide few answers. They were also a means of community organising and building a shared knowledge and language around HIV prevention and safer sex that men could take into their interactions with sex partners and friends.

The programme of workshops had the effect of including men who may not have been able to discuss HIV and their sexual practices with health care providers. The sex positive tone of the exercises was also a means of resisting the oppression and prejudice that many of us had experienced in different ways in family, work and social life. Moreover, the workshops were transgressive in the sense that sodomy remained a prosecutable sexual act until 1990 in Queensland (Robinson 2011). For all these reasons, the workshops were complicatedly situated at the intersection of the making of male homosexual life, legal proscription, and the need to respond to the newly spreading HIV pandemic. Stopping AIDS, then as it is now, necessitated practical address to life in particular circumstances to enable individual and collective action, a socio-political dimension of HIV prevention that is somewhat lost in the current turnings in discourse on the end of AIDS (Kippax and Stephenson 2016).

This example shows, too, that HIV prevention is not an absolute project, but one of gradual and reflexive adaptation of knowledge about how to take action on the risk and effects of HIV. Stop AIDS formulated a queer phronesis against threat to life; it helped to fashion practical responses to HIV that accounted for the sexual, legal, technological and relational means through which action was possible at that time. As the years passed, the Stop AIDS programme came to be replaced by other methods of community organising for HIV education and prevention as the response to the pandemic became more organised and as the HIV education able to be performed became more sophisticated through closer links with social and epidemiological research (Kippax and Race 2003). Significantly, Stop AIDS and workshop programmes like it were found in trials to show only weak evidence of attributable behaviour change (Robert and Rosser 1990). HIV prevention was found wanting in the particular scientific terms of behavioural theory, marking a likely early moment in the process where HIV educators were required to navigate different paradigms of scientific reasoning on how best to take action. Hindsight tells us, though, that the critical evaluation of Stop AIDS showed, not that the HIV prevention approach was flawed, but just that it was incomplete. The lesson that the evaluation of Stop AIDS afforded was that HIV prevention approaches are opened to the future in the sense that they are necessarily oriented to modification and improvement. The same can be said of any HIV prevention approach, including biomedical ones.

The narrow representations of the end of AIDS that currently imbue public and scientific discourse can be attributed to what Cindy Patton (2011) has referred to as the epistemological hegemony of particular biomedicalising approaches to HIV prevention and, in particular, particular methods of 'seeing' the pandemic. Patton argues that TasP, for example, frames HIV prevention in ways that can see only disease, and not illness:

> Witnessing illness requires the ongoing presence of the persons who are ill, as in the claims to dignity by the early persons with AIDS. Witnessing disease is the observation of the epidemic from the point of view of those who imagine themselves not subject to the disease, a disembodied meta-vision characteristic both of epidemiologists and research scientists who "see" the epidemic through statistical means, and also of the public officials who deploy that science as policy by speaking from the point of view of "the public" (Patton 2011, p. 255).

Some representations of TasP focus on disease and therefore do not benefit from the epistemological position afforded by witnessing the pandemic and how HIV can be prevented in ways that reflect the *social* realities of those affected. Patton notes, also, that biomedical HIV prevention is often predicated on the notion of right to health, but without the benefit of witnessing illness, it may be seen to reduce the freedoms of those affected by the pandemic. For Patton, therefore, viewing HIV prevention through a particular TasP lens makes it possible for wrongs to be committed in the language of rights.

In what follows, I want to explore biomedical HIV prevention in the light of Patton's and others' critiques. I consider a key feature of biomedicalised HIV prevention—mathematical modelling—to consider some of the assumptions about HIV prevention and its subjects built into these approaches. In particular, I will examine the growing literature that is helping to identify some of the blindspots of biomedical approaches to HIV prevention and consider how their effects could be extended in light of knowledge regarding the social and political action needed to prevent and moderate the impact of HIV amongst affected individuals and communities.

3.2   Algorithmic HIV Prevention

TasP as viable HIV prevention owes much to the mathematical modelling that has demonstrated at a population level how increased HIV diagnosis, treatment and reduced infectivity could considerably reduce the annual incidence of new infections (Granich et al. 2009; Kippax and Stephenson 2016). The models depend on the collection and combination of data about HIV diagnoses, treatment effects, viral loads, and HIV infectivity, HIV prevalence, sexual and drug using networks and risk behaviours; deepening a focus on particular forms of data as a source of truth-making and closely tying decision-making to data generation systems across clinical and community settings. HIV prevention policy frameworks feature largely quanti-tative targets, for example, UNAIDS's 90-90-90 programme (2014). Variations on the 90-90-90 targets have been proposed that add a 'fourth 90' focussed on psycho-social wellbeing (Lazarus et al. 2016, p. e94), but these conceptualisations of HIV prevention also reinscribe the underlying modelling logic of the TasP era. Axiom-atically, modelling orients public policy to the future, since the manipulation of key variables is assumed to lead to desired outcomes. TasP is therefore not simply the discovery of the HIV prevention properties of antiretroviral pharmaceuticals; it is an assemblage of the material, symbolic and temporal effects of data, mathematics, computational methods, the epidemiological gaze, diagnostic and pharmaceutical technologies, and many other actants (DeLanda 2016).

Modelling rationality and its application to TasP can be seen in the following fragment from an interview I conducted with a researcher based in North America[1]:

> Well, literally, you have equations that go into your model … like you just need, like let's say that you're going to assume that, in your model, this proportion of people get tested at least once a year. And that proportion might come from some community survey that's asked people: did you test in the last 12 months? So they'll have, let's say 80 per cent did for the sake of argument. So, you're gonna plug into your model that 80 per cent of people tested and then that goes into the mathematical equations. And then all along there's a lot of math. At another point in time, in the model, it might be: well what proportion of people who now have HIV and are in care, what proportion of them are on treatment? And that may come say from a cohort like ours or from a health administrative database or a clinical database. What proportion of people on treatment are suppressed? That could come from a whole other piece of evidence. So, you're able to bring information in from many different places and you create an environment where you first see how well your math can estimate what's really going on right now. Like does it calculate the right number of people with outcome X. And then, once you get that right, then you get to play and you get to say, "Well what if we got more people to test every year? What if we got more people on treatment? What if we had more people more of them undetectable? How does that affect the estimated infection rate that this model is pumping out, right?" So, and then people kind of associate cost with that. How much did it cost to do that kind of a health promotion program? What money do you save with healthcare savings? And people do all the math once it's … I think it can be very helpful for answering questions about … It's not the end-all of, it doesn't explain the human stories behind that but it has its, you know, benefits (2013).

The interview fragment shows rather clearly how variables—rates of testing, viral load measures and cost—are incorporated into models to assess their contribution to outcomes. It seems, however, that some—if not many—of the social dynamics and meanings that also shape HIV prevention (stigma, prejudice, homophobia, fear) may not get into the models because they are less easy to quantify.

In addition, the TasP approach and its models do not appear to engage with the reflexivity of their subjects, people affected by HIV. The creative and reflexive use of the knowledge generated by biotechnology has typified responses to HIV, for example, in relation to the practice of negotiated safety (Kippax et al. 1993), strategic disclosures of serostatus online to reduce exposure to prejudice (Davis and Flowers 2014), or accessing PrEP off prescription via online pharmacies (Nwokolo et al. 2017). Individuals, who gain knowledge of what TasP can do, are likely to incorporate that knowledge into their decisions and practices, thereby contributing to the effects TasP can have in lifeworlds. These hermeneutical aspects of TasP cannot be simply reduced to risk compensation, which supposes an actuarial and atomised approach to the risk of HIV transmission (Davis 2002). New kinds of risk considerations are likely to emerge through the reduction of existing ones that TasP is designed to moderate. Whether and how mathematical modelling will address these new futures is not clear and underlines some of the drawbacks of HIV prevention reductionism.

---

[1]The interview fragments come from the *Transformative HIV and Sexual Health Technologies* project, funded by a Monash Research Accelerator Grant (2013–2014). Ethics approval for this project was granted by Monash University Human Research Ethics Committee.

In addition, as with any mode of HIV prevention, the models that undergird TasP are incomplete even in the view of those who create them. As the interviewee above noted, 'It's not the end-all of, it doesn't explain the human stories behind that', showing that modelling and therefore TasP are only some of the components of effective HIV prevention, a point made by Kippax and Stephenson (2016). A similar provisionality emerges in the following fragment from an interview with a policy maker in the UK, who observed a shift in her reckoning of the value of modelling and its utility:

> Of course, I always defer to, you know, the experts but we're beginning to question that a little bit more. We think maybe the inputs into the modelling might have led us down a different path. .. one of the things that I realised, like the rise and rise of modelling happened during that time, and modelling is a very seductive kind of black art, you know, because it's about, it's a scientific crystal ball-gazing, you know. It says, you know, "This is what might happen in the future," and it has a real scientific base to it so you just, we love numbers. And they're very kind of convincing. You know, when this was being developed, I think I had far more of a blind faith in the modelling than I do now. This is nothing against the modellers 'cause they are fantastic people, working very hard and very, very smart, but I didn't, I s'pose I didn't have the nous or . . . this makes it sound it was all me . . . we didn't have the nous to say, "Hold on a second. Let's question the assumptions that go into it." We kind of assumed that all the inputs were appropriate. But I, to tell the truth, we didn't, probably didn't have the same accurate input then that we do now (2014).

The above account signals growing awareness of what models can and cannot do, leading to some reservations with regard to how they can be most profitably used. It shows in another way how TasP and related approaches can be opened to their futures, questioned and improved.

3.3   Multiplicity and Particularity

End of AIDS discourse and mathematical modelling, then, gloss over the social, technological and temporal multiplicities and particularities of biomedical HIV prevention in real life contexts. Paul Flowers (2001) developed an early account of the future of HIV prevention for gay men in light of emerging knowledge of what highly active antiretroviral treatment meant for people with HIV and their partners, including, emerging knowledge of viral load and its implications for infectivity and risk of reinfection that might compromise HIV treatment. Flowers's framing of biomedical HIV prevention argued for increased socio-sexual specificity due to the fragmentation of the risk management strategies of gay men as sero- and treatment-related self-understandings proliferated. At first, safer sex for gay men was predicated on unifying liberation identities and the extension of sexual agency for all (Watney 2000), during a period when the HIV test did not exist and then when it did, was not necessarily recommended given that for some time no HIV treatments were available. By the late 1990s, safer sex strategies had been transformed by biomedical knowledge and effects, so much so that Flowers argued, presciently, for a growing attention to fragmentation and therefore the deepening complication of HIV prevention approaches.

Corinne Squire's (2013) qualitative research in the UK and South Africa with people with HIV, establishes in other ways how living long term with HIV and transnational mobilities and differences nuances the prospects for biomedical HIV prevention. Based on experiential narratives, Squire shows that the rollout of access to ART is partial and that not everyone finds available medications unproblematic to take over the long term, particularly people who have used earlier, less effective forms of ARTs. Interviewees spoke of considerable ambiguities with regard to their status as no longer sick but not utterly free from illness and of enduring considerations of navigating family life, sexual life, work and in the cases of refugees, citizenship and health rights in the UK. These experiential perspectives demonstrate that the realities of the post-TasP situation are somewhat glossed over in public and expert discourse on the end of AIDS. The myriad ways in which lived experience does not fit the universalising talk of the end of AIDS led Squire to focus more fully on HIV particularities, that is, the ways in which lived experiences of people with HIV do not always accord with how the pandemic is framed in science and policy discourse.

Following Flowers and Squire, biomedical HIV prevention takes on a kaleidoscopic quality and in ways not always indicated by the mathematical and scientific models used to design it. Moreover, HIV prevention complexity appears to be in part an effect of biomedical approaches. In another example, Baral et al. (2019) have questioned some of the premises of the TasP approach through a critical reading of biostatistics and knowledge showing that the risk of onward transmission of HIV is not universal for couples *per se*, or static over time for any particular couple. They suggest that HIV prevention approaches focussed on universal access to treatment may miss some couples with high levels of transmission risk and thereby produce pockets of inequity for those who may be in most need of HIV prevention support. They argue, therefore, against blanket population—and therefore suboptimal—HIV prevention and for more tailored and specific approaches that reflect the prevention needs of particular couples. Furthermore, it also appears that TasP may work best for the regular partners of heterosexual and gay people with HIV, but not so well for gay men with multiple partners. This insight has to do with the knowledge that infectivity is highest during the initial phases of infection (Cohen 2019). For gay men with multiple partners, TasP may simply be too delayed to have an effect, whereas PrEP may be useful, a point of view foreshadowed by Flowers (2001).

Biomedical approaches may also distort HIV prevention in unhelpful ways. Niels van Doorn's (2012), ethnographic research with Black and Minority gay and bisexual men in Baltimore showed that biomedical HIV prevention promised to stop the spread and effects of the virus, but also left communities abandoned to racialised inequalities and homophobia due to underinvestment in the social and political dimensions of health care, drawing into question how sustainable TasP and PrEP could be in these communities. Biomedical HIV prevention may therefore be implicated in the undercutting of already precarious, under-resourced community mobilisation, upon which the long-term prevention of HIV is likely to depend. Van

Doorn helps to draw attention, therefore, to how some modes of biomedical HIV prevention can see disease but be blind to illness, as identified by Patton (2011), giving the impression in this form of HIV prevention that lives only gain significance to the extent that they pose a threat to public health.

Picking up on a thematic raised by Flowers (2001), biomedical HIV prevention has different implications for people with different HIV serostatus or at different stages in their treatment for HIV. For example, Brisson and Nguyen (2017) found that HIV positive gay men in Paris responded to PrEP in many ways, including by endorsing the expanded opportunities for education about HIV, biotechnology and HIV prevention, feeling reassured of safety for their sexual partners, and with indifference. Young et al. (2016) have noted that in Scotland, both TasP and PrEP are understood in light of pre-existing expectations that people living with HIV are responsible for preventing HIV, implying that TasP and PrEP are elided and that therefore biomedical HIV prevention confers responsibility on people with the virus. These responses to PrEP underscore the multiple and particular ways in which biomedicalised HIV prevention is taken into real life.

3.4   Biomedical HIV Prevention as Social Public Health

These complex responses to the prospect of biomedical approaches to HIV prevention show that, for it to be effective across real life contexts and over time, attention needs to be given to its inherent disease gaze (Patton 2011), and a related tendency to representation of the social as a barrier to its effectiveness. As Kippax and Stephenson (2016) have argued, a more thoroughly articulated social public health is the medium through which biomedical HIV prevention can fulfil its aspirations. They define their approach as follows.

> This social approach, which elsewhere has been termed a social public health (Kippax and Stephenson 2012), moves beyond reliance on individual capacities or social structures or drivers as separate entities, and recognises that individual capacities are intimately tied to the enabling (or disabling) character of social norms, practices and institutions, which are, in turn, understood to be transformed or modified by community mobilisation and social movements (Kippax and Stephenson 2016, p. 144).

As the foregoing discussion indicates, biomedical HIV prevention addresses itself to viruses in bodies and populations and less well to the social factors that shape how people are able to respond to HIV. In particular, the mathematical models used to design prevention methods like TasP are predicated on a disease gaze and therefore help to constitute particular truth claims about how HIV prevention can be effective. How, then, can biomedical HIV prevention be framed as social public health so that it can be optimised and the harms and drawbacks it may produce be avoided or mitigated? How could such 'biosocial HIV prevention' produce forms of power-knowledge that include the otherwise excluded and that expand options for action where they might have been closed off?

Some responses to these questions come from, perhaps, a surprising source. Researchers from the Dean Street sexual health clinic in London (Nwokolo et al. 2017) have been able to link a significant (29%) decline in the annual incidence of HIV diagnoses amongst gay men in London with a range of biomedical HIV prevention approaches, including: increased access to HIV testing; early treatment after diagnosis; and the use of PrEP. These findings, superficially, support biomedical HIV prevention and place the clinic at the centre of intervention, helping to 'privatise' and 'individualise' HIV prevention so as to close off collective action (Kippax and Stephenson 2016). But the researchers also linked decreases in HIV infections with other aspects of the services they provide, including: in recognition that gay men were accessing PrEP online and off prescription, a support and pill testing service to ensure the efficacy of their PrEP doses; priority access for clients at high risk of infection for STI screening and postexposure prophylaxis (PEP); and what is called 'tailored online support to reduce HIV transmission risk' (Nwokolo et al. 2017, p. e483). Their account of the services provided by the clinic suggests extensive knowledge about particular service users and their sexual lives, ease of access to services and support programmes, and a collaborative approach to user-driven access to PrEP and PEP. The success of the clinic may also be attributable to the relative privilege of the client group, although the social characteristics of service users is not available in the article concerned. However, the apparent success of the Dean Street approach situates biomedical technologies in what appears to be a client-centred and nuanced approach to HIV prevention, where the lives of service users are influencing how the clinic goes about its business. Further evidence for this approach to HIV prevention is warranted to support it and therefore increase its effectiveness, but it does suggest how the sexual health clinic can itself help to assemble social public health.

Researching TasP with people in sero-different relationships in Australia, Asha Persson (2016) offers another perspective on biomedical HIV prevention in social context. Interviewees asked to reflect on knowledge that HIV treatment reduces viral load and therefore the risk of HIV transmission made reference to the benefits for health, emotions and their relationships. They also spoke of the ways in which sexual practices, hitherto problematically in the HIV prevention 'spotlight', receded from view to be replaced by a focus on treatment and its management *per se*. In this reckoning of biomedical HIV prevention, sexuality was 'de-medicalised', slipping off the surveillance agenda to help shape a newly experienced freedom for intimacy among the couples. Persson cautions that these effects are not reason to suppose that biomedical HIV prevention does not have unwanted effects. In addition to some already discussed, Persson notes that TasP in particular might lead to moral imperatives on the patient for excellent treatment outcomes and sustained U=U status, pressure to dispense with condoms for penetrative intercourse, or sharper health inequities that arise for sero-different couples unable to access treatment and viral monitoring. Fine-grained analyses like these are needed to support those people who have to manage biomedical HIV prevention into their lives and relationships, another way in which the social public health basis for biomedical HIV prevention can be understood and exacted.

Biomedical HIV prevention is an important suite of tools and techniques, but its effective application will require social and political action. As one Sydney HIV clinician commented to me, the prospect of the end of AIDS sponsored by TasP is 'tantalising', but for them at least, understood to be idealised:

> It's an area where you can't help feeling, if you look at what the mathematical modellers do, they show that, if you get a certain proportion of the population with viral suppression then, theoretically, you could potentially see the end of the epidemic. And that's an ideal world, obviously, but it's tantalising (2014).

This practitioner's comment captures the challenge of translating the scientific knowledge of efficacy into effectiveness. Understanding how to make the ideal real, however, is a knowledge form that mathematical models seem unlikely to deliver. While clinical trials demonstrate what antiretroviral medications can do for infectivity and models what might be done for HIV transmission, they reveal very little about how to make these effects in myriad real-world contexts and in the long term. The social, therefore, is no barrier to biomedical HIV prevention, it is the medium of its realisation. The effective rollout of biomedical HIV prevention will require the practical knowledge generated in the life worlds of people affected by the pandemic. It is only through these means that we can discover how to end AIDS in light of what biotechnologies can be found to do.

Stopping AIDS was HIV prevention teleology before the pharmaceutical control of the virus became possible. Then, as now, imagining how to stop AIDS generated a shared knowledge, language and access to technologies, assembled to prevent infections and build collective action in ways meaningful and useful for people affected by the pandemic and fitted to the changing circumstances of their existence. If biomedical HIV prevention can stop AIDS it will be practical, situated social and political action that will make it happen.

Acknowledgements I am grateful for comments from Paul Flowers and Corinne Squire and the contributions made by interviewees. Research for this chapter was in part supported by a grant from the Monash University Research Accelerator Programme.

References

Baral, S., Rao, A., Sullivan, P., Phaswana-Mafuya, N., Diouf, D., Millett, G., et al. (2019). The disconnect between individual-level and population-level HIV prevention benefits of antiretroviral treatment. *The Lancet HIV, 6*(9), e632–e638.

Boseley, S., & Devlin, H. (2019, May 2). *End to AIDS in sight as huge study finds drugs stop HIV transmission. The Guardian.* Retrieved May 9, 2019, from https://www.theguardian.com/society/2019/may/02/end-to-aids-in-sight-as-huge-study-finds-drugs-stop-hiv-transmission.

Brisson, J., & Nguyen, V. (2017). Science, technology, power and sex: PrEP and HIV-positive gay men in Paris. *Culture Health & Sexuality, 19*, 1066–1077.

Cohen, M. (2019). Successful treatment of HIV eliminates sexual transmission. *The Lancet, 393*, 2366–2367.

Davis, M. (2002). HIV prevention rationalities and serostatus in the risk narratives of gay men. *Sexualities, 5*, 281–299.

Davis, M., & Flowers, P. (2014). HIV/STI prevention technologies and strategic (in)visibilities. In M. Davis & L. Manderson (Eds.), *Disclosure in health and illness* (pp. 72–88). Abingdon: Routledge.

DeLanda, M. (2016). *Assemblage theory*. Edinburgh: Edinburgh University Press.

Elford, J., Bolding, G., & Sherr, L. (2002). High-risk sexual behaviour increase among London gay men between 1998 and 2001: What is the role of HIV optimism? *AIDS, 16*, 1–8.

Flowers, P. (2001). Gay men and HIV/AIDS risk management. *Health, 5*, 50–75.

Granich, R., Gilks, C., Dye, C., De Cock, K. M., & Williams, B. G. (2009). Universal voluntary HIV testing with immediate antiretroviral therapy as a strategy for the elimination of HIV transmission: A mathematical model. *The Lancet, 373*, 48–57.

Kippax, S., & Race, K. (2003). Sustaining safe practice: Twenty years on. *Social Science and Medicine, 57*, 1–12.

Kippax, S., & Stephenson, N. (2012). Beyond the distinction between biomedical and social dimensions of HIV: Prevention through the lens of social public health. *American Journal of Public Health, 102*(5), 789–799.

Kippax, S., & Stephenson, N. (2016). *Socialising the biomedical turn in HIV prevention*. London: Anthem Press.

Kippax, S., Crawford, J., Davis, M., Rodden, P., & Dowsett, G. (1993). Sustaining safe sex: A longitudinal study of a sample of homosexual men. *AIDS, 7*, 257–263.

Lazarus, J. V., Safreed-Harmon, K., Barton, S. E., Costagliola, D., Dedes, N., & del Amo Valero, J. (2016). Beyond viral suppression of HIV – The new quality of life frontier. *BMC Medicine, 14*, 94.

Nguyen, V., O'Malley, J., & Pirkle, C. (2011). Remedicalizing an epidemic: From HIV treatment as prevention to HIV treatment is prevention. *AIDS, 25*, 1435–1441.

Nwokolo, N., Hill, A., McOwan, A., & Pozniak, A. (2017). Rapidly declining HIV infection in MSM in Central London. *The Lancet HIV, 4*, e482–e483.

Patton, C. (2011). Rights language and HIV treatment: Universal care or population control? *Rhetoric Society Quarterly, 41*, 250–266.

Persson, A. (2016). 'The world has changed': Pharmaceutical citizenship and the reimagining of serodiscordant sexuality among couples with mixed HIV status in Australia. *Sociology of Health & Illness, 38*, 380–395.

Robert, B., & Rosser, S. (1990). Evaluation of the efficacy of AIDS education interventions for homosexually active men. *Health Education Research, 5*, 299–308.

Robinson, S. (2011). Queensland labor and lesbian, gay, bisexual,transgender, intersex and queer policy. *Queensland Review, 18*, 207–215.

Rodger, A., Cambiano, V., Bruun, T., Vernazza, P., Collins, S., Degen, O., et al. (2019). Risk of HIV transmission through condomless sex in serodifferent gay couples with the HIV-positive PARTNER taking suppressive antiretroviral therapy (PARTNER): Final results of a multicentre, prospective, observational study. *The Lancet, 393*, 2428–2438.

Squire, C. (2013). *Living with HIV and ARVs: Three letter lives*. Houndmills: Palgrave Macmillan.

UNAIDS. (2014). *90-90-90: An ambitious treatment target to help end the AIDS epidemic*. Geneva: Joint United Nations Programme on HIV/AIDS.

van Doorn, N. (2012). Between hope and abandonment: Black queer collectivity and the affective labour of biomedicalised HIV prevention. *Culture Health & Sexuality, 14*, 827–840.

Watney, S. (2000). *Imagine Hope: AIDS and gay identity*. London: Routledge.

Young, I., Flowers, P., & McDaid, L. (2016). Can a pill prevent HIV? Negotiating the biomedicalisation of HIV prevention. *Sociology of Health & Illness, 38*, 411–425.

Chapter 4
PrEP, HIV, and the Importance of Health Communication

Josh Grimm and Joseph Schwartz

4.1 Introduction

> Like many cancer patients, a lot of the men [with AIDS] were convinced that there was some
> cure out there; they just hadn't been linked up with it. When they were, they'd beat this bug
> and it would just be some ugly nightmare that would fade slowly from their memory (Shilts
> 1987 p. 83).

In Randy Shilts' (1987) journalistic account of the barriers, prejudices, and outright failures that would ultimately lead to the AIDS pandemic in the United States (USA), the prospect of a cure is regularly discussed, a depressing ritual the reader decades later knows will be futile. And then, after roughly 32 million deaths since the start of the epidemic, it was discovered that a combination of two antivirals—tenofovir and emtricitabine (called pre-exposure prophylaxis and branded as 'Truvada')—which were formally used to treat HIV, could actually prevent it. Pre-exposure prophylaxis (PrEP) delivered the ability to prevent HIV infection in nearly 99% of cases, and given that the disease decimated an entire generation, its adoption among at-risk groups should be extremely high, if not universal.

And yet, in the USA, that was not the case. Knowledge, awareness and, most importantly, adoption of PrEP was slow, with many men who have sex with men (MSM) learning about PrEP not from doctors, public health campaigns, or news media outlets, but rather from friends and sexual partners. Slow adoption can be partially explained by institutional issues—barriers certainly exist, particularly in the USA, a country without universal health care and with systemic biases against

J. Grimm (✉)
Manship School of Mass Communication, Lousiana State University, Baton Rouge, USA
e-mail: jgrimm@lsu.edu

J. Schwartz
College of Arts, Media and Design, Northeastern University, Boston, USA

© Springer Nature Switzerland AG 2021   47
S. Bernays et al. (eds.), *Remaking HIV Prevention in the 21st Century*, Social
Aspects of HIV 5, https://doi.org/10.1007/978-3-030-69819-5_4

underrepresented populations. However, the lag in knowledge and awareness, which took years to begin to correct, suggests something more is happening. After all, clinical trials have shown that the medication is not the problem; the science is sound.

PrEP is essentially a case study of the important role that communication can play. Health communication has the ability to do more than merely raise awareness of a health issue, it can also 'influence perceptions, beliefs, and attitudes that may change social norms; prompt action; demonstrate or illustrate healthy skills; reinforce knowledge, attitudes, or behavior; show the benefit of behavior change; advocate a position on a health issue or policy; increase demand or support for health services; refute myths and misconceptions; and strengthen organizational relationships' (Freimuth and Quinn 2004, p. 3). Through communicating the severity of a health issue, the susceptibility of an individual or population, how a potential product or practice might benefit that individual or population, and what barriers might prevent those benefits from occurring, public health interventions can be successfully implemented. Health communication faces challenges in the United States, due in no small part to the uniqueness of the US healthcare system, which has no universal healthcare coverage. However, communication strategies can be an effective tool in mitigating health disparities and improving the overall health of a variety of populations.

We argue that issues involving communication—be it inaccurate, biased, or nonexistent— have hindered adoption of PrEP. While the USA is only one country, and every country has its own challenges and institutional barriers that make a single message or approach infeasible, hopefully this discussion will inform decision-making outside its borders. In this chapter, we will focus on how a lack of effective messaging likely damaged adoption in the USA, and we will also attempt to identify opportunities for improving communication surrounding PrEP moving forward. Specifically, the central question that this chapter aims to address is: How can insights from research in mass communication, interpersonal communication, and app-based communication be employed to increase awareness and adoption of PrEP among MSM?

4.2   Mass Media and PrEP

The case of PrEP is unique because, while this drug had implications that could have dramatically shifted the understanding of how HIV could be prevented, it also was aimed at a stigmatised population that raised the possibility of controversy, something healthcare corporations in the USA usually look to avoid. While some companies delay promoting newly-released pharmaceuticals for 6 months to help prevent doctors being inundated with patient requests for drugs that the physicians were unaware had been approved, it took Gilead over 4 years to release any type of promotional materials for PrEP. In an interview with the *New Yorker*, the director of legislative affairs for the San Francisco AIDS foundation explained that, 'In any other kind of F.D.A. approval, there would have been beautiful ads, lots of TV, and lots of press touting the fact that this was the new thing to keep people protected from HIV. Gilead chose not to do that' (Glazek 2013).

Perhaps as a result of this lack of marketing, PrEP adoption rates were low, and in 2016, Gilead launched its first branded advertising content. Even then, it wasn't a huge financial commitment. In 2016, the company spent $450,000 advertising Truvada, but $101 million in advertisements for its Hepatitis C treatment, Harvoni (Lee 2017). The company has since increased its mass media presence across a variety of mediums and outlets, ranging from dating/hook-up apps to television ads.

In the absence of an advertising campaign by Gilead, affected populations had to continue to rely on activists, which have long played a crucial role in the fight against HIV (Castro et al. 2019). Activist organisations in the USA—such as Gay Men's Health Crisis or the National Association of People with AIDS—have helped lead the way in providing information and support, advocating for policy change, and seeking access to health care. Without the involvement of communities and activists who are impacted by HIV, the chances of eradicating this disease are extremely low (Valdiserri and Holtgrave 2019).

In addition to marketing communication, mass media messaging, including Internet resources, can play an important role in disseminating information to a population in the hopes of altering attitudes and behaviour. Research demonstrates that MSM frequently search for health information online (Dahlhamer et al. 2017; Jabson et al. 2017). Internet health resources may be particularly valuable for young MSM because sex education in the USA often does not address LGBTQ health (Nelson and Carey 2016; Currin et al. 2017).

Given this research (Currin et al. 2017; Dahlhamer et al. 2017; Jabson et al. 2017; Nelson and Carey 2016), understanding how PrEP is being presented online is essential. In their study of online news coverage of PrEP, Schwartz and Grimm (2016) found that a substantial amount of news coverage contained a high level of uncertainty as journalists focused largely on potential side effects, cost, and conflicting information that suggested a general scepticism about how effective the Truvada drug trials actually were. Given the levels of uncertainty in news coverage—particularly when it came to articles that specifically discussed MSM—these have the potential to slow PrEP adoption. Patients who read news pieces that stressed uncertainty might be reluctant to discuss the drug with their primary care physician, or have a resistance to the idea of PrEP if it was brought up during a medical consultation.

The most straightforward solution of altering news coverage is complicated by newsroom norms and routines, as journalists do not see themselves as part of the public relations arm of Gilead. However, journalists also carry the responsibility of telling stories of at-risk populations, particularly with something as serious as health. The slow response of the press to inform vulnerable communities about the risk of HIV is a tragic, well-documented story (Shilts 1987), and there has to be a happy medium between shilling for a multinational biopharmaceutical company and ignoring a significant advancement in the field.

While these issues are something journalists need to address, other media sources might point to a new way of messaging to those who are seeking health information. A growing number of individuals at-risk for HIV, particularly young MSM, have turned to social media as a source of health information. Social media provide a particularly appealing platform for increasing awareness and adoption of PrEP. They are a highly-individualised source of information which allows its users to curate what they see. Individuals are more likely to pay closer attention to content related to one's health if the source of that information is similar to them in terms of race, gender, sexuality, or psychographics (Hirshfield et al. 2015), which, again, is ideal for social media. Because social media eliminate gate-keepers, content on social media is not restricted to journalists, allowing millions of individuals and organisations to post information. The potential here is that these outlets are not constrained by professional codes and norms, and while this can manifest itself in some particularly ugly discourse, it can also provide an opportunity for advocates to have a powerful voice to strenuously, consistently speak out about PrEP. Social media sites like Twitter allow individuals who might be hesitant to discuss health matters—particularly issues of sexual health—with family, friends, or even health care providers to have timely, succinct pieces of information.

When analysing messaging on Twitter about Truvada, Schwartz and Grimm (2017) found that tweets about the drug potentially reinforced barriers to adoption, as a substantial amount of messaging focused on different types of barriers, such as cost, side effects, adherence, and accessibility. It is unfortunate that this replicates some of the problematic findings from the online news analysis. Moreover, very few tweets focused specifically on some aspect of race, gender, or sexuality, which can decrease the likelihood of messages resonating with at-risk audiences. However, social media were able to demonstrate the potential for effectively communicating about PrEP as well.

On a more positive note, while health organisations and news outlets can play a role in mitigating misinformation, individuals have the ability to actively eliminate stigma, which is what Schwartz and Grimm's (2017) study revealed. Not only were individuals more likely than organisations to counter stigma or misinformation, but those anti-stigma messages were likely to be liked and retweeted. This anti-stigma messaging, combined with targeted messaging from health organisations—such as promoting available programmes that can assist patients with costs and other resources for acquiring PrEP—and general information from news outlets, could prove essential for informing the public about the latest developments in PrEP moving forward, particularly with injection updates, implants, and generic versions of Truvada. This information ecosystem can be particularly effective because, as the messaging moves to social media, those discussions become more focused on interpersonal communication, which can be particularly effective.

Entertainment-education involves placing health information into entertainment media, such as television shows and movies. Research suggests that it can be highly effective in reaching a large number of people (Foss and Blake 2019), especially those who may be resistant to traditional health campaigns. HIV has benefited greatly from this practice, whether it's from an HIV storyline in the plot of a soap opera that resulted in a spike in phone calls to the Center for Disease Control (Beck 2004) or developing arts-based HIV-prevention events that resulted in an improved understanding of condom use (Campbell et al. 2009). PrEP storylines remain a largely untapped resource, though recent programming suggests that might be changing; PrEP was woven into character storylines on HBO's *Looking*, and PrEP was also discussed (along with viral loads) on the hit television programme, *How to Get Away with Murder*.

In summary, mass communication is important to consider in studying PrEP because: (1) marketing communication can raise awareness of new innovations; (2) news media likely play a role in shaping audiences' perceptions of new innovations; (3) social media have emerged as a way for people to share information about new innovations without the constraints of traditional media gatekeepers; and (4) entertainment-education can be a valuable tool for providing large audiences with health information.

4.3 Interpersonal Communication

At a more micro level, research in interpersonal communication provides valuable insights into how MSM might be encouraged or discouraged from adopting PrEP. Interpersonal communication, in the form of doctor-patient communication, plays a significant role in health. Matusitz and Spear (2014) explained that 'doctor-patient communication is such a powerful indicator of health care quality that it can determine patients' self-management behavior and health outcomes' (p. 252). In fact, excellent doctor-patient communication is associated with positive health outcomes because it facilitates better treatment (Dasinger et al. 2001). Research has demonstrated that effective communication between patients and providers can result in increased medication adherence, increased compliance, better self-regulation and coping, and faster return-to-work rates (Dasinger et al. 2001). It is worth noting that like any skill, communication skills can be improved and in particular, healthcare providers are capable of 'modifying their communication style if there is sufficient motivation and incentive for self-awareness, self-monitoring, and training' (Ha and Longnecker 2010, p. 40).

The basis of effective communication between doctors and patients involves doctors' and patients' skill in information giving, information receiving, information verifying, and socioemotional communication (Cegala et al. 1998). Beyond these basic skills, a key component of excellent doctor-patient communication involves relationship building between doctors and their patients (Ha and Longnecker 2010), which occurs over time through communication (Dyche 2007). Relationships encourage doctors and their patients to reach a 'shared understanding of the patient's perspective on his or her health condition so that both can manage the problem itself' (Matusitz and Spear 2014, p. 254). Strong doctor-patient relationships also help patients navigate the uncertainty that is often inherent in medical tests, procedures, treatment, and aftercare (Brashers et al. 2002). In the next three sections, we discuss the role of interpersonal communication in MSM's health, including PrEP.

4.3.1   MSM and Doctor-Patient Communication

Compared to their heterosexual counterparts, MSM have more negative healthcare interactions and have a tendency to delay or avoid important medical care (Mayer et al. 2008; Lim et al. 2014; Hatzenbuehler and Pachankis 2016; Schwartz and Grimm 2019). Though there are a number of explanations for this, one reason is poor communication between MSM and their healthcare providers. For example, Fuzzell et al. (2016) found that many young LGBTQ patients' interactions with doctors were marked by 'awkwardness, discomfort, or judgmental attitude' (p. 1469). Similarly, Smith and Turell (2017) found that almost all participants in their focus groups reported 'healthcare provider discomfort with sexual health conversations' and 'healthcare provider expressions of discomfort' (p. 645). Interviews with health care providers have demonstrated that many health professionals actually are uncomfortable discussing sexual health with their MSM patients (St. Vil et al. 2019). Additionally, healthcare providers may have moral objections to sexual health interventions such as PrEP, and/or feel that their MSM patients are not interested in discussing sexual health with them (St. Vil et al. 2019).

Some MSM do not disclose their sexual identities and behaviours to their doctors (Durso and Meyer 2013; Kaiser Family Foundation 2014; Liu et al. 2014; Petroll and Mitchell 2015). This is a problem because a provider's knowledge of his or her patient's sexual identity and behaviours is essential for providing the best possible care (LGBT Health Education Center 2017). An individual's nondisclosure of sexual identity and sexual behaviours may be an attempt to avoid awkward or uncomfortable conversations (Smith and Turell 2017). Another possibility for nondisclosure could be MSM patients' concern that their healthcare provider may harbour discriminatory attitudes toward LGBTQ people. This concern would not be unfounded. In a study of thousands of healthcare workers, including doctors, nurses, and mental health providers, Sabin et al. (2015) found that heterosexual healthcare workers consistently expressed implicit preferences for treating heterosexual patients over LGBTQ patients, associating words such as 'awful' with LGBTQ patients and words such as 'happy' with heterosexual patients (p. 1834). The researchers pointed out that this is problematic because 'widespread provider implicit preferences about sexual orientation may contribute to health and health care disparities among sexual minority populations' (Sabin et al. 2015, p. 1836). Similarly, Eliason et al. (2011) conducted a survey of over 400 LGBTQ physicians. They found that in the workplace, 65% of respondents had heard derogatory comments about LGBTQ patients and 34% of respondents had observed discriminatory care of a LGBTQ patient.

The amount of time devoted to LGBTQ health in medical schools, including instruction on communicating with LGBTQ patients, tends to be low (Obedin-Maliver et al. 2011; Moll et al. 2014). In a study of 176 medical schools in the

USA and Canada, Obedin-Maliver et al. (2011) found that the median amount of time dedicated to LGBTQ health was five hours. Similarly, in a survey of over 4000 medical students, 67.5% of respondents rated the LGBTQ health-related curriculum at the medical school they attended as 'fair', 'poor', or 'very poor' (White et al. 2015, p. 256). Reflecting on the paucity of attention LGBTQ health receives in medical education, Bonvicini (2017) noted that 'there continues to be a deficiency of cultural competency education training specific to treatment of LGBTQ patients for members of the healthcare team across disciplines' (Bonvicini 2017, p. 2360).

4.3.2 PrEP, Communication, and MSM

The role of interpersonal communication in MSM's PrEP use and adoption is important to consider. A variety of studies demonstrate that ineffective, unpleasant, and/or stigmatising interactions with health care providers can discourage PrEP adoption (Halton et al. 2019; Schwartz and Grimm 2019; Sun et al. 2019). For example, Schwartz and Grimm (2019) interviewed 38 MSM about their experiences. Their findings showed that stigmatisation by healthcare providers was a common experience when discussing PrEP adoption. Additionally, Schwartz and Grimm found that many healthcare providers were ill-informed about PrEP or did not feel comfortable discussing it. As a result, to adopt PrEP, participants had to strongly advocate for themselves, which required high levels of health literacy and high levels of communication skill. These findings illuminated important communication-based barriers to PrEP adoption, given that most people have low levels of health literacy and or communication skill (Cegala et al. 2007; WHO 2016). Similarly, another interview study of MSM found that many interviewees described PrEP-related doctor-patient interactions as 'awkward' and 'condescending' (Brooks et al. 2019, p. 1969). The researchers noted that these types of encounters 'discouraged participants from openly communicating with medical providers about the sexual behaviors that make them appropriate candidates for PrEP' (Brooks et al. 2019, p. 1970).

Additionally, being on PrEP requires ongoing interactions with a healthcare provider. This is facilitated by a strong doctor-patient relationship, which is built through communication (Dyche 2007). The World Health Organization (WHO) recommends that patients on PrEP should be seen by their doctor every three months to monitor and assess side effects of the medication, to ensure adherence to the medication, and to test for sexually transmitted infections (WHO 2017). Research shows that patients who report that they trust and feel comfortable with their healthcare provider are more likely to adopt PrEP and maintain its use (Sun et al. 2019).

In summary, understanding the impact of interpersonal communication is critical in PrEP awareness and adoption. At its best, doctor-patient communication can facilitate PrEP adoption and help to improve an individual's health. At its all-too-common worst, doctor-patient communication can discourage PrEP adoption and actively harm an individual's health.

4.4   Dating/Hookup Apps

In the past decade, one of the fastest-growing areas of opportunity for improving MSM sexual health—in particular the prevention of HIV and the promotion of PrEP—has been dating/hookup apps. In this section, we outline research on apps and their potential for improving MSM's health and increasing PrEP adoption and awareness.

Grindr, one of the most-used dating/hookup apps for MSM (henceforth 'apps'), was launched in 2009 (Fox 2019). Grindr uses a smart phone's geolocation functionality to connect users who are nearby. Users are displayed in a grid of profile photos, ordered from nearest to farthest from the person using the app. Tapping on a photo allows users to see others' profiles, send messages and pictures, and permits an individual to share his precise location. After exploding in popularity, alternatives to Grindr, including Scruff, Adam4Adam, and Growler, were launched a few years later. Research has revealed dating/hookup apps play a substantial role in the dating and sexual lives of many MSM (Sun et al. 2015; Badal et al. 2018; Rosengren et al. 2019).

Health advocates have realised the possibilities of apps in health promotion, including the promotion of PrEP, and generally app users are amenable to these efforts (Hall et al. 2017; Kesten et al. 2019; Fields et al. 2020). For example, in their study of young Black MSM, Fields et al. (2020) found that sexual health messages on apps could be regarded positively if they clearly distinguished themselves from spam messages and if messages avoided stigmatisation of users by focusing exclusively on race or other demographics. Fields et al. (2020) noted that apps potentially provide opportunities to reach hard-to-find MSM outside of gay-related physical spaces. Similarly, Czarny and Broaddus (2017) found that MSM regarded health-related messages on apps acceptable, especially when apps offered sexual health resources, including information about PrEP, that users could access on their own terms.

Ventuneac, John, Whitfield, Mustanski, and Parsons (2018) conducted a survey of MSM on a popular app to determine how interested users would be in using a variety of sexual health resources if they were available on the app. Results showed that users were most interested in features designed to locate LGBTQ-friendly healthcare providers, receive lab results, schedule healthcare appointments, and contact healthcare providers. Ventuneac and colleagues noted that compared to in-person strategies, apps may offer a cost-effective way to reach a large number of MSM.

In an innovative study, Hall et al. (2017) employed Grindr as a tool for health promotion by having a health educator set up a profile advertising that he was available to answer questions about sexual health. Although the health educator was friendly and engaged in relationship-building strategies with users, he did not initiate conversations with users to 'be respectful of the culture of the app user community, as it is inappropriate to target users with unsolicited HIV-related messages' (p. 41). Users routinely asked questions about HIV and STI testing and other sexual health issues.

In summary, apps are a promising new way to communicate with MSM and MSM appear open to receiving information and resources through them. They have the potential to provide MSM with health information, including information about PrEP. Additionally, they are potentially an effective way to reach people who may not be reachable through other forms of communication.

4.5   Conclusion

Communication in a variety of forms provides an important resource for sharing information, reducing uncertainty, challenging stigma, and emphasising the benefits of PrEP. However, as Freimuth and Quinn (2004) pointed out, health communication efforts, whether mass media, impersonal, or app-based, cannot make up for a lack of healthcare access and will not be successful in an environment that does not support health.

This chapter has outlined three areas of communication research—mass media, interpersonal communication, and app-based communication—that can be drawn on to increase PrEP adoption and awareness. Mass media, including marketing communication, news, social media and entertainment media can be leveraged in a variety of ways to inform MSM about PrEP and to encourage them to discuss it with their healthcare provider.

Interpersonal communication can have a tremendous impact on individuals' health. Communication training for healthcare providers at all levels would help to increase PrEP adoption and positively impact MSM's overall health. Moreover, the fact that so many at-risk individuals first learned about PrEP from friends and sexual partners rather than a targeted public health campaign or news article speaks to the importance of that interpersonal communication. Additionally, empowering people who have adopted PrEP to discuss it with their social networks could also help to increase PrEP use and fight PrEP stigma.

Dating/hookup apps such as Grindr, Scruff and Growlr already provide some health information to users, but more could be done to increase their impact. In collaboration with users, messages about PrEP could be developed that are tailored to the individual based on variables such as health resources available in the users' area, frequency of app use, time of day, sexual behaviours, and substance use.

While a lack of coordinated communication likely slowed and disrupted the adoption of PrEP, as detailed in this chapter, communication offers a variety of avenues to help move toward the elimination of HIV. Through the effective use of communication, coupled with the latest innovations in medicine, a reality without HIV is within reach.

References

Badal, H. J., Stryker, J. E., DeLuca, N., & Purcell, D. W. (2018). Swipe right: Dating website and app use among men who have sex with men. *AIDS and Behavior, 22*, 1265–1272.

Beck, V. (2004). Working with daytime and primetime television shows in the United States to promote health. In A. Singhal, M. J. Cody, E. M. Rogers, & M. Sabido (Eds.), *Entertainment-education and social change* (pp. 207–224). Mahwah, NJ: Lawrence Erlbaum Associates.

Bonvicini, K. A. (2017). LGBT healthcare disparities: What progress have we made? *Patient Education and Counseling, 100*, 2357–2361.

Brashers, D. E., Goldsmith, D. J., & Hsieh, E. (2002). Information seeking and avoiding in health contexts. *Human Communication Research, 28*, 258–271.

Brooks, R. A., Landrian, A., Nieto, O., & Fehrenbacher, A. (2019). Experiences of anticipated and enacted pre-exposure prophylaxis (PrEP) stigma among Latino MSM in Los Angeles. *AIDS and Behavior, 23*, 1964–1973.

Campbell, T., Bath, M., Bradbear, R., Cottle, J., & Parrett, N. (2009). An evaluation of performance-arts based HIV-prevention events in London with 13–16 year olds. *Perspectives in Public Health, 129*, 216–220.

Castro, D. R., Delabre, R. M., Morel, S., Michels, D., & Spire, B. (2019). Community engagement in the provision of culturally competent HIV and STI prevention services: Lessons from the French experience in the era of PrEP. *Journal of the International AIDS Society, 22*, 72–74.

Cegala, D. J., Coleman, M. T., & Turner, J. W. (1998). The development and partial assessment of the medical communication competence scale. *Health Communication, 10*, 261–288.

Cegala, D. J., Street, R. L., Jr., & Clinch, C. R. (2007). The impact of patient participation on physicians' information provision during a primary care medical interview. *Health Communication, 21*(2), 177–185.

Currin, J. M., Hubach, R. D., Durham, A. R., Kavanaugh, K. E., Vineyard, Z., & Croff, J. M. (2017). How gay and bisexual men compensate for the lack of meaningful sex education in a socially conservative state. *Sex Education, 17*(6), 667–681.

Czarny, H. N., & Broaddus, M. R. (2017). Acceptability of HIV prevention information delivered through established geosocial networking mobile applications to men who have sex with men. *AIDS and Behavior, 21*, 3122–3128.

Dahlhamer, J. M., Galinsky, A. M., Joestl, S. S., & Ward, B. W. (2017). Sexual orientation and health information technology use: A nationally representative study of US adults. *LGBT Health, 4*(2), 121–129.

Dasinger, L. K., Krause, N., Thompson, P. J., Brand, R. J., & Rudolph, L. (2001). Doctor proactive communication, return-to-work recommendation, and duration of disability after a workers' compensation low back injury. *Journal of Occupational and Environmental Medicine, 43*, 515–525.

Durso, L. E., & Meyer, I. H. (2013). Patterns and predictors of disclosure of sexual orientation to healthcare providers among lesbians, gay men, and bisexuals. *Sexuality Research and Social Policy, 10*, 35–42.

Dyche, L. (2007). Interpersonal skill in medicine: The essential partner of verbal communication. *Journal of General Internal Medicine, 22*, 1035–1039.

Eliason, M. J., Dibble, S. L., & Robertson, P. A. (2011). Lesbian, gay, bisexual, and transgender (LGBT) physicians' experiences in the workplace. *Journal of Homosexuality, 58*, 1355–1371.

Fields, E. L., Long, A., Dangerfield, D. T., Morgan, A., Uzzi, M., Arrington-Sanders, R., & Jennings, J. M. (2020). There's an app for that: Using geosocial networking apps to access young black gay, bisexual, and other MSM at risk for HIV. *American Journal of Health Promotion, 34*, 42–51.

Foss, K. A., & Blake, K. (2019). "It's natural and healthy, but I don't want to see it": Using entertainment-education to improve attitudes toward breastfeeding in public. *Health Communication, 34*, 919–930.

Fox, C. (2019, March 25). *10 years of Grindr: A rocky relationship*. BBC News. Retrieved August 13, 2020, from https://www.bbc.com/news/technology-47668951.

Freimuth, V. S., & Quinn, S. C. (2004). The contributions of health communication to eliminating health disparities. *American Journal of Public Health, 94*, 2053–2055.

Fuzzell, L., Fedesco, H. N., Alexander, S. C., Fortenberry, J. D., & Shields, C. G. (2016). "I just think that doctors need to ask more questions": Sexual minority and majority adolescents' experiences talking about sexuality with healthcare providers. *Patient Education and Counseling, 99*, 1467–1472.

Glazek, C. (2013, September 30). *Why is no one on the first treatment to prevent HIV? New Yorker*. Retrieved August 13, 2020, from https://www.newyorker.com/tech/annals-of-technology/why-is-no-one-on-the-first-treatment-to-prevent-h-i-v.

Ha, J. F., & Longnecker, N. (2010). Doctor-patient communication: A review. *Ochsner Journal, 10*, 38–43.

Hall, W., Sun, C. J., Tanner, A. E., Mann, L., Stowers, J., & Rhodes, S. D. (2017). HIV-prevention opportunities with GPS-based social and sexual networking applications for men who have sex with men. *AIDS Education and Prevention, 29*, 38–48.

Halton, B. R., Roberts, J. N., & Denton, G. D. (2019). Factors associated with discussions of human immunodeficiency virus pre-exposure prophylaxis in men who have sex with men. *Ochsner Journal, 19*, 188–193.

Hatzenbuehler, M. L., & Pachankis, J. E. (2016). Stigma and minority stress as social determinants of health among lesbian, gay, bisexual, and transgender youth: Research evidence and clinical implications. *Pediatric Clinics, 63*, 985–997.

Hirshfield, S., Grov, C., Parsons, J. T., Anderson, I., & Chiasson, M. A. (2015). Social media use and HIV transmission risk behavior among ethnically diverse HIV-positive gay men: Results of an online study in three US states. *Archives of Sexual Behavior, 44*, 1969–1978.

Jabson, J. M., Patterson, J. G., & Kamen, C. (2017). Understanding health information seeking on the internet among sexual minority people: Cross-sectional analysis from the health information national trends survey. *JMIR Public Health and Surveillance, 3*(2), e39.

Kaiser Family Foundation. (2014). *HIV/AIDS in the lives of gay and bisexual men in the United States*. Retrieved August 13, 2020, from http://www.kff.org/report-section/hivaids-in-the-lives-of-gay-and-bisexual-men-in-the-united-states-section-4-condom-use-and-hiv-testing/.

Kesten, J. M., Dias, K., Burns, F., Crook, P., Howarth, A., Mercer, C. H., et al. (2019). Acceptability and potential impact of delivering sexual health promotion information through social media and dating apps to MSM in England: A qualitative study. *BMC Public Health, 19*, 1236.

Lee, J. (2017, May 3). Gilead slowly rolls out ads for Truvada for PrEP – 4 years after approval. *MM&M*. Retrieved August 13, 2020, from https://www.mmm-online.com/home/channel/campaigns/gilead-slowly-rolls-out-ads-for-truvada-for-prep-4-years-after-approval/.

LGBT Health Education Center. (2017). *Do ask, do tell: Talking to your healthcare provider about being LGBT*. Retrieved August 13, 2020, from https://www.lgbtqiahealtheducation.org/wp-content/uploads/COM13-067_LGBTHAWbrochure_v4.pdf.

Lim, F. A., Brown, D. V., Jr., & Kim, S. M. J. (2014). CE: Addressing health care disparities in the lesbian, gay, bisexual, and transgender population: A review of best practices. *AJN The American Journal of Nursing, 114*, 24–34.

Liu, A., Cohen, S., Follansbee, S., Cohan, D., Weber, S., Sachdev, D., & Buchbinder, S. (2014). Early experiences implementing pre-exposure prophylaxis (PrEP) for HIV prevention in San Francisco. *PLoS Medicine, 11*, 1–6.

Matusitz, J., & Spear, J. (2014). Effective doctor–patient communication: An updated examination. *Social Work in Public Health, 29*, 252–266.

Mayer, K. H., Bradford, J. B., Makadon, H. J., Stall, R., Goldhammer, H., & Landers, S. (2008). Sexual and gender minority health: What we know and what needs to be done. *American Journal of Public Health, 98*, 989–995.

Moll, J., Krieger, P., Moreno-Walton, L., Lee, B., Slaven, E., James, T., et al. (2014). The prevalence of lesbian, gay, bisexual, and transgender health education and training in emergency medicine residency programs: What do we know? *Academic Emergency Medicine, 21*, 608–611.

Nelson, K. M., & Carey, M. P. (2016). Media literacy is an essential component of HIV prevention for young men who have sex with men. *Archives of Sexual Behavior, 45*(4), 787.

Obedin-Maliver, J., Goldsmith, E. S., Stewart, L., White, W., Tran, E., Brenman, S., et al. (2011). Lesbian, gay, bisexual, and transgender–related content in undergraduate medical education. *JAMA, 306,* 971–977.

Petroll, A. E., & Mitchell, J. W. (2015). Health insurance and disclosure of same-sex sexual behaviors among gay and bisexual men in same-sex relationships. *LGBT Health, 2,* 48–54.

Rosengren, A. L., Menza, T. W., LeGrand, S., Muessig, K. E., Bauermeister, J. A., & Hightow-Weidman, L. B. (2019). Stigma and mobile app use among young black men who have sex with men. *AIDS Education and Prevention, 31,* 523–537.

Sabin, J. A., Riskind, R. G., & Nosek, B. A. (2015). Health care providers' implicit and explicit attitudes toward lesbian women and gay men. *American Journal of Public Health, 105,* 1831–1841.

Schwartz, J., & Grimm, J. (2016). Uncertainty in online US news coverage of Truvada. *Health Communication, 31,* 1250–1257.

Schwartz, J., & Grimm, J. (2017). PrEP on twitter: Information, barriers, and stigma. *Health Communication, 32,* 509–516.

Schwartz, J., & Grimm, J. (2019). Stigma communication surrounding PrEP: The experiences of a sample of men who have sex with men. *Health Communication, 34,* 84–90.

Shilts, R. (1987). *And the band played on.* New York, NY: St. Martin's Press.

Smith, S. K., & Turell, S. C. (2017). Perceptions of healthcare experiences: Relational and communicative competencies to improve care for LGBT people. *Journal of Social Issues, 73,* 637–657.

St. Vil, N. M., Przybyla, S., & LaValley, S. (2019). Barriers and facilitators to initiating PrEP conversations: Perspectives and experiences of health care providers. *Journal of HIV/AIDS & Social Services, 18,* 166–179.

Sun, C. J., Stowers, J., Miller, C., Bachmann, L. H., & Rhodes, S. D. (2015). Acceptability and feasibility of using established geosocial and sexual networking mobile applications to promote HIV and STD testing among men who have sex with men. *AIDS and Behavior, 19,* 543–552.

Sun, C. J., Anderson, K. M., Bangsberg, D., Toevs, K., Morrison, D., Wells, C., et al. (2019). Access to HIV pre-exposure prophylaxis in practice settings: A qualitative study of sexual and gender minority adults' perspectives. *Journal of General Internal Medicine, 34,* 535–543.

Valdiserri, R. O., & Holtgrave, D. R. (2019). Ending HIV in America: Not without the power of community. *AIDS and Behavior, 23,* 2899–2903.

Ventuneac, A., John, S. A., Whitfield, T. H., Mustanski, B., & Parsons, J. T. (2018). Preferences for sexual health smartphone app features among gay and bisexual men. *AIDS and Behavior, 22,* 3384–3394.

White, W., Brenman, S., Paradis, E., Goldsmith, E. S., Lunn, M. R., Obedin-Maliver, J., et al. (2015). Lesbian, gay, bisexual, and transgender patient care: Medical students' preparedness and comfort. *Teaching and Learning in Medicine, 27,* 254–263.

WHO. (2016). *Health literacy.* Retrieved August 13, 2020, from https://www.who.int/healthpromotion/conferences/9gchp/health-literacy/en/

WHO. (2017). *HIV/AIDS.* Retrieved August 13, 2020, from https://www.who.int/hiv/mediacentre/news/hiv-testing-prep/en/.

Chapter 5
Anticipating Policy, Orienting Services, Celebrating Provision: Reflecting on Scotland's PrEP Journey

Ingrid Young

5.1 Introduction

Scotland made pre-exposure prophylaxis (PrEP) available through National Health Service (NHS) sexual health services in July 2017. As the first country in the UK to make PrEP available through state-funded health services, free at the point of access, there was much celebration. Scotland was heralded as a leader in HIV prevention (Boseley 2017; Nandwani 2017). Scotland's journey to PrEP has been shaped in no small part by global HIV debates, international research and health policies (WHO 2014; McCormack et al. 2016), governance and cost-effectiveness debates in health policy and provision (Khan et al. 2017; Sandset and Wieringa 2019), and promissory biotechnological narratives about the end AIDS (Kippax and Stephenson 2012; Duncombe et al. 2019). But what should we make of this journey? While it is important to consider how we got 'here', it is also important to understand what 'here' is. What does the journey to and celebration of PrEP in Scotland tell us about what this new HIV biotechnology is, how it could be made available within and across communities, and how its access and use is oriented by activist, research and policy work?

Adams, Murphy and Clarke argue that anticipation, or 'thinking and living toward the future' (Adams et al. 2009, p. 246) has become characteristic of daily life. Anticipation as an 'affective state', they argue, is 'not just a reaction, but a way of actively orienting oneself temporally... [towards a] future that may or may not be known for certain, but still must be acted on nonetheless.' (p. 247). These anticipatory regimes shape health, prevention and risk practices in efforts to avoid or enable imagined futures. Anticipatory regimes configure technoscience and biomedical

I. Young (✉)
Centre for Biomedicine, Self and Society, Usher Institute, University of Edinburgh, Edinburgh, UK
e-mail: ingrid.young@ed.ac.uk

© The Author(s) 2021
S. Bernays et al. (eds.), *Remaking HIV Prevention in the 21st Century*, Social Aspects of HIV 5, https://doi.org/10.1007/978-3-030-69819-5_5

practices by orienting actors and networks towards a particular or hoped for future by making demands in the present. It is important, then, to examine how and where these anticipatory regimes emerge and shape imagined futures through the imperative to act—or react—in the present. Others have drawn on this work to explore shifting technoscientific methods, such as the role of adaptive trials (Montgomery 2017), and HPV vaccinations (Moldanado 2017) and the 'end of AIDS' (Lloyd 2017). The journey to PrEP in Scotland allows us to examine how activist practices, clinical and policy debates and investments in particular biotechnological orientations work towards a particular future. Within this chapter I explore the Scottish PrEP journey as a site of anticipatory regimes, oriented towards a particular imagined PrEP future, invested in specific systems of health provision, and community sexual and activist practices.

5.2   A Note About Methods

This chapter charts the PrEP journey based on my research, observation and participation in PrEP engagement, debate and policy between 2011 and 2020. As a qualitative researcher, invested in working collaboratively with community and clinical partners, I have undertaken multiple qualitative PrEP research projects in Scotland: anticipating PrEP provision (Young et al. 2014); considering the critical HIV literacy demands of PrEP (Young 2019); exploring UK PrEP activism; and evaluating Scottish PrEP services. I have also worked with community, clinical and policy partners in Scotland and England through numerous engagement activities, working groups, writing groups and committees in relation to PrEP decisions and policy during this time (Nandwani et al. 2016; Brady et al. 2018; HPS and ISD 2019). This chapter, then, is grounded in the perspectives and concerns of someone who has both observed and been a part of the PrEP journey in the UK; that is, it is academically grounded, reflexively situated and community invested.

The UK does not have one central health system; health policy and provision fall under the jurisdiction of the separate health systems of England, Scotland, Wales and Northern Ireland, each of whom have varying levels of 'devolved' powers or self-governance. In this chapter, the Scottish journey is charted alongside key PrEP developments in England, a country whose health developments dominate UK national media coverage and with which most devolved UK country health policies are compared. This is not intended to sideline Wales or Northern Ireland in their efforts to make PrEP available, but to focus on the Scottish community, activist and policy experiences in relation to its larger neighbour. Original quotations, where presented in this chapter, come from focus group participants made up of PrEP activists, as part of the Sex, Drugs and Activism project (2018–2019) that explored PrEP activism in the UK.[1]

5.3 Anticipating Policy, 2012–2015

The early years of PrEP in Scotland could be characterised as quiet contemplation. Although PrEP globally emerged as one of two tools heralded to bring an 'end to AIDS' (Havlir and Beyrer 2012) with considerable buzz around its potential at international conferences in the run up to and following the 2012 FDA approval, this enthusiasm was not shared amongst very many HIV stakeholders in Scotland. One community HIV activist described excitement about PrEP at the 2012 AIDS conference but found little engagement upon return.

> . . .so that was 2012 AIDS Conference, I came back and I couldn't find people to talk to about PrEP in Scotland. . .we'd be talking about it in the office and keeping our heads out to see is anyone having this conversation in any way and what we found routinely was either people having no idea what we were talking about or very aggressive no's, so not wanting to discuss it. We started raising it with HIV clinical leads for several years trying to get them to make a statement about it, even if their statement was 'we have no statement' like something. Nothing.

Noting either the silence or rejection of PrEP, community activists described the considerable labour they put into getting PrEP recognised as something to discuss in relevant HIV and/or sexual health fora. After repeated failed attempts to get PrEP 'on the agenda', one HIV activist summarised what they considered to be the attitude from Scottish policymakers to PrEP:

> I . . . said 'this is outrageous we have been raising PrEP for the longest time you could have a two-hour meeting on PrEP alone' and then we were responded to and told this is not considered a significant enough matter and it won't be discussed.

Although PrEP within international HIV circles had been gaining traction, with increasing attention paid to how it might be implemented, the repeated rejection of early community attempts to get PrEP on the agenda meant any critical discussion of what PrEP could be was done in isolated pockets of community and clinical activists,

---

[1]As part of this project, I organised and took part in interactive focus groups/oral history 'workshops' with PrEP 16 community activists across Scotland and England. These workshops featured discussions of PrEP 'activist artefacts', explorations of PrEP activist strategies and reflections on the PrEP journeys in and across both countries. Participants were invited from a range of community organisations who had been involved in PrEP activism and advocacy in some way. These workshops were co-facilitated by a social science researcher and a community practitioner, both of whom were familiar with the HIV activist, research and policy field in the UK. Ethics approval was provided by the Usher Institute Ethics Research Group at the University of Edinburgh. Given the small size of PrEP activists in the UK, no identifying features have been indicated for extracts presented in this article to protect the anonymity of workshop participants. This research was supported by a Wellcome Trust Seed Award Sex, Drugs and Activism (207928/Z/17/Z).

and often amongst those with connections to other UK or international networks of HIV activists.

In their 2012 joint statement, the British HIV Association (BHIVA) and the British Association of HIV and Sexual Health (BASSH) (McCormack et al. 2012) declared there was insufficient evidence that PrEP would work in a UK context. This statement—offered in advance of FDA approval and in the context of growing enthusiasm—officially established a 'lack of evidence' as the primary reason for not considering PrEP implementation across the UK. Scottish community activists described multiple conversations with HIV clinicians, policy makers or others who might be in a position to make decisions about PrEP provision where they were repeatedly told 'there's not enough evidence on this and we're not sure.' This uncertainty is important to note. What is 'enough evidence'? Or perhaps more accurately, on whose bodies should PrEP evidence be based (Epstein 2007)? While FDA approval was based on evidence from multiple trials with heterosexual men and women, and gay and bisexual men, concerns surrounding the failure—or flat results—of PrEP trials with women played an important role in shaping how reliable this evidence was for UK clinicians.

> I remember having a conversation with [an HIV clinician] at that point and [the clinician] going 'if the, was it the Voice trial the one that failed, if the Voice trial had just worked…

Implying that just *one more trial* with results might have convinced UK—including Scottish—clinicians and policy makers seems at odds with the claims made in the joint statement that there was not enough evidence for *UK specific* services. Regardless of whether it was the gendered bodies who 'failed' to comply with PrEP adherence (van der Straten et al. 2014), or the (non-Global North) national health system contexts of PrEP users who did comply with PrEP adherence, policy actors in the UK—including Scotland—required further evidence of PrEP's effectiveness.

Results from the PROUD trial released in 2015 dramatically shifted PrEP narratives. PrEP had been shown to reduce risk of HIV transmission in gay and bisexual men by 86% (McCormack et al. 2016). On the basis of these results, PrEP in a UK context was hailed as a 'game-changer' with activists and clinicians now openly calling for it to be made available now that robust evidence had been provided (Young et al. 2020). Most UK media focused on the plans of the larger health services in England. There was limited coverage of the PROUD trial results in Scottish-specific media, with only one article including any Scottish voices. Amongst statements by London-based clinicians and policymakers, HIV Scotland's CEO stated that PROUD confirms PrEP effectiveness and that there was an obligation for NHS Scotland to make PrEP available.

> We are calling for action and asking the Scottish Government and the NHS to expedite making PrEP available. The evidence on PrEP is clear; time after time it is a highly effective prevention initiative. (Valiotis as cited in Tufft 2015).

Although this call was not in relation to a specific population, the article proceeded to focus on the benefits for gay and bisexual men. Here we see a dominance of England-based voices for a UK-wide issue that would eventually affect health provision in four distinct UK health systems; with an increasing focus on PrEP as an intervention for gay and bisexual men emerging from PROUD, and the framing of this 'game-changing' PrEP evidence nationally, the anticipation of what PrEP is (an effective, robust HIV prevention intervention), who it is for (gay and bisexual men) and where it should be accessed (NHS *England*), began to take shape.

PrEP activism in England became more visible following the release of the PROUD results. PrEP was a key feature of London Pride in 2015, and two activist groups launched in October 2015: PrEPster and Iwantprepnow.com. Multiple third sector organisations, activist groups and individuals formed the #united4prep coalition in early 2016 to advocate for PrEP on the NHS, consolidating a coalition of community actors more publicly advocating for PrEP (Portman 2017). Scottish-based activists described an absence of this community activism and expressed frustration at what they perceived as attempts to stifle PrEP activist efforts in Scotland.

> We just said 'we're going to promote it, we don't really care what your response is we're just going to promote it' and then they actually took it on board. But it's that, they come up with excuses and you hear them in conversations 'well if somebody got HIV and we would be held accountable and we're not quite feeling secure enough yet to send out that message'.

The frustration in lack of policy action shaped English PrEP activism and was made visible through seemingly coordinated online and physical #united4prep activities and campaigns driven by a network of HIV and LGBT community activists, third sector leaders and HIV researchers. Where policy hesitancy was identified, there also appeared to be a collective response to this gap from this group. In contrast, frustration around hesitancy of existing policy makers, clinicians and community organisations to coordinate PrEP advocacy in Scotland continued to shape *individual* activist efforts; those who sought to make PrEP a health and human rights issue in Scotland continued to work in isolation and/or in collaboration with largely non-Scottish-based partners.

5.4 Orienting Services 2016–2017

With a growing community activist movement in England and a solid clinical and cost-effectiveness evidence-base, the decision of NHS England in March 2016 to not fund PrEP came as a surprise to many (Lancet 2016). Although ultimately defeated, this decision was seen to reflect health policy views that PrEP was ultimately a 'lifestyle' drug for gay men to have risky sex (Mowlabocous 2019). Court challenges by the National AIDS Trust (NAT) and subsequent media debates centring on deserving citizens and homophobic rhetoric (Mowlabocous 2019) helped to consolidate the gendered framing of PrEP as an HIV intervention for gay and bisexual men instead of a tool for anyone at risk of HIV. A British Broadcasting Corporation

(BBC) documentary cast this controversy as the 'people' vs the NHS, setting the needs of gay and bisexual men, haunted by a long history of HIV trauma as in particular need of this 'game-changing' HIV prevention tool (Henderson 2018; Jones et al. 2020). That activists responded (rightly) to the ongoing homophobic responses by defending PrEP use of gay and bisexual men as responsible also helped to shape not only who PrEP was for, but how it might be used effectively. Moreover, this framing of PrEP as a viable and responsible clinical option for gay and bisexual men was further bolstered through visible coalitions of gay community *and* clinical activists, primarily in England (Portman et al. 2016; Portman 2017).

Although debates concerning the NHS England decision centre largely on how gay and bisexual men's health needs were seen to be problematically viewed by health policy makers, (Mowlabocous 2019), we also need to consider the governance structures which contribute to or enable these policy decisions. Khan et al. (2017) outline how the re-organisation of NHS Services in England following the 2012 Health and Social Care Act shifted responsibility for services and treatment and the allocation of funding. Confusion, overlap and debate about where or with whom responsibility lies for the commissioning of PrEP services—either within clinical health services or by local authorities now responsible for public health—illustrates how PrEP provision is shaped by the very services and policy that make it available. In Scotland, HIV prevention policy and provision fall to NHS Scotland and is overseen by the Scottish Government's Sexual Health and Blood Borne Virus (SHBBV) Framework (Scottish Government 2011). This Framework has driven a significant shift in Scottish policy and funding of sexual health services since 2011 to improve sexual health and wellbeing (Scottish Government 2015). Framework governance was directed at this point by the Executive Leads group, comprised of HIV and sexual health clinical stakeholders, Scottish Government and third sector representatives. In 2016, the SHBBV Framework Executive Leads agreed to a PrEP Short Life Working Group (SLWG) to consider if and how PrEP might be made available in Scotland. An observer described how despite a lack of consensus at policy level about PrEP, a few members of this group successfully argued for and actioned the SLWG in anticipation of Scottish provision: '"actually we need to be prepared" and I don't think there was agreement in the room but [the chair of the meeting] just said "this needs to be prepared"'. The mechanisms of the Framework, enabled here by leadership within the structure of Framework governance, rather than consensus, allowed for the decision to be made to prepare for PrEP provision. It also shaped how this preparation was undertaken.

While the SHBBV Framework enabled action on PrEP, it also shaped the possibilities of provision. The PrEP SLWG, which ran from March—October 2016, was comprised of sexual health and HIV practitioners, community pharmacists, third sector actors, academics, community members and observers from the Scottish Government and the Scottish Medicines Consortium (SMC). Apart from a community pharmacist, no non-sexual health and/or HIV practitioner participants took part. The parameters of group discussions and the final report focused on the provision of PrEP almost entirely by sexual health services; the lack of specific sexual health services in the smaller health boards meant PrEP would be exceptionally delivered through primary care, in line with existing provision of sexual health care in these areas. A 'lack' of quantitative PrEP acceptability evidence on which to base estimates of potential uptake meant the SLWG report drew on research with and referenced gay and bisexual men only, reflecting ongoing disparities in sexual health research with diverse populations (e.g. trans* communities, black and ethnic minority communities). Finally, the recommended eligibility criteria drew heavily on the PROUD trial protocols; only an additional category of equivalent risk was added after *significant* discussion and debate to address PrEP use for those who did not fit into these clinical criteria based on research with gay and bisexual men (Nandwani et al. 2016).

The acceptance of this report in October 2016 meant that PrEP was approved for provision in Scotland, subject to the licensing of Truvada (emtricitabine tenofovir disproxil) for PrEP use (requiring the patent holder Gilead filing an application with the Scottish Medicines Consortium (SMC)). Concerns were aired at the meeting that this decision could encounter the same 'homophobic' media attack seen during the NHS England decision and subsequent court battles (Mowlabocous 2019).

> [Someone] at the meeting said: 'we can't let what's happened in England happen here, we need to be on top of it, we need to go to the media and control the message and say this is what we're doing' and then [this proactive media strategy] was completely pulled back.

While one of the approving members advocated for directly addressing the anticipated negative media coverage—assuming that PrEP would be seen as an HIV intervention for gay and bisexual men—there was sufficient *opposition* to this proactive approach. This meant there were no formal plans for the SHBBV Framework leads or NHS services to actively engage with the media about the potential PrEP and homophobic stigma at this stage However, HIV Scotland—an HIV and human rights policy organisation—in collaboration with other third sector, academic and clinical partners, organised a series of PrEP community to generate discussion, interest and engagement amongst communities who might benefit from PrEP. These events held across the country in November and December 2016 featured a screening of the Proud Study film (Feustal 2015) which explained PrEP and described experiences of its use, and a panel comprised of an academic (myself), clinical practitioners, policy and gay men's sexual health activists who could answer questions about and provide evidence on PrEP. Although attempts were made by organisers and local partners to include a wide range of communities affected by HIV, the events were almost exclusively attended by—and ultimately geared towards—gay and bisexual men and some sexual health professionals. An absence of diverse community participation meant that discussions focused on now well-rehearsed debates about reduced condom use and PrEP, and featured arguments between 'older' and 'younger' gay men about what responsibility was and if and how PrEP challenged community histories of safer sex strategies. Panel and attendee responses largely positioned PrEP use as an act of responsibility in the changing world of HIV prevention and emphasised the need to draw on this narrative to challenge existing—and anticipated—PrEP stigma. Interwoven in these discussions were debates not only about what PrEP was, but what gay community itself was *and could be* in light of potential new HIV prevention options.

In April 2017, the SMC approved Gilead's submission to licence Truvada for use as PrEP. This meant that NHS Scotland was obliged to offer PrEP by July. This announcement was met with celebration and reflection. Dr. Rak Nandwani, chair of the PrEP SLWG, described the role of activism and collaboration in making PrEP a reality in the Scottish context, claiming that 'Scotland now also has the advantage of a firmly established community alliance built on the back of the PrEP work' (Nandwani 2017, p. 239). As in other parts of the UK, well-established collaborations between Scottish community organisations have been constrained due to reductions in and fragmentation of HIV funding over the past 10 years. Although previous collaborative HIV work between organisations had historically been undertaken, the PrEP work helped to strategically focus newly imagined collaborative endeavours. While significant in its contribution to the SMC community consultation, this community alliance included organisations who work in and across HIV, but did not include other community specific voices, such as those working with or lived experience of sex work, trans* communities, and/or people who use drugs (SMC 2017). The alliance built through leadership of key community organisations and actors to navigate a complex regulatory system should not be under-valued, but also highlights how these processes and existing organisational capacity can exclude those already marginalised voices and experiences. Nandwani situates this policy achievement in the wider context of Scottish nationalism in relation to sexual rights.

> There is an emerging sense of Scotland seeing itself as a forward-looking nation. Part of this is the shedding of homophobia, sometimes aligned to strongly held faith views. In 2016, Scotland found itself as a country where four of the leaders of its six main political parties were out as lesbian, gay, or bisexual. (Nandwani 2017, p. 238).

That LGBT rights and a sense of Scottish identity as a nation is used to frame the PrEP decision is significant; in opposition to the battles of NHS England and ongoing homophobia, the Scottish PrEP decision became something to celebrate as an achievement for a progressive, LGBT-inclusive Scottish health system, further pointing to the imagined primary beneficiaries of this new biotechnology. PrEP was made available in Scotland through NHS sexual health services in July 2017, with no additional funding for either the medication or additional services that PrEP provision would entail.

5.5   Celebrating PrEP 2017–2019

The provision of PrEP in Scotland was celebrated across UK media. This coverage often framed Scottish PrEP provision in contrast to the lack of provision in England. PrEP became a tool to illustrate not only the differences between the two national health systems, but to influence and shame health policy makers in England.

> This game-changing prevention tool has the potential to massively reduce HIV rates and turn Scotland into a model internationally of how to do HIV prevention well. The speed and decisiveness of the Scottish process contrasts starkly with delays in the other three UK nations (Gold, as cited in Boseley 2017).

The first-year report on PrEP provision (HPS and ISD 2019) was also met with simultaneous celebrations of Scottish efforts and disdain for the lack of progress in England. News coverage and statements by HIV organisations drew on Scottish data to further illustrate *English* failure, with one article in a mainstream national newspaper entitled: 'Scotland's introduction of HIV drug PrEP "puts England to shame"' (Brooks 2019). The release of the second year Scottish PrEP report resulted in similar commentary on limited progress in England, this time including a statement by a new CEO of HIV Scotland that addressed many of the ongoing achievements of PrEP provision, highlighted ongoing gaps, but ended with a strike at the lack of PrEP provision in England. 'It's high time NHS England. . .followed Scotland's lead and makes PrEP available on the NHS' (Sparling 2019). Within the first few years of provision, Scotland's PrEP programme has been repeatedly drawn on to illustrate not only PrEP's effectiveness, but the wider impact on sexual health.

> Scotland is leaps ahead, having made PrEP available through the NHS several years ago. That's another crucial lesson that we've learned from the earlier implementation of PrEP in Scotland: offering the drug brings people into sexual health services who otherwise wouldn't be using them. PrEP in Scotland has become a wonder intervention that also draws people towards HPV vaccination, hepatitis testing and treatment, and psychosexual services (Nutland 2020).

The mobilisation of and enthusiasm for Scottish PrEP provision by UK activists as a '*wonder intervention*' highlights how provision itself and the imagined effect it could have on sexual health was the cause of celebration. But beyond celebrating PrEP *provision,* there has been little interrogation of how well that provision has been implemented, sustained and who is—and is not—able to access PrEP under these conditions. In other words, while these national 'celebrations' point to presence of health policy, they do not engage in what resources, support and efforts are needed for its effective implementation or impact.

Within the Scottish health sector, the experience of PrEP provision was not *entirely* celebratory. In spite of the praise in the national press, PrEP activists were again stymied in their attempts to announce the provision of PrEP within Scotland itself.

> When we agreed that [PrEP] would be made available and we were talking about doing a big PR exercise, the public health said no, absolutely not. One because they didn't want to embarrass themselves to pretend that they weren't already on it, but underneath all that it was really clear they weren't on it, they didn't know how to respond if the press got in touch with them. And we said we should be talking to the media and the press but they wouldn't do it, they would not. They blocked us at every avenue.

The absence of a campaign—or even a plan—about the launch of PrEP provision was in contrast with the launch of the HPV vaccination for boys that took place at the same time (Scottish Government 2017). Activists felt that the lack of a PrEP campaign was not only about lack of resources or coordination, but an ongoing uncertainty of PrEP itself, and what it might mean for services.

> I think it really was down to a lot of people in the public health sector not having a scooby about PrEP, they just didn't know how it worked, they didn't know who it would affect, what the criteria was, it was about their own insecurities...

That there were no national campaigns to publicly launch PrEP in July 2017 did not stop local activists and services from telling those they worked with about PrEP. Community service providers, and especially those working with gay and bisexual men actively campaigned about PrEP within their outreach and support work. Again, those involved in PrEP campaigning before the official decision largely worked in or had specific roles in organisations supporting HIV and sexual health for gay men. The absence of national campaigns that might support PrEP use across communities affected by HIV, such as Black African men and women, trans* communities, people who use drugs and people who sell sex were noticeably absent from the discussions and engagement.

5.6   Postscript: After the PrEP Party

Reports from the first two years of PrEP provision highlight much higher numbers of PrEP prescriptions for gay and bisexual men than originally anticipated (HPS and ISD 2019). The higher than predicted numbers continue to challenge services, with a constant demand and no sign of levelling off of new PrEP users (HPS 2019). Significant numbers of gay and bisexual men prescribed PrEP were new and/or lapsed sexual health service users (HPS 2019; HPS and ISD 2019). The 'success' of PrEP for communities of gay and bisexual men should not be underestimated, and the anticipation of PrEP as an intervention for gay and bisexual men has indeed been borne out; data from the first two years of PrEP services report that *less than 1 per cent* of people prescribed PrEP in this time period were *not* gay or bisexual men. (HPS 2019) So what does this mean? An absence of PrEP access by women, trans* communities and those from Black African communities certainly points to an orientation of provision which maintains or exacerbates existing sexual health inequalities; people who are diagnosed with HIV from these communities continue to be affected by higher rates of 'late diagnosis' and in some cases, difficulties in maintaining an undetectable viral load (Brown et al. 2017; O'Halloran et al. 2019). This confirms (again) that provision of a new biotechnology would not—in and of itself—respond to the complex sexual health and wellbeing needs of such communities.

The absence of access to PrEP in the UK by diverse communities has not gone unnoticed. Discussions and eventually campaigns about access for PrEP for women, trans* and Black African communities began to emerge from around 2017 (AVAC 2017; Sophia Forum 2017; PrEPster 2019) and there has been a growing push for PrEP information and support to be *adapted* to suit the needs of these communities.

Here we see how PrEP provision—and support—is premised on a 'universal' PrEP user, where clinical criteria maps neatly onto the gendered and sexualised bodies of gay men. While the growing activism by communities themselves in relation to PrEP has begun to be supported in England (Positive East 2018; Africa Advocacy Foundation 2019; GMI Partnership and PrEPster 2019; My Genderation 2019) there has been, to date, little activity or support in Scotland. In an attempt to move past the generic 'what about women' or #prep4women trope that has emerged in UK PrEP activism, a Scottish workshop in September 2018 brought together community, clinical and academic stakeholders to consider which women we were talking about and what specific needs might be (Young and Calliste 2019). This workshop identified how Black African women, women who engage in sex work, women who use drugs and trans* communities (including women, men and non-binary people) more broadly see and experience (sexual) health services as hostile environments that reinforce discrimination, prejudice and exclusion on the basis of race, gender, drug use and sex work. While conversations and strategies to address some of these issues within existing sexual health services began to take place at this workshop, participants agreed that attention to language, exploring multiple forms of peer support and offering PrEP through non-traditional or outside of sexual health services (including but not limited to general practice), could go some way to encouraging discussion, access and improved support. It is unclear, however, if any of these specific issues have been taken on board by Scottish health services; structural change to address these considerable—and longstanding—health inequality issues have not explicitly been on the agenda for those making policy decisions about PrEP at a local service and surveillance level. The only exception to this has been the introduction of the option to record gender different to that at birth within the Scottish National Sexual Health System (NaSH), an electronic records system which is used in 11 of the 14 territorial health boards in Scotland (ISD 2016). That trans* communities may now have their (binary) gender identity accurately recorded, however, has not addressed the wider barriers of access to services, nor clarity around eligibility criteria for PrEP for those who do secure a consultation.

5.7 Conclusion

The Scottish PrEP journey has been particularly gendered, nationalised and embodied specific sexual—and health—practices. It has been shaped by debates around *sufficient* and *appropriate* clinical evidence, opportunities for and mechanisms of leadership in health governance and policy, assertions of national identities through championing sexual rights, and sustained community activist efforts. The orientation of provision and the configuration of community networks who lobbied for and might access PrEP suggest how anticipatory regimes of biomedical HIV prevention shape and are shaped by existing structural forces which prioritise specific forms of evidence, imagined PrEP users and biomedical hierarchies. Although Scotland provided PrEP through state-funded health services before other UK countries, it is not currently 'ahead' in how it imagines and enables access to PrEP for more 'diverse' communities of those who may benefit from it. This raises key questions around PrEP futures imagined in community activism. With PrEP provision the ultimate goal, PrEP became an object to be added to and enhance existing health structures, whose primary beneficiaries were gay and bisexual men, rather than the means to reimagine and re-orient HIV prevention in ways that might engage with heterogeneous communities affected by HIV. As PrEP in Scotland continues to evolve, and begins to engage more widely with those beyond the 'usual suspects', we will need to continue to pay attention—and respond—to how ongoing anticipatory regimes shape and enable particular promissory PrEP narratives.

References

Adams, V., Murphy, M., & Clarke, A. (2009). Anticipation: Technoscience, life, affect, temporality. *Subjectivity, 28,* 246–265.

Africa Advocacy Foundation. (2019). *PrEP and Prejudice.* Retrieved March 1, 2020, from https://www.prepandprejudice.org.uk.

AVAC. (2017). *Concensus statement on women and PrEP.*

Boseley, S. (2017, April 10). People at risk of HIV in Scotland to be given PrEP drug on NHS. *The Guardian.*

Brady, M., Rodger, A., Asboe, D., Cambiano, V., Clutterbuck, D., Desai, M., et al. (2018). *BHIVA/ BASHH guidelines on the use of HIV pre-exposure prophylaxis (PrEP).* London: British HIV Association; British Association of Sexual Health and HIV.

Brooks, L. (2019, February 27). Scotland's introduction of HIV drug PrEP "puts England to shame." *The Guardian.*

Brown, A., Rawson, S., Kelly, C., Nash, S., Kall, M., Enayat, Q., et al. (2017). *Women and HIV in the United Kingdom data to end of December 2017.* London: Public Health England.

Duncombe, C., Ravishankar, S., & Zuniga, J. (2019). Fast-track cities: Striving to end urban HIV epidemics by 2030. *Current Opinion in HIV and AIDS, 14,* 503–508.

Epstein, S. (2007). *Inclusion: The politics of difference in medical research.* Chicago: University of Chicago Press.

Feustal, N. (2015). *The proud study [documentary].* Hamburg: Georgetown Media.

Forum, S. (2017). *PrEP for Women* [leaflet]. *London: i-base.*

GMI Partnership & PrEPster. (2019). *PrEP champion project final report.* London: Public Health England Innovation Fund.

Havlir, D., & Beyrer, C. (2012). The beginning of the end of AIDS? *New England Journal of Medicine, 367,* 685–687.

Henderson, M. (2018, June 22). *The people vs the NHS: Who gets the drugs? [Television broadcast].* London: BBC.

HPS. (2019). *Implementation of HIV PrEP in Scotland: Second year report.* Glasgow: Health Protection Scotland.

HPS & ISD. (2019). *Implementation of HIV PrEP in Scotland: First year report.* Edinburgh: Health Protection Scotland, Information Services Division.

ISD. (2016). National Sexual Health System (NaSH). NHS National Services. https://www.ndc.scot.nhs.uk/National-Datasets/data.asp?SubID=104

Jones, C., Young, I., & Boydell, N. (2020). The people vs the NHS: Biosexual citizenship and hope in stories of PrEP activism. *Somatechnics, 10*(2), 172–194.

Khan, T., Kieslich, K., & Littlejohns, P. (2017). Why was a judicial review required to allow the English National Health Service to commission pre-exposure prophylaxis for HIV? *The Lancet, 390*, S5.

Kippax, S., & Stephenson, N. (2012). Beyond the distinction between biomedical and social dimensions of HIV prevention through the Lens of a social public health. *American Journal of Public Health, 102*, 789–799.

Lancet. (2016). UK PrEP decision re-ignites HIV activism. *The Lancet, 387*, 1484.

Lloyd, K. (2017). Centring 'being undetectable' as the new face of HIV: Transforming subjectivities via the discursive practices of HIV treatment as prevention. *BioSocieties, 13*, 470–493.

McCormack, S., Fidler, S., Fisher, M., & BHIVA, BASHH. (2012). The British HIV Association/ British Association for Sexual Health and HIV position statement on pre-exposure prophylaxis in the UK. *International Journal of STDs and AIDS, 23*, 1–4.

McCormack, S., Dunn, D., Desai, M., Dolling, D., Gafos, M., Gilson, R., et al. (2016). Pre-exposure prophylaxis to prevent the acquisition of HIV-1 infection (PROUD): Effectiveness results from the pilot phase of a pragmatic open-label randomised trial. *The Lancet, 387*, P53–P60.

Moldanado, O. (2017). Evidence, sex and state paternalism: Intersecting global connections in the introduction of HPV vaccines in Colombia. In E. Johnson (Ed.), *Gendering drugs* (pp. 199–244). London: Palgrave.

Montgomery, C. (2017). From standardization to adaptation: Clinical trials and the moral economy of anticipation. *Science as Culture, 26*, 232–254.

Mowlabocous, S. (2019). "What a skewed sense of values": Discussing PrEP in the British press. *Sexualities*. https://doi.org/10.1177/1363460719872726.

My Genderation. (2019). *Trans people taking PrEP*, London.

Nandwani, R. (2017). Pre-exposure prophylaxis is approved in Scotland. *Lancet HIV, 4*, e238–e239.

Nandwani, R., Valiotis, G., & Scottish HIV Pre-Exposure Prophylaxis Short Life Working Group (2016). *PrEP in Scotland*. Scottish Health Protection Network (SPHN). https://www.hiv.scot/ Handlers/Download.ashx?IDMF=3552380c-0e28-472e-be2e-49eecc40d6ed

Nutland, W. (2020, February 22). If I can be protected against HIV, others should be too. *The Guardian*.

O'Halloran, C., Sun, S., Nash, S., Brown, A., Croxford, S., Connor, N., et al. (2019). *HIV in the United Kingdom: Towards zero HIV transmissions by 2030 2019 report*. London: Public Health England.

Portman, M. (2017). Pre-exposure prophylaxis: Making history. *BMJ Sexually Transmitted Infections, 93*, 7.

Portman, M., Owen, G., Quinn, K., Craddock, A., Thomspon, M., Nwoloko, N., et al. (2016). Clinician and community collaboration on PrEP in the UK – A narrative. *BMJ Sexually Transmitted Infections, 91*, P229.

Positive East. (2018). *Mama says*. London: Positive East. https://www.youtube.com/watch? v=dj0W9DZs-zg&feature=emb_title.

PrEPster. (2019). *MobPrESH*. Retrieved June 16, 2019, from https://prepster.info/mobpresh/.

Sandset, T., & Wieringa, S. (2019). Impure policies: Controversy in HIV prevention and the making of evidence. *Critical Policy Studies, 0*, 1–16. https://doi.org/10.1080/19460171.2019.1661865.

Scottish Government. (2011). *Sexual health and blood borne virus framework 2011–2015*. Edinburgh: Scottish Government.

Scottish Government. (2015). *Sexual health and blood borne virus framework 2015–2020 update*. Edinburgh. Scottish Government

Scottish Government. (2017). *New vaccination programme begins*. Retrieved March 1, 2020, from https://www.gov.scot/news/new-vaccination-programme-begins/

SMC. (2017). *Minutes of the SMC Meeting held on Tuesday 7 March 2017*.

Sparling, N. (2019). *Two years on: The drug that revolutionised prevention*. https://www.hiv.scot/ news/two-years-on-the-drug-that-revolutionised-prevention

Tufft, B. (2015, December 2). HIV charity in call for NHS to prescribe drug. *The Herald,* 10.

van der Straten, A., Stadler, J., Montgomery, E., Hartmann, M., Magazi, B., Mathebula, F., et al. (2014). Women's experiences with Oral and vaginal pre-exposure prophylaxis: The VOICE-C qualitative study in Johannesburg, South Africa. *PLoS One, 9,* E89118.

WHO. (2014). *Consolidated guidelines on HIV prevention, diagnoses, treatment and Care for key Populations.* Geneva: World Health Organisation.

Young, I. (2019). *Making the case for HIV literacy: A developing HIV literacy report.* Edinburgh: University of Edinburgh.

Young, I., & Calliste, J. (2019). *PrEP and women in Scotland roundtable: A community report.* Edinburgh: University of Edinburgh.

Young, I., Flowers, P., & McDaid, L. M. (2014). Barriers to uptake and use of pre-exposure prophylaxis (PrEP) among communities most affected by HIV in the UK: Findings from a qualitative study in Scotland. *BMJ Open, 4,* e005717. https://doi.org/10.1136/bmjopen-2014-005717.

Young, I., Boydell, N., Patterson, C., Hilton, S., & McDaid, L. (2020). *Configuring the PrEP user: Framing Pre-exposure Prophylaxis in UK newsprint 2012–2016.* Culture, Health and Sexuality in Press.

Open Access This chapter is licensed under the terms of the Creative Commons Attribution 4.0 International License (http://creativecommons.org/licenses/by/4.0/), which permits use, sharing, adaptation, distribution and reproduction in any medium or format, as long as you give appropriate credit to the original author(s) and the source, provide a link to the Creative Commons license and indicate if changes were made.

The images or other third party material in this chapter are included in the chapter's Creative Commons license, unless indicated otherwise in a credit line to the material. If material is not included in the chapter's Creative Commons license and your intended use is not permitted by statutory regulation or exceeds the permitted use, you will need to obtain permission directly from the copyright holder.

Chapter 6
Fighting for PrEP: The Politics of Recognition and Redistribution to Access AIDS Medicines in Brazil

Felipe de Carvalho Borges da Fonseca, Pedro Villardi, and Veriano Terto Jr

6.1 Introduction

By challenging market and moral structures, HIV/AIDS activism has played a significant role in turning a major public health crisis into remarkable public health victories. Understanding the innovative features of such activism is a necessary exercise to explore contemporary repertoires of insurgency against several forms of injustice and oppression.

In this article, we use the frameworks proposed by Nancy Fraser and Axel Honneth (Fraser 1995; Fraser and Honneth 2003; Honneth 2003) to analyse HIV/AIDS activism in the field of access to medicines in Brazil. These authors emphasise the need to aggregate socio-political-cultural recognition policies to the traditional policies of economic redistribution. In this chapter, we will argue that the emergence of new HIV/AIDS biomedical prevention technologies offer an opportunity to re-energise access to medicines activism, for the sake of notions of identity and equity.

This opportunity however, emerges against a backdrop in which HIV/AIDS activism is at the verge of oblivion due to a complex web of challenges that range from a crackdown of the HIV/AIDS funding landscape to the deterioration and privatisation of public health systems; from the fragmentation of the HIV/AIDS social movement to the rising of conservative governments.

Nancy Fraser (1995) proposes a theoretical framework differentiating two conceptions of injustice, the socio-economic injustice and the cultural/symbolic injustice, for which redistribution and recognition are the remedies, respectively. Fraser explores connections and interferences that arise in the interaction of redistribution

F. de Carvalho Borges da Fonseca (✉) · P. Villardi · V. Terto Jr
Brazilian Interdisciplinary AIDS Association, Rio de Janeiro, Brazil
e-mail: felipe@abiaids.org.br

© Springer Nature Switzerland AG 2021
S. Bernays et al. (eds.), *Remaking HIV Prevention in the 21st Century*, Social Aspects of HIV 5, https://doi.org/10.1007/978-3-030-69819-5_6

and recognition agendas, pointing out the need for them to be 'harmonized programmatically and made to synergize politically' (Fraser 1995, p. 149).

Thinking about HIV/AIDS activism within this framework may provide some interesting insights. In the early days of the HIV/AIDS epidemic, the context of misinformation and moral panic made people affected by the disease a target of both symbolic injustice and socio-economic injustice. The very first struggles were thus against invisibility and silence, associated with exclusion and death. Breaking invisibility and silence meant talking about life with HIV/AIDS instead of death, transforming the symbolic/cultural perception of the disease. At the same time, it meant the creation of policies to ensure the fulfilment of rights for people living with HIV/AIDS in order to change the social-economic structures of exclusion.

There is an additional perspective from which it is possible to look into HIV/AIDS activism. Some authors see in HIV/AIDS a concrete example of the emergence of a biological citizenship (Rose 2007), or a politicised biology (Biehl 2004), according to which embracing the seropositive identity means a sort of 'rebirth' (Comaroff 2007) and a legitimacy to navigate scientific and political discourses critically. Especially the fight for access to the means of survival that arises out of, and forges identities around, a politicised biology, creates a dynamic whereas the biopower that condemns bodies and beings to a sub-level of humanity is also the fuel that fosters the emergence of identities aimed at exposing the deleterious effects of such exclusion, in a process of 'counterbiopolitics' (Comaroff 2007), a concept we will also explore.

The authors of this chapter are part of the access to medicines movement in Brazil and have been living and producing this field from both activist and academic fronts. On one hand, it is fair to say that the information used to develop this work comes from a privileged position, since the authors have been in the forefront of many actions and campaigns that will be discussed here. On the other hand, this work can also be seen as a self-reflection effort. Therefore, there is no intent to have any distancing from the object. Rather, as insiders, we write this text with passion, updated information and responsibility.

6.2   Recognition Through Redistribution in the Access to Medicines Agenda

In the 1990s, Brazil's response to HIV/AIDS became widely recognised by the enactment of a free and universal access to treatment policy. It is important to note that this policy was the culmination of an advocacy agenda by civil society, that developed new political concepts to merge the agendas of recognition and redistribution. Among those concepts, we can name two, both coined by the activist Herbert Daniel: 'civil death' describes the process of exclusion and loss of citizenship that emerged from the seropositive identity; and the 'ideological virus', referring to the stigma and other forms of structural violence that surrounded HIV positive people, threatening their lives in the social sphere as much as the virus did in the biological sphere (Daniel 2018).

Both Daniel and Herbert de Souza (also a leading Brazilian activist early in the epidemic) were strong defenders of a politics of solidarity (Parker 1994), based on whether society as a whole responds to the epidemic at all levels, thus creating a favourable environment for the restoration of the broken link between HIV positive identity and citizenship (de Souza 1994; Daniel 2018). Universal access to treatment, offered through a public health system sustained by all citizens through their taxes, was thus seen as a very important tool to create a collective ownership over the response to the epidemic and also a sense of dignity for people living with HIV/AIDS, greatly supporting their struggle for recognition. Therefore, although universal access to treatment can be perceived primarily as a redistributive policy, in Brazil it went beyond that, leading to important gains in terms of recognition.

In that regard, one of the greatest contributions by Brazilian civil society was to frame the response to HIV/AIDS as a human rights issue, rather than just a technical, biomedical one. This contributed to the process of 'contemporary politicization of HIV/AIDS' (Comaroff 2007) and opened space for important debates in the field of recognition, helping to include in the programmatic dimension of governmental programmes topics such as sexuality, gender, religion and drug use, among others. Access to treatment was also seen as a matter of human rights, given its relevance for the realisation of the right to health and, above all, of the right to life.

As noted, by creating a narrative of solidarity, inclusion, human rights and citizenship, Brazilian civil society created strong and innovative justifications for a universal access to medicines policy that went far beyond biomedical and socio-economic justifications. This was instrumental for generating recognition through redistribution, or, in other words 'redistribution as an expression of recognition' (Fraser 1995, p. 73).

6.3 Recognition for Redistribution: Occupying the Intellectual Property Arena

Following the signature of the TRIPS (Trade Related Aspects of Intellectual Property Rights) agreement in 1995, the adoption of a new patent law in Brazil became mandatory, putting at high risk one of the pillars of Brazil's HIV/AIDS response: the local generic production, by state-owned laboratories, of the first generation of HIV/AIDS drugs. Such production was possible because Brazil's legislation excluded food and medicines from patentability, but the TRIPS agreement determined that all technological fields should be included in the new global patent regime, creating uncertainty around the price of future generations of antiretroviral treatments in Brazil. Intense lobbying by the pharmaceutical industry in Brazil's parliament resulted in the approval of an unbalanced patent law that included very few of the health protective measures that Brazil as a developing country could have adopted. As documented by Nunn et al. (2007), the costs of the Brazilian universal treatment programme exploded as soon as patented antiretroviral drugs (ARVs) started to be included in the guidelines. According to their research, total annual drug expenditure on ARVs doubled between 2001 and 2005, reaching US$414 million in 2005. 'Patented ARVs accounted for between 60 and 70% of total costs from 2001 to 2003 but then jumped to 80% of total costs in 2004 and 2005' (Nunn et al. 2007, p. 1807). In 2005, the government issued an official note declaring that the treatment programme was at risk of discontinuity because of the high price of patented medicines.

Concerned with this sustainability issue, civil society groups started to monitor the impact of patents on the circulation of cheap, generic versions of ARVs. The Working Group on Intellectual Property (GTPI) was born from this effort, as part of the Brazilian Network for the Integration of Peoples (REBRIP). GTPI brought together activists, NGOs and social movements to develop an advocacy agenda in all fields in which intellectual property could harm social policies, including knowledge, agriculture and health. However, the urgent need to preserve the sustainability of the HIV/AIDS programme made the group more specialised in access to medicines and led it to be predominantly composed of HIV/AIDS organisations, including its secretariat which has been based at the Brazilian Interdisciplinary AIDS Association (ABIA) from GTPI's creation to the present.

GTPI's first challenge was a battle for recognition as a relevant stakeholder on intellectual property debates. Following a trend also observed in other countries, civil society and patient groups were not considered relevant parties in the formulation of patent policies and decisions. GTPI had to confront the view that intellectual property is a field reserved only for industry experts and lawyers, and ensure its democratisation by involving people affected by drug monopolies in the conversation. This effort brought the recognition debate to an unusual arena, turning people living with HIV/AIDS into intellectual property stakeholders dedicated to removing barriers for access to treatment.

Some of the actions developed by the group contributed to this sort of political recognition. For example, inspired by the protagonist role of Thai and Indian civil societies, beginning in 2006 GTPI started to use patent oppositions as a strategy to reduce the price of essential drugs. Patent opposition means a direct intervention in the patent examination process, providing to patent examiners technical arguments that can serve as basis for the rejection of a patent application. If the arguments are considered valid and a rejection follows, it means that civil society could avoid a monopoly over an essential drug, opening space for generic competition, price reduction and scale-up of universal access public policies. It also means that civil society groups perform a role as interested parties in the patent examination process, contributing to the politicisation of the intellectual property arena, based on an innovative combination of recognition and redistribution.

From 2006 to 2019, GTPI filed 20 patent oppositions, achieving remarkable results, such as the rejection of patents on the essential HIV/AIDS drug tenofovir (Viread), including for its combination with emtricitabine (Truvada), which is used for prevention purposes. As a consequence, tenofovir and tenofovir/emtricitabine were never under monopoly in Brazil and could be produced locally in generic versions, generating huge savings for Brazil's public health system and the maintenance of the universal treatment policy that, as we have explored, serves as a policy of both redistribution and recognition.

Honneth (2003), in his theory of the fight for recognition, conceives subjectivity as something built in a conflictive world, marked by asymmetric power relations between individual and collective subjects. The conflicts around access to medicines and, in particular, the disputes in the IP arena, are marked by profound power asymmetries. Civil society organisations were nonetheless able to intervene upon a substantial engine of the HIV/AIDS market, such as the monopoly over the drug tenofovir, marketed by the US pharmaceutical giant Gilead Sciences. This is not an ordinary achievement, considering that between 2008 and 2013, more than 80% of Gilead's revenue has been linked to TDF-containing products (Walwyn 2013).

Following Honneth's thought, we can consider that the power asymmetry is counterbalanced by the logic of moral conflict, which has a central stage in forging both identities and social transformation agendas. Lack of access to a given treatment, or the risk of losing access, forges an individual experience of disrespect, that by its turn feeds a collective political mobilisation, strong enough to challenge the structural market violence that sustains poor access to treatment.

6.4   Biocapital and Structural Violence

Sharing knowledge about treatment to empower people in regards to their options and choices was a strong mark of HIV/AIDS activism in Brazil. Under this approach, access to treatment is not limited to a biomedical strategy aimed at containing the virus, it is also destined to promote quality of life, so people should be able to choose what treatment better suits their needs and lifestyle, considering dosage, side effects, food restrictions etc. (Cerqueira and Terto 2015).

People living with HIV/AIDS in Brazil thus fought not only for accessible treatments, but also for rapid incorporation of new treatment options. This approach, however, is constantly under threat for various reasons. Firstly, the government often refuses to update the treatment guidelines as mandated by law; secondly, international agencies may often recommend a standard treatment regimen for developing countries, based on a 'one size fits all' approach that ends up being too reductionist and blind to the challenges people may face in relation to adherence; and thirdly, the big pharmaceutical companies are constantly re-launching the high price/poor access crisis that marked the beginning of the epidemic, backed by ever-expanding patent monopolies, which are by their turn secured by increasingly unbalanced patent laws. Therefore, better treatment options are constantly out of reach for developing countries, creating a world divided into treatment regimens for the rich and treatment regimens for the poor. This is an example of the potential association between biotechnology and structural violence as discussed by Comaroff (2007), when looking at Brazil's case:

Even as activists, NGOs, and the state collaborate to provide medication on a national scale, new lines of exclusion spring up to separate those worthy of salvation from those condemned to death camps. Biotechnology here thrives alongside structural violence (Comaroff 2007, p. 208).

Debunking the intellectual property system myth and exposing it as a source of structural violence is thus a fundamental tactic, that ranges somewhere between affirmative and transformative redistribution (Fraser 1995). At a granular level, it deals with moving targets, as normally activists work on a case by case approach, targeting different drug monopolies one at a time. When these tactics are combined with treatment literacy,[1] they promote a deeper transformation on power relations, as access to drugs is translated into the language of rights, accountability, transparency, social participation, in a way that drugs or other health goods can no longer be reduced to commodities as dictated by the logic of biocapital. Going even further, the agenda of reforming the intellectual property system points towards expanding health protective measures on patent laws and international treaties or even to the suspension of the TRIPS agreement for essential health technologies.[2] This macro agenda is a way for 'redressing distributive injustice by deep political-economic restructuring, as opposed to surface reallocations' (Fraser 1995, p. 84).

As an example of granular 'counterbiopolitics', we can refer to the 'first steps workshops on intellectual property and access to medicines' organised by GTPI, that bring together both treatment literacy and intellectual property criticism. Between 2013 and 2019, GTPI organised 15 workshops in 13 different cities throughout the country.

This experience revealed the need to generate awareness about treatment options and empower grassroots organisations and healthcare professionals to challenge the power structures that impose sub-optimal treatment practices, leading to poor adherence and abandonment of treatment. These workshops also served as laboratories for campaigns that lead to the incorporation of new drugs in Brazil's public health system, despite initial reluctance from government officials, international organisations and parts of the medical community. Such reluctance is normally based in the defence of medical protocols that select a few cost-effective treatment options aiming to ensure universal distribution, but without acknowledging individual needs that would be better addressed if a wider range of treatments was available at accessible prices. Therefore it's 'an approach aimed at redressing injustices of

---

[1]Treatment literacy is an education strategy that understands medicines as more than just a biomedical tool or a product. It is a strategy that takes into account the multiple meanings of the treatment to a person or a group of persons, placing medicines in the center of a political, economic and cultural dynamics. Treatment is not a static thing. Rather, its meanings are produced by patients and activists. The implication of this is that each individual or collective will have different approaches towards their own treatment, but always considering it not only as a simple good. This concept is similar to 'Prevention Literacy', in the sense discussed in Parker and others (2015). For more, please consult the ITPC Act Toolkit (ITPC 2014).

[2]This proposal was made in the report HIV and the Law: https://hivlawcommission.org/report/ and at the people's summit held at the sidelines of the 2017 WTO Conference in Buenos Aires: https://fueraomc.org/final-statement/.

distribution that can thus end up creating injustices of recognition' (Fraser 1995, p. 85).

In this regard, an important example is the drug dolutegravir, incorporated in Brazil only after significant pressure from civil society, based on the understanding that the previous treatment options standardised by global and national protocols created particular adherence challenges for young populations. However, many important treatment options remain out of reach for people living with HIV/AIDS in Brazil, especially fixed-dose combinations.

This situation can be intensified by the so-called 4.0 industrial revolution, that is reshaping healthcare and directing the biopharmaceutical industry to the paradigm of individualised medicine that is, by definition, a complete turnaround from the mass treatment era. For example, Roche Brazil's president affirmed that out of the 100 molecules under research by the company, only two or three are directed to mass treatment, the rest are focused on rare diseases and conditions (Ediane 2019). The HIV/AIDS treatment itself is moving towards the class of monoclonal antibodies (mAb), whose production rely on advanced biotechnology techniques that are dominated by very few companies. In 2018, ibalizumab, the first mAb was approved by the FDA for HIV/AIDS treatment, indicated for multi-drug resistant cases. The listed price announced in the US was US$118,000 per patient/year.

6.5 Fighting for PrEP

Since 2012, when the Food and Drug Administration (FDA) approved the drug tenofovir/emtricitabine - TDF/FTC (Truvada) for HIV pre-exposure prophylaxis (PrEP), civil society organisations in Brazil have been pushing the government to consider its incorporation for that indication. In 2016, at the 21st International AIDS Conference, when Brazil's government finally declared publicly its intention to initiate PrEP as a public policy, through the roll out of TDF/FTC (2 years after the World Health Organization (WHO) had recommended it as an effective prevention method for men who have sex with men (MSM)), two major interconnected concerns arose: what limitations would be imposed by patents and high price of this drug and how conservative forces would oppose the adoption of such method. To address these challenges together, GTPI started a campaign called 'Free Truvada', claiming that the drug should be free of both patents and prejudice, based on the understanding that expanded access to this and other prevention technologies depends on the fight against both moral and market barriers. Also, the connection between choice of prevention method and individual autonomy was part of a larger attempt to 'establish institutionally and culturally expanded forms of mutual recognition' (Honneth 2003, p. 156), through which deeper normative societal transformations can follow.

The moral barriers became clear during the TDF/FTC incorporation process, which had several delays associated with registration bureaucracies and also came with conservative views about the right to prevention. Rumours indicated that some members of the technical committee that oversees drug incorporation for the public health system had argued it would be immoral to invest in a drug to be used in association with sexual practices.

Such rumours coincide with an overall perception by the HIV/AIDS movement that an evangelical morality is shaping public policies in many levels, including the technical sphere. This moral barrier risks undermining even the biomedical arguments that indicate positive impacts of new prevention technologies in the reduction of new transmissions and other important indicators. HIV/AIDS activists, in their turn, pushed the discussion beyond the biomedical sphere, claiming that the social and political dimensions of prevention technologies such as TDF/FTC need to be discussed, considering that they provide a great opportunity to raise important conversations about sexuality, sex behaviours, sex spots, that are all relevant for comprehensive prevention policies. These three views were under dispute around the process of TDF/FTC's incorporation in Brazil. We can identify in this context a moral conflict for recognition (Honneth 2003) in which the non-availability of more effective HIV/AIDS prevention methods stands as a disrespect for vulnerable populations and in which public policies that address sexuality stands as a disrespect for religious segments of society.

Civil society organisations closely monitored the technical meetings that discussed the incorporation of TDF/FTC and voiced concerns through the press about delays and the lack of transparency. In early 2017, a public consultation was launched to decide on the incorporation and thanks in part to the 'Free Truvada' campaign and the efforts made under the 'first steps workshops', a huge number of civil society organisations contributed, sending submissions in favour of the incorporation. This consultation reached 3543 submissions (CONITEC 2017), one of the highest numbers ever recorded, favouring the approval of the protocol for use of TDF/FTC as PrEP, despite opposition by conservative forces. Among the contributors there was also the Federal Public Defender Office (DPU, acronym in Portuguese) from the state of São Paulo, that some months before had organised an event in which many specialists and civil society groups participated, including GTPI. Based on the event discussions, the DPU made a submission that not only defended PrEP as a useful and necessary sanitary tool, but also as a means to promote the right to sexual freedom and to express human dignity (DPU (SP) 2017). The incorporation was approved in early 2017 and in December 2017, PrEP service was implemented in 36 public health units across 22 cities, primarily for high-risk populations.

The fight against patent barriers was also successful and actually started in 2010 when a patent opposition was first filed by GTPI. At that time, TDF/FTC was approved only for treatment, but studies on its potential for prevention were already happening. Considering this dual relevance, GTPI filed arguments against the granting of the patent, which was found to be a mere combination of two known substances thus failing the inventive step criteria. GTPI submitted additional arguments to the patent office in 2016 to highlight the lack of inventive step in the patent application. These arguments served as the basis for the rejection of Gilead's application in January 2017 and are cited in the first paragraph of the decision published by the patent office. Just after GTPI's opposition, in November, a local generic producer announced its intention to enter the market.

At some point between November 2016 and January 2017, the Indian generic company Hetero also applied for registration in Brazil. These moves evidence that the opposition by GTPI sent strong signs to generic producers and increased pressure over Gilead. All of these events increased the government's negotiation power and forced Gilead to reduce its price from US$752 to US$276 per patient per year (a 63% reduction).

Price reduction in this context meant the sustainability of the prevention policy and its further expansion. It also minimised the impact of the argument that public money would be wasted to provide drugs to be used in a sexual context. The economic argument still exists and it is linked with the notion that, in a constitutional perspective, the right to health is only implemented as a right to treatment not as a right to prevention, and that medicines should be provided only to ill people not to healthy individuals. The fight for PrEP challenges this view in favour of an expanded notion of rights.

It is important to note that there are many divergent opinions about PrEP policies among civil society groups in the Latin America. Some think that a medicalised approach to prevention is part of a broader medicalisation strategy that favours pharmaceutical companies and that there is not enough knowledge on what effects the regular use of an ARV has for a healthy person, in terms of side effects or resistance patterns. Also, there is concern about pushing for the roll-out of a drug for prevention while a lot of people in the world still lack access to treatment.

On the other hand, those who advocate for the roll-out of TDF/FTC as a universal PrEP policy argue that prevention methodologies are outdated and becoming less effective, which leads to increased infection rates. Therefore, any option that effectively helps people to have safer sex practices should be considered as a relevant tool to reinvigorate prevention policies, as inaction also has a significant impact on people's health. In conclusion, the costs and risks associated with PrEP are much lower than the cost of inaction. Also, data from many countries shows that a successful roll-out of PrEP can have very significant results in reducing transmission. Finally, the call for states to offer a broader range of prevention tools contributes to promote the notions of citizenship and dignity, as it implies the recognition that individuals should be entitled to the freedom of making their sexual options with autonomy and choose the prevention method that better suits their existential needs. For those groups that defend access to PrEP as a matter of right to health and right to freedom, the concern with the concentration of power by pharmaceutical companies can be circumvented by confrontational strategies to improve access to medicines, such as patent oppositions, that in the case of Brazil were very effective, enabling generic producers to enter the market and keep prices at a sustainable level, which was essential to ensure the continuation of the public policy.

6.6   Austerity Measures and Necropolitics

As discussed so far, the fight for PrEP has many dimensions and it is inherently connected to the political environment. One aspect of such an environment is the combination of biomedicalisation and conservatism, leading to a reduced policy space for the human rights agenda. Another aspect is the lack of support for civil society organisations combined with the growing fragmentation of the HIV/AIDS movement that has as one of its main origins the overall scarcity of funds for civil society organisations, especially those engaged in advocacy activities.

For many years now, 'traditional' donors have stepped back from Latin America, based on the false premise that much progress had been made in access to treatment and social policies. This is partially true, as the fruits of such progress were not at all equally shared and as the fragility of the victories required more long-term commitment to civil society work in order to protect them.

The void created in funding for civil society is being occupied by private actors, especially pharmaceutical corporations. According to FCAA (2020), in 2018, the company Gilead was the second largest philanthropic funder and the top corporate funder for HIV/AIDS. Gilead is also the top philanthropic funder of PrEP related activities. This is particularly problematic as the access to medicines movement was founded to confront power abuses by pharmaceutical companies and relied on the mobilisation capacity of the HIV/AIDS movement to achieve huge wins. However, now many HIV/AIDS NGOs have disappeared, and others are running after funding coming from any source, including pharmaceutical companies, compromising the ability of the movement to hold pharmaceutical companies accountable for their patent and price abuses.

This is not an isolated trend, the idea that private actors have a major role to play is everywhere across the healthcare spectrum. One of the major agendas promoted by the World Health Organization (WHO) today is the so-called Universal Health Coverage (UHC), aimed at ensuring everyone has access to health without enduring any financial hardship (de Noronha 2013; Tangcharoensathien et al. 2020). While this goal may be a motivation for countries that lack the most basic health services, it may be a setback for countries that have well established public health systems, such as Brazil, based on progressive social policies and solidarity principles. UHC has a premise that sustaining health systems that provide all levels of service, integral approaches and that act on social determinants of health is not sustainable, therefore governments should commit only to a minimum package of services and should seek partnerships with the private sector (Giovanella et al. 2018). In the field of HIV/AIDS the minimum package of services is quite clear when we think of the biomedical strategies such as 'test and treat' that come without any component of psychosocial assistance, promotion of rights, education, etc.

UHC is part of a larger agenda of reforming the state for the sake of efficiency and establishing austerity measures for the sake of economy. By proposing more participation of private actors, the main argument is reduction of bureaucracy and improvement on efficiency. The reductionist 'package of services', by its turn, comes along with the idea that a large state structure wastes too much money and that healthcare costs must be optimised, by sharing responsibilities with private insurance market (Lima 2015), that will promote low cost options, advancing in the territory of what were once free, universal and integral services. A study analysing Latin American countries that applied the UHC model concluded that the coverage targets haven't been met, the package of services are inequitably offered and the fragmentation of the healthcare system intensified. Therefore, there is no evidence in the region that UHC has more effective results, in comparison to the universal systems that were established in most of the countries (Giovanella et al. 2018).

The World Bank is a major stakeholder in the UHC agenda and has its own package, which includes public-private partnerships, use of public or pooled funds to pay private providers, and adjusting public expenditures to austerity measures (Lima 2015). These agendas create more space for private actors that at the same time also receive loans from World Bank to make mergers and acquisitions, expanding their reach in countries where public health systems are being shrunk by such policies (IFC and World Bank 2018). This mosaic of contradictory policies comes under the umbrella of the UHC paradigm, although they risk disrupting health systems capacities where they are based in a different set of principles.

However, Brazil is not only aligned with cutting social policies and de-investing in the public health system, but is also poised to implement the most socially regressive austerity package in the world (the Constitutional Amendment 95), in the words of the UN special rapporteur on extreme poverty and human rights, Philip Alston (Watts 2016). According to the UN senior official, the package is 'an attack on poor people'. It was approved in 2016 and effectively freezes federal government spending for two decades in areas such as health, education and infrastructure, among others. The so-called 'ceiling' on public expenditure establishes that the spending cap can only increase by the rate of inflation in the previous year, which means in real terms that expenditure in all these areas remains frozen at 2016 levels until the year 2037, despite obvious increasing need in healthcare, for example, given the aging of the population.

The relationship between austerity and structural violence becomes evident considering that one of the targets is the Unified Health System (SUS), created as a major expression of solidarity and democracy and turned into the largest public health system in the world in terms of coverage (Lima et al. 2005; Castro et al. 2019). The freezing of the budget for health, the degradation of a universal public health system into a universal coverage model driven by the market and the reductionist approach to services in fields such as HIV/AIDS unequivocally point towards people paying with their lives for these adjustments. The environment in which rights are violated is built-up via state led policies, but companies also play a key role. Pharmaceutical companies can also be seen as offenders of the public health budget, as they often charge extortionate prices for drugs that are to be distributed by SUS, backed by their patent monopolies, and that are, quite often, undeservedly granted. Without sustainable prices, the SUS's access to medicines programmes can no longer survive, nor will the people who rely on them. In summary, the population's rights are being reduced every day, while for companies there is an untouchable architecture of impunity. This is a structural violence that GTPI has been trying to address in some international forums such as the Inter-American Court of Justice,[3] UN working Group on Business and Human Rights[4] and the Global Campaign to Dismantle Corporate Power and Stop Impunity.[5]

The structural violence imposed by the constitutionalised austerity and by the deliberate dismantlement of the public health system, however, is not the only factor leading to the naturalisation of social exclusion. Since the 2018 presidential campaign, Brazil has submerged into a climate of omnipresent violence. The elected president, during his campaign, made several aggressive statements about authorising the police to undertake extrajudicial killings, about reducing the protections to the rainforest and the traditional people living there and about scrutinising NGOs to force them to stop their activities (Daniels 2019). As his mandate started, the violence towards minorities has been stimulated along his support base and authoritarian proposals have become priorities for the government, such as alleviating the police force from responsibility for killings during their duty, creating a climate of war against crime that is inherently a war on the poor.

As regards HIV/AIDS, the government issued a presidential decree in early 2019 that establishes a new structure for the Ministry of Health. As a result, the former Department of STIs, AIDS and Viral Hepatitis is now named the 'Department of Chronic Illnesses and Sexually Transmitted Diseases' (free translation). The name change can be understood as an indication of intentions to reduce the effort to tackle HIV/AIDS and a move towards a de-prioritisation and neglect of a disease that still kills around 12,000 people in Brazil every year. New HIV infections are increasing in the country, especially among populations who experience stigma and discrimination, increasing their challenges to access prevention and treatment services. This decree makes those people even more marginalised (Parker 2020).

In early 2020, another attitude by the president reinforced symbolic violence against people living with HIV/AIDS. In a live interview on television, trying to defend the sexual abstinence policy announced by the Minister of Women, Family and Human Rights in early 2020, he stated that 'a person with HIV is an expense for everyone here in Brazil'. The main lesson after 40 years of fight against HIV/AIDS is that stigma and discrimination are the greatest barrier to controlling the epidemic. In saying that people living with HIV/AIDS cause harm to society, the president harms years of gains on recognition and tacitly authorises stigma, discrimination and the violation of their human rights.

The loss of rights is not merely fruit of political preferences, they are part of 'politics of death' or 'necropolitics' (Mbembe 2018), which means the exercise of the power of dictating who must live and who should die, that derives from an

---

[3]Denounce available here: http://deolhonaspatentes.org/wp-content/uploads/2018/02/relatorio_gtpi2017_final_WEB.pdf.

[4]Submission available here: https://deolhonaspatentes.org/punicao-de-transnacionais-por-violacoes-de-direitos-humanos-em-debate-na-onu/.

[5]Website: https://www.stopcorporateimpunity.org/.

'generalized instrumentalization of human existence' (Mbembe 2018, p. 10). Under this logic, the biophysical elimination of the other is seen as something that reinforces the 'potential of life and security' (Mbembe 2018, p. 20) for a certain group. The elimination of people living with HIV/AIDS reinforces security of those who are seronegative, the elimination of the poor reinforces the security of those who are rich, and so on. By putting the debate in terms of survival, a biopolitical rationality is activated, in which economic structures also have authority to perform such elimination.

The issue of patents is exemplary. The ideological argument that sustains the patent system claims that high prices are necessary to sustain investments in the next generation of drugs, that will save many lives. Therefore, monopolies ensure the future of biomedical R&D. Given that one of the main conditionalities for the consumption of medicines is related to wealth (Hasenclever et al. 2010), this ideological argument basically states that medicines must be out of reach for populations from poor countries in order to ensure that the biopharmaceutical industry can save lives in rich countries; and that any change in this equation will risk the lives of the rich. This argument puts the debate in terms of survival of one population in direct relation to the genocide of the other, similar to what Foucault (1988) referred to as 'be capable of killing in order to go on living' to describe the atomic conflict context.

The same is true for the UHC approach, pushed forward to expand private markets, without any evidence that this will improve health outcomes; on the contrary, other countries' experiences show that it will actually mean deterioration of services and exclusion, especially of poor people and marginalised populations. As 'necropolitics' advance at a rapid pace as an institutionalised functioning, the capacity to build redemptive politics of citizenship and 'counterbiopolitics' is severely damaged by lack of funds, authoritarian regimes and co-optation by the private sector.

6.7 Conclusion

As discussed in this chapter, in the context of access to medicines and the response to HIV/AIDS, socio-economic injustice driven by austerity, privatisation and patent abuses promotes and naturalises structural violence that reinforces exclusion, especially of those that are already targeted by the cultural/symbolic injustices derived from conservatism and 'necropolitics'. Redemptive politics of solidarity that unify the social demands around identity and equity are extremely needed. Therefore, civil society action must emphasise the moral justification for normative revindications, as proposed by Honneth (2003) and make recognition and redistribution synergise politically, as proposed by Fraser (1995).

Preserving the lessons learned through access to medicines struggles and sustaining the fight for PrEP and all its potentialities for the expansion of human rights-based politics is thus a crucial agenda. The mere resistance of a PrEP public policy in

Brazil in such a challenging environment could be considered a great achievement, but it is not sufficient. The policy by itself may be affirmative, but it shall not be transformative unless it is used as a tool to reverse state violence and stigmatisation processes that take people from their condition of subjects of their own lives and rights. Beyond that, any further attempt to confront this worrisome web of violence must be aimed at challenging the very notion that asymmetries in human development and inequality are deemed to be normal facts. This is why any health technology or medical intervention, as well as any health policy, must be held accountable to notions of citizenship that do not separate biology from political subjectivities, but rather connect it with human dignity on its highest standards.

References

Biehl, J. (2004). The activist state: Global pharmaceuticals, AIDS, and citizenship in Brazil. *Social Text, 80*, 105–132.

Castro, M. C., Massuda, A., Almeida, G., Menezes-Filho, N. A., Andrade, M. V., de Souza Noronha, K. V. M., Rudi Rocha, R., et al. (2019). Brazil's unified health system: The first 30 years and prospects for the future. *The Lancet, 394*(10195), 345–356. https://doi.org/10.1016/S0140-6736(19)31243-7.

Cerqueira, O., & Terto, Jr., V. (2015). Sobre a construção da agenda de acesso a tratamentos para o HIV/AIDS no movimento social de AIDS no Brasil. In *Prêmio GTPI Jacques Bouchara de produção acadêmica voltada para o ativismo*. Prêmio GTPI 1. Rio de Janeiro: Associação Brasileira Interdisciplinar de AIDS (ABIA). https://issuu.com/gtpi/docs/premio_gtpi_web.

Comaroff, J. (2007). Beyond bare life: AIDS, (bio) politics, and the neoliberal order. *Public Culture, 19*(1), 197–219. https://doi.org/10.1215/08992363-2006-030.

CONITEC (Comissão Nacional de Incorporação de Tecnologias no Sistema Único de Saúde). (2017). *Consulta pública Para elaboração de PCDT Para profilaxia pré exposição (PrEP) ao HIV*. Brasília - DF. http://conitec.gov.br/images/Consultas/Contribuicoes/2017/CP_CONITEC_04_2017_PCDT_Profilaxia_pr%C3%A9-exposi%C3%A7%C3%A3o_ao_HIV_PrEP.pdf.

Daniel, H. (2018). *Vida antes da morte*. 3ª. Rio de Janeiro: Associação Brasileira Interdisciplinar de AIDS (ABIA). http://abiaids.org.br/wp-content/uploads/2018/12/VIDA_ANTES_DA_MORTE_LIFE_BEFORE_DEATH_site.pdf.

Daniels, J. P. (2019). Populism threatens Brazil's HIV/AIDS response. *The Lancet/HIV, 6*(10), e650–e651. https://www.thelancet.com/journals/lanhiv/article/PIIS2352-3018(19)30301-7/fulltext.

de Noronha, J. C. (2013). Cobertura Universal de Saúde: Como Misturar Conceitos, Confundir Objetivos, Abandonar Princípios. *Cadernos de Saúde Pública, 29*(5), 847–849. https://www.scielo.br/pdf/csp/v29n5/03.pdf.

de Souza, H. (1994). *A cura da AIDS/the cure of AIDS*. Rio de Janeiro: Relume Dumará. http://www.abiaids.org.br/_img/media/A%20Cura%20da%20AIDS.pdf.

DPU (SP). (2017). *Parecer: inclusão das novas tecnolgias de profilaxia pré-exposição (PrEP) na política pública para HIV/AIDS - direito à PrEP*. https://www.defensoria.sp.def.br/dpesp/repositorio/0/Parecer%20-%20PrEP%20-%20Defensoria%20Publica.pdf.

Ediane, T. (2019). *Para o laboratório que mais investe em P&D no mundo, a indústria farmacêutica precisa se reinventar*. Revista Época, April. Available at: https://epocanegocios.globo.com/Empresa/noticia/2019/04/para-o-laboratorio-que-mais-investe-em-pd-no-mundo-industria-farmaceutica-precisa-se-reinventar.html. Accessed 21 June 2020.

FCAA. (2020). *Philanthropic support to address HIV/AIDS in 2018*. Funders concerned about AIDS, January 2020. Washington, DC. https://www.fcaaids.org/wp-content/uploads/2020/02/Philanthropic-Support-to-Address-HIVAIDS-in-2018-web-version-2.0.pdf. Accessed 12 Aug 2020.

Foucault, M. (1988). *História da Sexualidade I – A vontade de saber*. Rio de Janeiro: Graal.

Fraser, N. (1995). From redistribution to recognition? Dilemmas of justice in a 'post-socialist' age. *New Left Review, 212*, 68–93.

Fraser, N., & Honneth, A. (2003). *Redistribution or recognition? A political-philosophical exchange*. New York; London: Verso.

Giovanella, L., Mendoza-Ruiz, A., Pilar, A. d. C. A., da Rosa, M. C., Martins, G. B., Santos, I. S., et al. (2018). Sistema universal de saúde e cobertura universal: desvendando pressupostos e estratégias. *Ciência Saúde coletiva, 23*(6), 1763–1776. https://doi.org/10.1590/1413-81232018236.05562018.

Hasenclever, L., Fialho, B., Klein, H., & Zaire, C. (2010). *Economia industrial de empresas farmacêuticas*. Rio de Janeiro: E-papers.

Honneth A. (2003). *Luta por reconhecimento: a gramática moral dos conflitos sociais*. São Paulo: Editora 34.

IFC (Internacional Finance Corporation) and World Bank. (2018). *Better-managed hospitals in Brazil offer remedy to thousands*. Available at: https://www.ifc.org/wps/wcm/connect/news_ext_content/ifc_external_corporate_site/news+and+events/news/impact-stories/better-managed-brazilian-hospitals. Accessed 22 June 2020.

ITPC. (2014). *Advocacy for Community Treatment – ACT Toolkit: Strenghthening community responses to HIV treatment and prevention*. Available at: https://itpcglobal.org/wp-content/uploads/2015/02/ACT-Toolkit-2.0.pdf. Accessed 22 June 2020.

Lima, J. C. F. (2015). O Banco Mundial, a Organização Mundial de Saúde e o "novo universalismo" ou a "cobertura universal de saúde". In J. M. M. Pereira & M. Pronko (Eds.), *A demolição de direitos: Um exame das políticas do Banco Mundial Para a educação e a saúde (1980–2013)* (pp. 233–253). Rio de Janeiro: EPSJV.

Lima, N. T., Gerschman, S., Edler, F. C., & Suárez, J. M. (2005). *Saúde e democracia: história e perspectivas do SUS*. Editora FIOCRUZ.

Mbembe, A. (2018). *Necropolítica*. São Paulo: N-1 edições.

Nunn, A. S., Fonseca, E. M., Bastos, F. I., Gruskin, S., & Salomon, J. A. (2007). Evolution of antiretroviral drug costs in Brazil in the context of free and universal access to AIDS treatment. *PLoS Med, 4*(11), e305. https://doi.org/10.1371/journal.pmed.0040305.

Parker, R. (1994). *A Construção da Solidariedade: AIDS, Sexualidade e Política no Brasil*. Rio de Janeiro: ABIA, IMS/UERJ Relume-Dumará.

Parker, R. (2020). Brazil and the AIDS crisis. *Oxford Research Encyclopedia of Latin American History*. https://doi.org/10.1093/acrefore/9780199366439.013.865.

Parker, R., Gavigan, K., Ramirez, A., Prerez-Brumer, A., Terto Jr., V., e Vagner de Almeida. (2015). Prevention literacy: Reinventing HIV prevention for the 21st century. *GAPW Policy Brief*. http://gapwatch.org/wp-content/uploads/2015/11/PolicyBrief_2015nov.pdf.

Rose, N. (2007). *The politics of life itself: Biomedicine, power, and subjectivity in the twenty-first century*. Princeton: Princeton University Press.

Tangcharoensathien, V., Mills, A., Patcharanarumol, W., & Witthayapipopsakul, W. (2020). Universal health coverage: Time to deliver on political promises. *Bulletin of the World Health Organization, 98*(2), 78–78A. https://www.who.int/bulletin/volumes/98/2/20-250597/en/.

Walwyn, D. (2013). Patents and profits: A disparity of manufacturing margins in the tenofovir value chain. *African Journal of AIDS Research, 12*(1), 17–23. https://doi.org/10.2989/16085906.2013.815407.

Watts, J. (2016, December 9). Brazil's austerity package decried by UN as attack on poor people. *The Guardian*. Available at: https://www.theguardian.com/world/2016/dec/09/brazil-austerity-cuts-un-official. Accessed 22 June 2020.

Part II
Pleasure, Agency and Desire

Chapter 7
The Beatification of the Clinic: Biomedical Prevention 'From Below'

Kane Race

7.1 Experimental Subjects

Can the history of AIDS ever be told without repeating dichotomies—medicine versus culture and politics—that were set up as the epidemic emerged and developed? (Engelmann 2018, p. 217).

Collective (self)-experimentation with bodies, pleasures, drugs, modes of intimacy and relations of care has been a critical element in the processes through which gay men and their communities have grappled with the exigencies of HIV since the beginning of the epidemic. These experiments have been a significant feature, not only in the emergence of modern gay communities and the sexual ecologies within which the virus was first found to proliferate and rapidly spread, but also (and just as importantly) in the wide-ranging innovations in community mobilisation, disease prevention, care practices, clinical relations, patient advocacy, peer education and institutional re-arrangements that have constituted this unprecedented response to a public health emergency. In this paper I argue the frame of collective experimentation is good for troubling familiar narratives that frame the recent biomedical turn in HIV prevention as a straightforward imposition of biomedical authority and technoscientific mandates on unwitting communities and populations (prevention 'from above'), and for drawing out the ways in which community mobilisation, (sub)cultural innovation and collective self-fashioning have shaped and transformed HIV ontologies.

'Working on heuristic rules about the world is a deeply embedded feature of human interaction and should be encouraged, not condemned,' HIV researcher Peter Davis once proposed (Davies 1993, p. 279). His remarks were made in the context of a discussion about the invention of gay men's practices of 'negotiated safety'—a

K. Race (✉)
Department of Gender and Cultural Studies, University of Sydney, Sydney, Australia
e-mail: kane.race@sydney.edu.au

© Springer Nature Switzerland AG 2021 91
S. Bernays et al. (eds.), *Remaking HIV Prevention in the 21st Century*, Social Aspects of HIV 5, https://doi.org/10.1007/978-3-030-69819-5_7

practice that social scientists identified in collaboration with gay community educators back in the early 1990s. 'Negotiated safety' is usually claimed as a social innovation, and so it was; but one might nonetheless concede that the process of 'working on heuristic rules about the world' has more than social (or even human) coordinates and implications. It entails the experimental labour of testing habitual associations between technologies, objects, sociomaterial relations, cultural associations and the world (diagnostic tests, relationship structures, conventions of intimacy and sexual urges) in a process that gives rise to new practices, objects, and knowledges that transform the nature of realities and the reality of natures in material ways. Ontological politics, in other words.

Another example of affected communities 'working on heuristic rules about the world' consists in the forms of community activism that converged around drug development and approval practices in the USA and beyond under the banner of HIV treatment activism. By vigorously contesting 'the formats of treatment research, clinical trial procedures, the distribution of medications, and so on' (Papadopoulos 2018, p. 155), community treatment activists transformed relations among human and non-human actors (doctors, patients, medications, clinical assays) and brought new biomedical practices and pharmaceutical objects into being (Epstein 1996). As Papadopoulos maintains, this collective experimentation preceded and exceeded the terms of HIV treatment activism, encompassing a diverse array of activities that span from the redesign of care services and educational modes to the invention and reinvention of sexual practices; from intervening in media representations to lobbying local authorities, from negotiating new subjectivities, solidarities and affective bonds, to 'extensive experimenting with one's own body and (not officially approved) drugs' (Papadopoulos 2018, p. 156):

> Gay men became a community and engaged in AIDS activism as a way of understanding and managing this ontological encounter. AIDS activism is the attempt to create a material, biochemical, medical, social and cultural space in which the relation of the human body and HIV could be reshaped after the initial outbreak of the epidemic (p. 157).

In paying due attention to a whole range of intimate experiments in his account of these 'compositional practices', Papadopoulos produces a welcome symmetry across diverse activities that neatly sidesteps what A.N. Whitehead calls the 'bifurcation of nature' (Whitehead 1920). This phrase refers to the modernist tendency of dividing the world up into two discrete disciplinary domains: the privileged realm of primary qualities (natural laws and objective facts), the determination of which is normally entrusted to hard scientists; and the realm of secondary qualities (the variable terrain of subjective meanings and cultural values) that social scientists and humanists are left to muddle over, explain and interpret. With a few notable exceptions, critics and advocates of HIV biomedical prevention alike tend to abide by the disciplinary terms of this bifurcation, characterising the new prevention paradigm, for example, as 'a striking re-medicalization of our approach to the HIV epidemic' that conceives the epidemic as 'a medical problem best addressed by purely technical, biomedical solutions whose management should be left to biomedical professionals and scientists,' (Nguyen et al. 2011). In this discourse, biomedical approaches to prevention are charged with the crime of subordinating grassroots initiatives and collective activism to the juggernauts of 'biomedical triumphalism', 'techno-eschatology', and top-down solutions to public health problems. While there can be no doubt that 'professional knowledge systems in HIV have invested heavily in biomedical technologies' over recent decades (Adam 2011, p. 6), the bifurcation of HIV prevention into these primary and secondary domains reduces the range and scope of community mobilisation and social interventions in problematic ways. Specifically, it reduces their terrain of operation to the 'merely cultural' or 'primarily social', and risks neglecting the material dimensions and ontological impacts of these forms of collective experimentation.

This chapter explores the significance of experimentality, pleasure and play in recent developments taking place under the rubric of biomedical prevention. It considers the emergence of community-based clinics in a number of urban gay precincts around the world that aim to optimise the outcomes of biomedical prevention by offering services such as rapid HIV testing, STI screening and treatment referral in community settings. These initiatives have led to new kinds of collaboration between affected communities and clinical actors that take the situated experience of the sexual self as a significant and valued source of information in clinical services design. But they are especially distinctive in their proposal to address barriers to prevention and care on the part of the communities they seek to engage through cultural interventions that include the aesthetic stylisation and re-design of clinical practices and spaces. This demonstrates the emergence of a relatively new object in community-based strategic and programmatic responses to HIV prevention which I call the beatification of the clinic.

7.2 On Beatification

When I first conceived this chapter I was under the impression the Catholic ritual of canonisation involved a step called *beautification*, and since this term also refers to aesthetic interventions it had the kind of double meaning that suited my argument about community clinics. Readers familiar with Catholic hagiography will no doubt retort that beautification is not the same thing as beatification and the two terms should not be confused, since the latter has a technical meaning that refers to something more than (or at least different from) questions of beauty and mere aesthetics. It is a step in a formal ritual whereby the Pope declares a deceased person venerable enough to have entered a state of bliss, usually on the basis of some miracle they have performed (or that God has caused to work through them). So it would indeed be a mistake to conflate these terms or confuse their meanings, as my title would have us do. But while this chapter's title was conceived in error, premised on a semantic confusion of proximate terms, the dissonance this error creates may nonetheless be generative for thinking through different tendencies in the present era of HIV prevention.

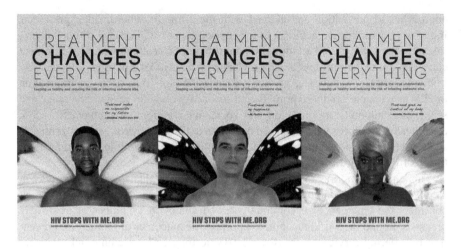

Fig. 7.1 Posters from the *HIV Stops With Me* Campaign (New York State Department of Health 2017)

Certainly, the mood of 'biomedical triumphalism' that pervaded discourses of biomedical prevention from the early 2010s typically invested biomedicine with miraculising potential, venerating the clinic as a privileged scene of HIV prevention on a global scale. The joyous incantation of a 'prevention revolution' and the heady promise of an 'AIDS-free generation' commonly assumed a jubilant tenor and near-apostolic form. A campaign produced by the State of New York in 2017 can serve as a ready example of this trend: its posters featured PLWHA of various genders, sexualities and ethnicities sprouting the wings of butterflies beneath a pealing slogan: 'TREATMENT CHANGES EVERYTHING'. In the smaller, less shouty, fine-text this claim was expanded upon: 'Medications transform our lives by making the virus undetectable, keeping us healthy and reducing the risk of infecting someone else' (Fig. 7.1).

This iconography invests treatment with consecrating power, turning the technical affordances of medication into an occasion for ecstatic rapture. Treatment is framed as a catalyst for redemption, self-transformation and resplendent self-completion; bearing the capacity not merely to heal those affected by HIV but *change everything*; overhaul the subject and make them new again. With its promise to turn people with HIV into impeccable subjects of HIV prevention, treatment emerges here as nothing less than a mechanism for moral, emotional and physical self-transformation, turning grubs into butterflies, making saints out of sinners. We are summoned to bear witness to—or better yet, participate in—a miracle: the beatification of the clinic.

This imagery of personal salvation and miraculous self-transformation is altogether different from the experimental operations this chapter takes as its primary focus. The experiments I have in mind are far less grandiose and sanctifying in nature, and much more pragmatic, modest and secular by comparison: they neither promise nor demand a purification of the soul. To better grasp these differences and their significance for my argument we might turn to Foucault's work in *The Use of Pleasure* on the historical formation of subjects through practices of problematisation and stylisation (Foucault 1985).

Foucault introduces his study by proposing an approach that seeks to 'define the conditions in which human beings 'problematize' what they are, what they do and the world in which they live' (1985, p. 10). He proposes analysing 'the *problematizations* through which being offers itself, necessarily, to be thought— and the *practices* on the basis of which these problematizations are formed' (1985, p. 11). In directing this approach to the formation of ethical subjects in antiquity, he observes 'problematization was linked to a group of practices that have been of unquestionable importance in our societies: I am referring to what might be called the "arts of existence"':

> What I mean by the phrase are those intentional and voluntary actions by which men not only set themselves rules of conduct, but also seek to transform themselves, to change themselves in their singular being, and to make their life into an *oeuvre* that carries certain aesthetic values and meets certain stylistic criteria (Foucault 1985, pp. 10–11).

These aesthetics of existence interested Foucault because they 'functioned not as standards by which to normalize populations but as elements in a procedure that a few people might adopt with the aim of living what they considered a beautiful and praiseworthy life' (Halperin 1995, p. 68). Rather than involving disciplinary subjectification and the wholesale conversion of subjects to social norms, they raise the possibility of stylising one's relation with oneself and the conditions in which it materialises according to deliberately chosen criteria of value. Writing at the beginning of the AIDS crisis, one of Foucault's concerns when undertaking this work was how to adapt and direct the power exercised by medical and moral experts in the time of the epidemic (Foucault 1993). As he disclosed in an interview, 'the idea of the *bios* as a material for an aesthetic piece of art is something that fascinates me' (Foucault 1984, p. 348).

In Foucauldian sociology, aesthetics of existence are generally used to refer to neoliberal technologies of the self. But in this chapter I approach the experimental practices of gay men and their communities as innovations that subject matters of HIV prevention to problematisation and propose certain stylisations of existence and its relations on this basis. The target of aesthetic labour in this instance is not the individual *per se* but the socio-material arrangements that make HIV prevention as practicable, pleasurable and accessible as possible. Gay men and their communities continue to be involved in problematising HIV transmission and crafting distinctive, stylised responses to it. The body of this chapter is devoted to exploring how collective aesthetic experimentation is participating in the realisation of HIV pre- vention objects among gay men in the present context of biomedical prevention. The community-based clinics that have recently emerged in urban gay precincts in various parts of the world constitute a primary focus. Before this, I work through a number of other pertinent examples to further substantiate my claim about the exemplary power of attending more carefully to histories of biomedical prevention 'from below'.

Since the performative turn in sociologies of science, technology, economics, medicine, sexuality and knowledge it has become commonplace to claim that research does not simply represent realities, but is actively involved in their making. On this view, medical, sexual and economic realities are not simply given but *provoked into being* by research practices and other framing devices, to borrow Fabian Muniesa's (2014) terminology. In the following section I do not claim to provide an exhaustive account of 'biomedical prevention from below': the examples I give are merely schematic and suggestive. They are provocative in intent, selected for their pragmatic and illustrative value and not at all comprehensive in their empirical rendering. But this could be said of any experiment.

7.3   Biomedical Prevention from below: Some Provocations

Steven Epstein's study of the early years of HIV treatment activism recounts the crucial role that community treatment activists played in the contestation of clinical endpoints used by research scientists to evaluate the efficacy of antiretroviral drugs. The acceptance of viral load test results as a surrogate measure for determinations of drug efficacy, the progression of HIV disease, and eventually as a proxy for bodily infectivity might not have occurred so readily or even taken place in the mid-1990s were it not for this legacy of critical engagement with bioscientific technicalities on the part of community activists. Indeed, one might claim that the very premises of biomedical prevention (specifically, its predication on notions of viral suppression) are built on foundations laid by the collaborative work of community activists, lay experts and research scientists.

While the invention and deployment of viral load assays within the heterogenous field of HIV science has yet to be documented in sufficient historical detail to establish whether this argument holds merit, it nonetheless became apparent to Australian social scientists as early as 2001 that HIV-positive gay men were incorporating the results of these tests into their sexual practices and prevention repertoires, dispensing with condoms in certain circumstances on the basis of having an undetectable viral load (Rosengarten et al. 2000; Race 2003). This took place a full decade before clinical trials finally corroborated the reliability of these vernacular hypotheses, preceding the emergence of U=U as a popular slogan and basic rallying point for community advocacy enthusiasts by an even longer shot (about 16 years).

As one of the social researchers involved in the process of documenting these prevention innovations and brokering their legitimacy, I found Foucault's framework proposed in *The Use of Pleasure* very useful for making these vernacular innovations ethically intelligible. By framing various tactics of HIV prevention— condom use, negotiated safety, strategic positioning, etc.—as *ethics,* i.e. 'practical techniques adopted for the achievement of certain implicit and explicit goals' (Race

2003, p. 371) it became possible to render practices that were typically taken to be breaches of public health norms as historically variable experiments in HIV prevention rather than instances of moral transgression. 'Foucault flags the possibility of bringing a certain amount of care and attention to self-practice that is not automatically disqualified from intelligibility on the basis of its non-adherence to prescribed norms,' I later reflected. The distinction between ethics and overarching moral norms produces 'the possibility of conceiving de-pathologizing modes of care, education and service-provision' (Race 2008, p. 417), allowing us to draw out how affected groups evaluate, test and put to work the possibilities of new products of knowledge.

Cooper and Waldby coined the term 'clinical labour' to account for forms of embodied labour that are central to biomedical innovation but 'rarely considered as labour' such as participation in clinical trials (Cooper and Waldby 2014). The mass participation in clinical research to test the efficacy and affordances of HIV antiretroviral drugs on the part of gay men and other affected groups are surely part of the story of biomedical prevention 'from below' on this account. Their provocation can be taken further if we consider the forms of labour that take place outside the official frameworks of clinical research but tacitly inform its propositions and hypotheses: what I call *experimental labour*. The risk reduction practices discussed above are one example of such experimental labour: a full decade before clinical researchers 'discovered' that the antiretroviral suppression of viral load eliminated the risk of HIV transmission, gay men were trialling this proposition and putting it into practice. Similarly, the evaluation and approval of Pre-Exposure Prophylaxis (PrEP) was most probably informed by the calculated risk-taking of sexual actors undergoing Post-Exposure Prophylaxis (PEP). The sexual experiments of those receiving PEP provided a vernacular proof of concept that research scientists appropriated and formalised as a basis for PrEP trial protocols, to test whether certain antiretroviral combinations might protect HIV-negative individuals from becoming infected despite their ongoing exposure to risk. Meanwhile, the idea of PrEP 'on demand' or 'intermittent dosing'—which has been subject to a number of clinical trials recently—seems predicated on a situation in which intended users plan their sexual escapades some time in advance, rather than sex 'just happening' (as was often once the case in urban gay culture). The habit of arranging casual sex some time in advance—in the form of weekend sex sessions, for example—is a unique affordance of the digital sex infrastructures that have emerged as a prominent feature of gay men's sexual arrangements over the past two decades, and with which they have experimented (Race 2018). To frame these social precedents for trial hypotheses as a kind of experimental labour is to acknowledge the productive effects and potential value of people's risk-taking and vernacular experiments that occur prior to, and inform, the hypotheses and designs of official clinical trials.

Indeed, the experimental labour entailed in using drugs that are not officially approved has a longer history within gay culture. A 1999 article in the *Village Voice* entitled 'Higher and Higher: Drug Cocktails—Pleasures, Risk and Reasons' delved into the use of drugs on gay dancefloors—from antiretroviral medications to illicit stimulants and psychoactive compounds—and the mix of recreational and therapeutic purposes behind it:

> This weekend, and every weekend on dance floors across the city, thousands of teeth-grinding subjects [...] engage in an underground research project. Amid flashing lights and pounding music, untutored freelance pharmacologists conduct experiments on their own bodies to determine what happens when one consumes a bewildering array of pills and powders in the confined and humid setting of a nightclub (Owen 1999).

Today, most of the drugs the article discusses are being investigated for therapeutic purposes. Ecstasy, marijuana, LSD and ketamine are among the drugs being tested to address conditions such as Post-Traumatic Stress Disorder, anxiety and depression in largescale clinical trials. But this a topic for another paper (Race forthcoming).

The introduction of combination antiretroviral therapy in 1996 in Western countries is commonly narrated as a normalisation of responses to HIV/AIDS.[1] But such interpretations miss something important about the persistence and ongoing significance of forms of experimental labour and subcultural innovation that make it possible to tell an alternative story of *biomedical prevention from below*. The dominant narrative of normalisation overlooks the active participation of affected communities in the shaping and application of biomedical strategies and their possibilities. It expropriates the labour of experimental subjects and casts it as the exploitable property of biomedicine and pharmaceutical companies. This buttresses the monopoly of biomedical authority over public health policy at the very moment that antiretroviral and diagnostic technologies are becoming subject to necessarily heterogenous forms of socialisation.

7.4   The Stylisation of the Clinic

The ratification of Treatment as Prevention and PrEP is commonly narrated in terms of the rise of pharmapower and biomedicalisation. In the previous section I argued such narratives overlook the experimental labour of affected communities in the crafting of new prevention strategies. Indeed, the main drivers for the development of PrEP were public health and the gay community, rather than Big Pharma, as Karsten Schubert has pointed out (Schubert 2019).[2] Indeed, gay community-based HIV organisations have been among some of the most enthusiastic proponents of biomedical prevention. To use the parlance of a later epidemic (COVID-19), the

---

[1] An article entitled 'the normalization of AIDS in Western European countries' describes how the 'exceptional innovations in prevention, patient care, health policy and questions of civil rights' that characterised the initial emergence of AIDS gave way to a state of normalisation in health policy at this moment (Rosenbrock et al. 2000, p. 1607).

[2] 'The development of PREP was spearheaded by an interaction between the gay and public health communities through an integration of gay stakeholders in the processes of the three most important PREP-MSM studies iPrex, Ipergay and Proud' (Schubert 2019, p. 137)

endorsement of treatment as prevention in largescale clinical trials provided an opportunity to develop a much-wanted 'exit strategy' (Petersen et al. 2020) from the restrictive and frustrating demands of physical distancing (i.e. using condoms). This has prompted organisations to direct the bulk of their recent prevention efforts toward the technical reorganisation of clinical services to maximise access and uptake of HIV testing and treatment. Sexual practice no longer constitutes the sole target of community HIV prevention initiatives: rather, new forms of engagement with biomedicine are conceived to produce healthier sexual citizens. But this is not merely a case of intensified biomedicalisation, as standard accounts would have it. These initiatives can be framed in alternative terms as a *sexual enculturation of the clinic*.

Community-based organisations have long drawn on their familiarity with specific sexual cultures to equip those participating in these cultures with ways to reduce risk. Longstanding efforts to make condoms and educational resources available in sex-on-premises venues is but one example of such work, which can be characterised as a kind of experiment with the sexual infrastructures of gay culture that achieves its ends by engaging with given discourses and structures of sexual pleasure rather than opposing them. The new genre of gay community-based clinics can be understood in similar terms: as an infrastructural experiment that draws on its fluency in gay cultural and sexual pleasures to make the use of certain prevention technologies more accessible, practical and possible. In particular, it seeks to counter some of the confronting aspects of HIV diagnostic testing by affirming the legitimacy of gay sexual pleasures and practices.

I first encountered this new genre of community-based clinics as a tourist in San Francisco walking through the Castro district one evening in the early 2010s. One of the shops that caught my attention had a large metallic wall within, with brightly coloured alphabet magnets on it—fridge magnets that many of us grew up with as children. I found this invitation to participate in creative and pedagogical play striking enough to want to stop and find out more. What I discovered was that this was not some trendy café or social venue as I had assumed, but a drop-in sexual health clinic called Magnet that offered rapid HIV testing and STI screening. Especially interesting were the aesthetic and ludic dimensions of the appeal this storefront made to passers-by. The design of the space was playful and engaging enough to make me want to linger on my stroll through an already colourful neighbourhood. A 2015 article from the *New York Times* captures some key aspects of the clinic's design:

> The Magnet Clinic [. . .] did 9600 H.I.V. tests last year. It lies in the heart of the Castro, the city's rainbow-flag-bedecked gay mecca, and resembles a cheery cell-phone store: The waiting room has couches, flowers, disco music and photographs of the Sisters of Perpetual Indulgence, a campy drag troupe. A mobile of smiling penis toys dangled over one examination table. "We didn't want it to feel like a jail cell," said the nursing director, Pierre-Cedric Crouch, wearing the clinic's signature "No Blame/No Shame" T-shirt. "And we have no stigma. You can come in saying you just slept with 20 guys and don't know what a condom is, and we don't criticize you. We help you out" (McNeil 2015).

As this passage indicates, community-based clinics seek to counter barriers to HIV testing by promoting a non-judgmental, sex-positive, gay-friendly clinical experience.

Since that first encounter, I have visited similar initiatives in urban gay centres around the world. Dean St Express is a self-service clinic run by Britain's NHS located in London's Soho area and draws on 'the colourful vibe of the surrounding neighbourhood' to create an appealing and engaging ambience that foregrounds pleasure and convenience and 'departs entirely from the sterile, dingy aesthetic ubiquitous in the sector' (Van Gilder Cooke 2014).

> The screening rooms are all based on a different shop in the area, each with unique décor and signage. The waiting room features cinema seats for waiting visitors, while the reception area includes a large window where patients can watch scientists in the lab analysing their samples. In addition, NHS Dean St features cutting-edge technology, including iPads for registration and a pneumatic vacuum that whisks samples straight to an on-site laboratory.

As with Magnet, designers have sought to make the space welcoming and inviting to the communities it seeks to engage. By making an aesthetic feature of the techniques and devices of pathology testing (normally left backstage), it encourages new modes of engagement between consumers and biomedicine.

In Australia the design of community-based clinics has enlisted a variety of methods, from speculative design research to commissioning the work of community artists to decorate the clinical premises. Again, the overall effect is to make these spaces feel more like sex-positive community or leisure spaces than medical centres. Promotional material for these clinics draws on urban gay cultural and subcultural sensibilities to produce HIV testing as a routinised part of participation in gay life. The promotional video for Thorne Harbour Health's Pronto Clinic, first established in inner north Melbourne in 2015, was directed by a local gay party promoter Nik Dimopoulos and adopts a gay subcultural aesthetic that features tattooed gay and transmasculine models in jockstraps showcasing the pinprick HIV diagnostic test alongside latex gloves, gay fetish gear, condoms, and PrEP, all to the beat of an underground electronic soundtrack (Fig. 7.2). The minimalistic text accompanying the video reads:

> Whether you're protected or unprotected, if you fuck, get tested four times a year—summer, winter, autumn and spring—for peace of mind. It's quick, results in 15 minutes. PRONTO: Gay run service, Trans inclusive.

The overall effect is to embed clinical procedures such as rapid HIV-testing within a trendy gay subcultural vernacular repertoire; as convenient means of equipping and protecting the modern gay sexual actor.

7.5 Flipping Stigma, Reframing Diagnosis

Jeanne Ellard (2015) has identified a number of things community-based clinics are doing to make HIV and STI testing easier for clients in Australia. These include:

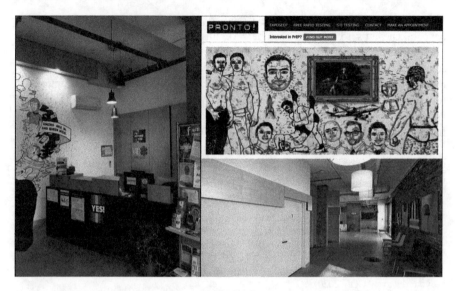

Fig. 7.2 Thorne Harbour Health's Pronto Clinic in Fitzroy, Melbourne

- Locating services in inner city areas where many gay men live
- Making the appointment process easy, for example offering on-line bookings
- Offering rapid HIV tests
- Providing HIV and STI testing free of charge
- Staffing services with skilled peer educators
- Delivering a non-judgmental service
- Working in partnership with clinical services and individual clinicians to ensure appropriate clinical governance procedures are followed.

This is a useful articulation of the strategic rationale behind these services, but public health reporting conventions hardly do justice to the aesthetic dimensions of the work entailed in pursuing these objectives. Community-based sexual health services are ontological experiments that seek to create new forms of access and engagement between biomedicine and affected communities in the name of prevention and care. They are distinctive in how they incorporate community knowledges, aesthetics, tastes and participants into the service-design and service-delivery process. Framing these activities in terms of *sexual enculturation* highlights how these infrastructural experiments are informed by the specific sexual and social cultures produced and inhabited by affected groups. At the same time, it brings into view a potential shortcoming of these strategies: the particularisation of the clinic through this kind of aesthetic work may make the clinic a more appealing space to those who identify with these cultures but is just as likely to alienate those who disidentify with their aesthetic forms. In this respect, it is best to approach the beautification of the clinic as an evolving project that is best informed by data on the cultural orientation of those groups found to be less likely to access HIV testing and treatment. It is noteworthy that in Australia, where surveillance data indicates that gay men from

Asian countries are less likely to test regularly for HIV, community-based clinics have taken steps to involve members of this demographic in their design and promotional activities. While they have largely been elaborated in Western gay settings to date, community-based HIV clinics can be understood as a 'fluid technology' that may be adapted to serve the needs of different cultures and communities (de Laet and Mol 2000). The founders of Magnet report having worked with community-based educators in many other countries including Peru, Spain and India to develop culturally appropriate clinics for affected communities.

One of the striking things about these community-based efforts to optimise the effectiveness of biomedical prevention that contrasts sharply with a previous moment in HIV prevention is their de-dramatisation of the prospect of HIV diagnosis. The online campaign materials for Australia's *Ending HIV* campaign state:

> You may have heard that HIV treatments can be a hassle to take and have bad side effects. In the past, that was the experience for many people but it's much less the case these days. The variety of new treatments that are available today are far more effective against HIV, far better tolerated and pose minimal side effects. People starting modern treatment take a few tablets once or twice a day, some only needing one pill once a day. Discuss your options with your doctor (ACON 2020).

Similar claims are made in the promotional material for similar services around the world. This is a far cry from how HIV treatment was represented in prevention campaigns of a previous era, when community educators were inclined to dramatise the difficulties associated with treatment in efforts to promote HIV prevention behaviours. For example, San Francisco's *HIV is No Picnic* billboard campaign of 2002 depicted PLWHA experiencing some of the more gruesome side-effects of treatment—night sweats, distended abdomens, pronounced facial wasting and diarrhoea—in its bid to tackle increases in sexual risk-taking. Where prevention specialists once thought it appropriate to arouse and amplify fears and anxieties about HIV and STI infection to promote behavioural change, community-based clinics have adopted a strategy that represents almost a complete reversal. They seek to de-escalate fear and de-dramatise infection to expand their reach and do their work; i.e. to encourage more people to come forward and engage in regular testing.

7.6 Conclusion

> Social transformation is difficult if not impossible to achieve in the clinic (Kippax and Stephenson 2012, p. 796).

Community-based clinics are based on a certain problematisation of the circumstances in which gay and other men who have sex with men avoid HIV testing. They act on these circumstances by stylising the clinic as a sex-positive, non-judgmental, culturally appealing space that equips gay men with practical and convenient ways of managing their HIV status. These initiatives can be approached as experiments that 'attempt to create a material, biochemical, medical, social and cultural space in which the relation of the human body and HIV [can] be reshaped' and the impact of the virus on people's sexual and social lives is minimised (Papadopoulos 2018, p. 157). In this sense they are continuous with a longer history of community mobilisation and cultural intervention that newly articulates relations between bodies, technologies and sexuality to produce new gay subjectivities. Where some commentators frame recent developments in terms of the biomedicalisation of sexuality, I have argued we are also seeing a sexual socialisation of biomedicine.

Recent work in sexuality studies has begun to explore the value of framing sex in terms of playfulness and play. Not only is play a term of choice within diverse sexual cultures; it also captures something of general significance about the framing of sex within leisure markets. Susanna Paasonen suggests a 'focus on play makes it possible to highlight improvisation driven by curiosity, desire for variation and openness towards surprise as things that greatly matter in sexual lives' (Paasonen 2018, p. 9). The notion of playfulness 'intermeshes and overlaps with those of improvisation, exploration, curiosity and experimentation, yet it also stands apart from them in foregrounding pleasure and bodily intensity as key motivations for sexual activity' (p. 2). Paasonen conceives play as central to the transformations associated with sexual activity: As pleasure moves us 'towards different scenes, fantasies, bodies and objects, and becomes attached to them, its forms are reorganized, and so is one's sense of self,' she writes (2018, p. 3).

The experimental activities of bodies and their pleasures can produce new ways of feeling, new relations, new communities and new forms of care. They have produced many innovations in HIV prevention, from the popularisation of safe sex, to negotiated safety to the invention of new risk reduction practices in the context of innovations in medicine. The sexual body is an extraordinarily generative creator of new associations, relations and attachments, not only between people but also between bodies and objects, technologies and settings. These can serve as a source of novelty and excitement, reconfiguring the practices they involve in unexpected ways (Race 2019). The reorganising and transformative potential of sex, pleasure, experimentation and play is evident in these perversions and reconfigurations of biomedical objects and practices, and it provides some basis for imagining a counter-history of the beatification of the clinic. Social transformation might be difficult if not impossible to achieve in the clinic, as Kippax and Stephenson have argued (Kippax and Stephenson 2012, p. 796), but this does not mean the clinic is not subject to socio-cultural transformation.

References

ACON. (2020). *Ending HIV campaign*. Retrieved June 27, 2020, from https://endinghiv.org.au/.

Adam, B. D. (2011). Epistemic fault lines in biomedical and social approaches to HIV prevention. *Journal of the International AIDS Society, 14*(S2), S2.

Cooper, M., & Waldby, C. (2014). *Clinical labour*. Durham, NC: Duke University Press.

Davies, P. M. (1993). Safer sex maintenance among gay men: Are we moving in the right direction? *AIDS, 7*(2), 279–280.

De Laet, M., & Mol, A. (2000). The Zimbabwe bush pump: Mechanics of a fluid technology. *Social Studies of Science, 30*(2), 225–263.

Ellard, J. (2015). *Community-based HIV testing approaches for gay and bisexual men.* Sydney: Australian Federation of AIDS Organisations.

Engelmann, L. (2018). *Mapping AIDS.* Cambridge: Cambridge University Press.

Epstein, S. (1996). *Impure science: AIDS, activism, and the politics of knowledge.* Berkeley: University of California Press.

Foucault, M. (1984). On the genealogy of ethics. In P. Rabinow (Ed.), *The Foucault reader* (pp. 340–372). New York: Pantheon.

Foucault, M. (1985). *The history of sexuality 2: The use of pleasure.* (R. Hurley, Trans.). London: Penguin Books.

Foucault, M. (1993). About the beginning of the hermeneutics of the self. *Political Theory, 21*(2), 198–227.

Halperin, D. M. (1995). *Saint Foucault.* Oxford: Oxford University Press.

Kippax, S., & Stephenson, N. (2012). Beyond the distinction between biomedical and social dimensions of HIV prevention through the lens of a social public health. *American Journal of Public Health, 102*(5), 789–799.

McNeil, D. (2015, October 28). San Francisco is changing the face of AIDS treatment. *The New York Times.*

Muniesa, F. (2014). *The provoked economy.* Abingdon: Routledge.

Nguyen, V. K., Bajos, N., Dubois-Arber, F., O'Malley, J., & Pirkle, C. M. (2011). Remedicalizing an epidemic: From HIV treatment as prevention to HIV treatment is prevention. *AIDS, 25*(3), 291–293.

Owen, F. (1999, July 21). Higher and higher: Drug cocktails – Pleasures, risks and reasons. *The village voice.*

Paasonen, S. (2018). *Many splendored things: Thinking sex and play.* London: Goldsmiths College Press.

Papadopoulos, D. (2018). *Experimental practice.* Durham, NC: Duke University Press.

Petersen, E., Wasserman, S., Lee, S., Go, U., Holmes, A. H., Al-Abri, S., et al. (2020). COVID-19 – We urgently need to start developing an exit strategy. *International Journal of Infectious Diseases, 96*, 233–239.

Race, K. (2003). Revaluation of risk among gay men. *AIDS Education and Prevention, 15*(4: Special issue), 369–381.

Race, K. (2008). The use of pleasure in harm reduction. *International Journal of Drug Policy, 19* (5), 417–423.

Race, K. (2018). *The gay science: Intimate experiments with the problem of HIV.* London: Routledge.

Race, K. (2019). What possibilities would a queer ANT generate? In A. Blok, I. Farias, & C. Roberts (Eds.), *The Routledge companion to actor-network theory* (pp. 168–180). London: Routledge.

Race, K. (forthcoming). A lifetime of drugs. In L. Wallace & S. Herring (Eds.), *Longterm: Essays on queer commitment.* Durham, NC: Duke University Press.

Rosenbrock, R., Dubois-Arber, F., Moers, M., Pinell, P., Schaeffer, D., & Setbon, M. (2000). The normalization of AIDS in Western European countries. *Social Science & Medicine, 50*(11), 1607–1629.

Rosengarten, M., Race, K., & Kippax, S. (2000). *Touch wood, everything will be ok.* Sydney: National Centre in HIV Social Research, University of New South Wales.

Schubert, K. (2019). The democratic biopolitics of PrEP. In H. Gerhards & K. Braun (Eds.), *Biopolitiken–Regierungen des Lebens heute* (pp. 121–153). Wiesbaden: Springer VS.

Van Gilder Cooke, S. (2014, April 30). Don't call the doctor: Stylish clinic uses DIY testing. *LSN Global.*

Whitehead, A. N. (1920). *The concept of nature.* Cambridge: Cambridge University Press.

Chapter 8
New Potentials for Old Pleasures: The Role of PrEP in Facilitating Sexual Well-being among Gay and Bisexual Men

Bryan A. Kutner, Adam Bourne, and Will Nutland

8.1 Introduction

For 40 years, HIV has cast a shadow over the sexual expression of many gay, bisexual and other men who have sex with men (GBMSM). The complexity inherent in all sexual conduct has been amplified by this community's experience of death, societal stigma, demonising media discourse about gay sex and political neglect with regard to HIV. Even within countries willing to acknowledge and affirm the rights of men to have sex with other men, a torrent of sex education interventions, public health campaigns and media messaging have portrayed such sexual contact as intrinsically risky and dangerous. However, GBMSM have by no means been passive recipients of this mischaracterisation of human sexuality. Many have sought ways to celebrate and assert their rights to rich and satisfying expression of sexual diversity. To counter the early threat to sexual health posed by HIV, many GBMSM developed their own public health discourse to describe pragmatic and realistically achievable approaches, what researchers came to term 'risk-reduction strategies', behavioural tactics such as negotiated safety (Kippax et al. 1997), strategic positioning (Van de Ven et al. 2002), or serosorting (Parsons et al. 2005). Such efforts came

B. A. Kutner (✉)
HIV Center for Clinical and Behavioral Studies, New York State Psychiatric Institute and Colombia University, New York, USA
e-mail: bak2133@cumc.columbia.edu

A. Bourne
Australian Research Centre in Sex, Health and Society, La Trobe University, Melbourne, Australia

Kirby Institute, UNSW Sydney, Sydney, Australia

W. Nutland
Department of Public Health, Environments and Society, London School of Hygiene and Tropical Medicine, London, UK

© Springer Nature Switzerland AG 2021
S. Bernays et al. (eds.), *Remaking HIV Prevention in the 21st Century*, Social Aspects of HIV 5, https://doi.org/10.1007/978-3-030-69819-5_8

in addition to, rather than instead of, relentless work to promote and facilitate condom use for those where this risk management strategy made sense. These attempts to accommodate to life under a long-term epidemic ameliorated understandable anxieties about HIV while also balancing that fear with opportunities for sexual and emotional pleasure and intimacy (Rhodes and Cusick 2000; Frost et al. 2008). However, GBMSM were also consistently criticised (often by public health professionals but also other members of the gay community) for engaging sexually in ways that were deemed to only *reduce* risk, rather than to eliminate it, as the use of a condom was (presumptuously and wrongly) assumed to accomplish (Eaton et al. 2007; Golden et al. 2008; Smith et al. 2015). This push and pull pitted public health against sexual pleasure, prioritising protection against infection as though these two goals were mutually exclusive.

Biomedical interventions that reduce HIV incidence have the potential to disrupt this historically stigmatising approach to public health messaging (Landers and Kapadia 2020). Pre-exposure prophylaxis (PrEP), in particular, has already reframed HIV for many GBMSM. By radically reducing the risk of HIV acquisition, PrEP has expanded public discourse to include not just the need for risk reduction but for health and pleasure as well (Grace et al. 2018). In doing so, biomedical innovations such as PrEP have the potential to facilitate a re-engagement with core sexual health principles, which have often proved hard (or impossible) for policy makers and health practitioners to embrace when addressing HIV among GBMSM. In 2006, the World Health Organization (WHO) defined sexual health as, '.. . a state of physical, emotional, mental and social well-being in relation to sexuality. .. not merely the absence of disease, dysfunction or infirmity' (WHO 2006). By this definition, sexual health requires a positive and respectful approach to sexuality as well as the possibility of explicitly encouraging pleasurable and safe sexual experiences, free of coercion, discrimination, and violence. Despite being cited in the preamble of numerous sexual health strategies across the globe (e.g. Hartney et al. 2015; An Roinn Sláinte/Department of Health 2015; Queensland Department of Health 2016), much health promotion, education and social marketing directed toward GBMSM has principally focused on ensuring the avoidance of infection or disease (Lorimer et al. 2013; French et al. 2014), rather than embracing the holistic understanding of sexual health recommended by WHO—and necessitated by the actual values and priorities of GBMSM (Bourne et al. 2013).

Within this chapter we first seek to describe how new experiences with PrEP have reshaped longstanding potentials for sexual satisfaction and pleasure among GBMSM and to articulate the ways in which PrEP has facilitated a renaissance in messaging about broader sexual health and well-being. Cognisant of such evidence, and of the long-standing WHO definition of sexual health, we examine how global and national PrEP-related policies or guidance documents shape health services design and delivery in a variety of country contexts, typically neglecting opportunities to leverage a holistic portrayal of sexual health for the sake of prioritising messages about infection prevention and control. This examination is accompanied by an exploration of PrEP-related communication created by and targeted at GBMSM. Taking a strengths-based approach, we examine three case studies of health promotion programmes that have sought to acknowledge and promote pleasure as a central facet of PrEP use. We conclude by exploring ways in which pleasure could, or should, be elevated within this latest phase of the HIV epidemic while contrasting such a proposal with the structural and cultural forces that seek to deny pleasure as a feature of the sex lives of GBMSM (and others). While as individual researchers and scholar activists, we seek to elevate the impact of HIV among transgender men and we firmly acknowledge the role that PrEP could play in their lives, our chapter focusses on cisgender men due to a distinct lack of available data and literature on additional male-identifying populations. Similarly, while efforts have been made to draw from across the spectrum of country income levels, much of our review speaks to high-income countries. This reflects continuing challenges faced in many low- and middle-income countries to recognise and affirm gay sexual practice in research and policy practices. We return to these limitations in our concluding remarks, asking who has structural access to pleasure in this latest phase of the HIV epidemic?

8.2 Evidencing Pleasure and PrEP

The notion that pleasure is central to health promotion is not new, but the advent of PrEP has stimulated a substantial reexamination of the role of pleasure in HIV prevention. Historically, accounting for sexual pleasure in the design and advancement of interventions to promote sexual health has been strongly recommended (Donovan et al. 1994; Nath et al. 2019), including to promote condoms and safer sex (Crosby and Mena 2017; Siegler et al. 2019). Indeed, sexual pleasure is a well-documented motivator of sexual behaviour across social contexts around the globe (Ekstrand 1992; Gold and Rosenthal 1998), from South Africa (Kiguwa 2015) to Lebanon (Aunon et al. 2015) to the Central African Republic (Simaleko et al. 2018). PrEP is a newer technology that prevents HIV without the impediments to pleasure evinced by many GBMSM who have found condoms difficult to use consistently.

Whether in pill or another form like a rectal microbicide gel, PrEP appeals to GBMSM interests in experiencing greater sexual pleasure while simultaneously reducing HIV-related anxiety (Calabrese and Underhill 2015; Giguere et al. 2015). Indeed, researchers find consistent signals that pleasure and anxiety reduction motivate PrEP initiation and maintenance. In Australia, GBMSM who use PrEP report lower HIV-related anxiety than eligible non-PrEP users (Keen et al. 2020) and note its capacity to help them overcome fear and enhance sexual pleasure (Holt et al. 2019; Philpot et al. 2020). Likewise in Switzerland, motivations toward PrEP use include the option to engage in sex with less worry and less anxiety (Gredig et al. 2016). GBMSM in France and Canada describe greater intimacy and an improved quality in their sex lives, consistent with findings in the USA (Gamarel and Golub 2015), and report less of the anxiety ordinarily induced by the perception of condoms as a barrier to pleasure and desire (Mabire et al. 2019). This may not be a universal pattern, as some GBMSM experience a decrease in anxiety without concomitant increases in satisfaction, but overall GBMSM on PrEP appear to experience meaningful improvements in their psychological health (Whitfield et al. 2019). The causal pathways to reduced anxiety and increased pleasure may not yet be absolutely clear, but this patterned shift in sexual health, as defined by WHO, appears to be intimately linked to changes in HIV-related stigma. Qualitative data from the USA suggest that PrEP users experience greater confidence discussing HIV status as well as their preferences with regard to condoms, and less stigma in relation to sexual partners living with HIV (Pantalone et al. 2019). However, the opposite may also be true in that the presence of PrEP may result in less communication about HIV and the status of respective partners given that PrEP (or an undetectable viral load) dramatically reduces the possibility of infection. Typical binaries of positive and negative may thus assume less significance in the context of biomedical technologies that render the risk of HIV acquisition very unlikely, a promise never quite achieved with consistent condom use alone (Smith et al. 2015).

8.3 Pleasure in PrEP Policy and Programme Planning

Despite the mitigating effects of PrEP on anxiety and the motivations to use PrEP that include pursuit of sexual health and pleasure, policy and practice guidelines rarely, if ever, note these motivations or draw upon them to promote uptake. A variety of organisations and agencies generate ongoing guidance related to the use of PrEP and its role within a broader HIV prevention and care landscape. This includes global health bodies, such as WHO and UNAIDS, whose guidelines frequently feature in the policies and practices adopted at a national level, as well as guidance produced at that national level which attends to local epidemics and health service circumstances. A review of relevant materials on PrEP and its recommended use among GBMSM in Australia, the United Kingdom, Kenya and Malaysia illustrates dominant framings or omissions in the promotion of anxiety reduction and sexual pleasure.

The 2016 WHO consolidated guidance on the use of antiretrovirals drugs for treating and preventing HIV infection (WHO 2016) have been referenced within most national PrEP prescribing guidelines issued by Ministries of Health, or similar delegated bodies, around the world. The document makes no reference to sexual pleasure, enjoyment or satisfaction, nor does it acknowledge the role that PrEP could play in reducing HIV-related anxiety. However, in a section termed 'Research gaps' for clinical guidelines, the report goes so far as to acknowledge how PrEP could improve sexual health and well-being:

> The implementation of PrEP in diverse situations will provide opportunities for understanding how PrEP influences sexual practices, which may include improved sexual health and emotional well-being, reduced stigma and discrimination against people living with HIV or increased use of other HIV prevention methods. (WHO 2016, p. 60).

Such an evidence base has indeed now been firmly established (as referenced above), however the omission of a holistic sexual health narrative within the consolidated guidance (published by the same organisation that crafted an expansive definition of sexual health) highlights the siloed nature of discussion between public health policy makers and practitioners who elevate the pursuit of certain outcomes (i.e. disease avoidance) over others (i.e. sexual health more broadly defined).

Building on this in 2019, WHO released guidance on the provision of event driven PrEP for GBMSM, the so called '2 + 1 + 1' approach (WHO 2019). In reviewing the evidence relating to the efficacy and impact of PrEP on GBMSM globally thus far, the document makes no reference to the emergence of evidence that the presence of the medication facilitates and enhances sexual pleasure, satisfaction and enjoyment. A section that details users' preferences for event based versus daily dosing of PrEP (p. 13) makes reference to the choice itself being valued (speaking to fundamental principles of health promotion) but includes no discussion of how either event driven or daily PrEP can facilitate a broader sense of well-being. The potential benefits of event driven PrEP use are articulated only in economic terms and with reference to pill-taking burden with all other concerns seemingly secondary.

At the level of the nation state, guidelines produced by the Australasian Society of HIV, Viral Hepatitis and Sexual Health Medicine (ASHM) aim to support the prescribing of PrEP and to 'assist clinicians in their evaluation and risk assessment of patients seeking PrEP' (ASHM 2019, p. 6). Such a framing immediately places emphasis on notions of infection avoidance, rather than fostering a sense of how the provision of PrEP might facilitate sexual well-being in its broader sense. The guidelines include a detailed account of risk factors for seroconversion, to guide risk assessment, further reinforcing a solidly infection avoidance framing. In suggesting that clinicians collect a sexual and drug use history from presenting patients, no attendance to satisfaction or enjoyment of sex is included, and proposals of PrEP initiation are framed entirely in terms of the risk of HIV acquisition.

Such omissions are replicated in other country contexts. The British HIV Association and British Association of Sexual Health and HIV (BHIVA/BASHH) guidelines on the use of HIV pre-exposure prophylaxis (PrEP) (British HIV Association and British Association for Sexual Health 2018) make no reference to sexual pleasure, satisfaction or enjoyment, nor do they acknowledge any role that PrEP may play in mitigating HIV related anxiety. Recommendations for baseline risk-assessment are entirely framed around the potential for seroconversion and allow no space for the attending clinician to acknowledge how sexual pleasure, or even the mitigation of sexual concerns, factor into PrEP initiation. In Malaysia, there is no national policy or guidance documents specific to PrEP but it features within the Strategic Plan for Ending AIDS 2016–2030 (Ministry of Health 2015). At no point, however, are concepts of sexual pleasure or satisfaction attended to and all framings of sexual health fall solidly within a disease avoidance paradigm. Likewise, the indications for PrEP outlined in the guidelines on use of antiretroviral drugs for treating and preventing HIV Infection in Kenya are all framed in terms of disease avoidance and not in facilitating a sense of sexual well-being (Ministry of Health and National AIDS & STI Control Programme 2016).

This collective lack of attendance to pleasure is troubling and may represent a missed opportunity to embrace the WHO definition of sexual health in its entirety, to frame PrEP use in sex positive ways that increase uptake among those GBMSM who stand to benefit the most. Policy documents guide health related funding, coordination and practice, in both clinical and community contexts and their framing has the potential to dramatically shift the narrative and revamp current prevention efforts. However, despite our criticism, we also remain mindful of the extraordinary effort some states, organisations and individuals have gone to in ensuring *any* mention of PrEP. Others within this edited collection have noted that the politics of PrEP provision are complex and layered with stigma (Guise this volume; Young this volume). Many of the authors (and publishing organisations) of the policy and guidance documents reviewed here have been staunch supporters of PrEP provision, helping to ensure adoption and integration into national health systems. Their efforts are to be applauded. We recognise the complex political and cultural circumstances in which they are written and the fact that they often have to attend to politically palatable language, especially in light of the hostile media reporting about PrEP noted elsewhere (Jaspal and Nerlich 2016).

8.4 Communicating Pleasure

Despite policy environments that often impinge on promoting sexual health holistically, populations who experience a range of benefits from new biomedical technologies may force public health programmes to re-engage with basic principles of health promotion. Health promotion includes the right to sexual pleasure in itself, beyond its role in helping to promote reductions in infectious disease (Underhill 2015; Landers and Kapadia 2020) to empower GBMSM both to make autonomous choices as well as to intervene with public health processes that typically impede that empowerment (Gruskin and Kismödi 2020). Globally, PrEP policy and practice have continued to perpetuate an arguably authoritarian and instruction-giving tone. In the past, instructions on condom use, particularly advice to use them consistently and carefully regardless of the diversity of sexual partnerships, perpetuated biocitizenship narratives of 'good' and 'bad' gays (Rangel and Adam 2014; Girard 2016). The potential now exists for educators to add PrEP to the list of HIV prevention methods that *should* be used (including how PrEP must be used daily rather than event driven), thereby prioritising the elimination of HIV and disregarding the additional benefits of PrEP like sexual satisfaction and pleasure.

Early research on the potential acceptability of PrEP (Nutland 2016), designed to inform strategic planning at a large HIV organisation in England, foreshadowed that sexual health needs beyond HIV prevention should be taken into account in prescribing and educating GBMSM about PrEP. These needs included reductions in anxiety and stress as well as physiological desires, such as forgoing the use of condoms to maintain erections more easily during sex. PrEP Facts, a US-based moderated Facebook group has maintained and promoted an ethos that discussions move beyond purely HIV prevention (Manley 2017). The administrators of this peer-education group dissuade use of instruction giving 'should' statements, instead encouraging participants to acknowledge the diverse, holistic health benefits of PrEP. It is not uncommon for members to celebrate the exchange of semen, particularly among GBMSM who grew up during an era when such behaviour was stigmatised as disregarding HIV prevention. Within these posts, GBMSM report feeling freed from the anxiety of seroconversion and exploring a fuller ranger of human sexuality (e.g. group sex, bottoming after years of only topping, sex with older men) that they could not have imagined had PrEP not been available.

Additional community-based efforts have deliberately challenged public health discourse about PrEP and sexual pleasure. PrEPster, a London-based peer health promotion programme, led by PrEP users and people living with HIV, explicitly prioritises the added sexual health benefits of PrEP. Their 2017 film *PrEP17* seeks to empower PrEP use among HIV affected communities in the UK (Feustel 2017). In the film, participants discuss not only how PrEP has provided greater certainty in their efforts to prevent HIV, but also its additional benefits. 'Bobby' focuses on how PrEP use has reduced stress and anxiety ['There's definitely a lot less stress, post-stress … so much stress, so it definitely minimizes all that stress'], while 'Winnie' articulates how PrEP provides an essential option, which allows them to take control of their HIV prevention. PrEPster has also made an intentional decision to reposition pleasure throughout their HIV health promotion materials. In their series of blogs about PrEP use, My PrEP Story, writers discuss and describe the additional benefits of PrEP. For example, Louis writes: 'I've been taking it for a couple of months, and you know what? Sex for me is great! Have my anxieties significantly reduced? Yes!' Their approach deliberately portrays PrEP users as empowered rather than vulnerable, allowing them to celebrate their sexuality and autonomy rather than be forever constrained by the HIV epidemic (PrEPster 2020).

In comparison to PrEP Facts and PrEPster, *Love Lazers*, a collective of grass roots health educators across Zurich, Germany and Columbia, is less emphatic about sexual pleasure. Instead, they highlight the 'psychological relief' that using PrEP can bring, including reducing stress around sex (Love Lazers 2015). Their informational materials normalise the challenges of discussing safer sex (for reasons that might include the lack of skills in doing so, or the incapacity of doing so due to alcohol or drugs, for example) and the HIV risk behaviours that may ensue. They note how PrEP promotes open discussion by not only protecting GBMSM against HIV acquisition but by also forging pathways to discuss sex, intimacy and risk more forthrightly as compared to more limited discussion about safer sex in the past.

8.5 Pathways for Pleasure

The policy and community responses to the advent of PrEP demonstrate that new biomedical HIV prevention technologies have the potential to exacerbate authoritarian approaches to sexual health, but also to liberate communities from this discourse. Pleasure and sexual satisfaction, including the relief from HIV-related anxiety and stigma that have accompanied adoption of PrEP, are likely central factors that will influence the uptake and sustained use of new HIV prevention technologies in the future. PrEP itself has inspired civil society groups to embrace the entirety of sexual health more forthrightly, and not simply the more limited benefits of disease reduction. That public health policymakers and programmers have been less inclined to consider the inclusion of pleasure-related topics within HIV prevention services is not surprising (e.g. Wohlfeiler et al. 2013), but the movement of advocacy groups, including their actual experiences with PrEP, may encourage public health officials to consider the benefits to health apart from the reduction of infectious disease. The motivations of GBMSM (including their attendance to pleasure) are not insignificant, in part because GBMSM continue to be sub-optimally engaged in PrEP, as established by recent PrEP cascades (akin to the HIV treatment cascade) (Holt et al. 2020). Policies and practices for the implementation of PrEP, including those which have been community-generated rather than policy-mediated, have served a crucial role in improving health promotion, particularly in the extent to which they harness motivations among GBMSM to engage in PrEP not simply as a tool to reduce HIV-related anxiety but to enhance their sexual expression and aspirations for sexual health in a more holistic sense. Among people living with HIV, sustained viral suppression likewise reduces the risk of HIV transmission to sexual partners, effectively to zero—and has been smartly promoted through the community-driven social marketing campaign 'U=U', or 'undetectable equals untransmissible.' In a similar way, the low-hanging fruit for public health policymakers could be the ability to tout these scientific advances, both in PrEP and U=U, as ways to leverage engagement among GBMSM. We hope our reflections on PrEP suggest the wisdom of voicing support for sexual health more broadly, because the message of infection control will inevitably lose its potency as the epidemic threat (hopefully) wanes. However, the motivation to engage in sexual expression in pleasurable, intimate and satisfying ways is much more intrinsic to human sexuality and is more likely to result in sustained conversation between public health and GBMSM populations.

In many countries, and within countries with inequitable access to healthcare, the availability of a new biomedical prevention technology like PrEP should not exacerbate existing inequalities. In these contexts, the social and psychological benefits of PrEP have the potential to land more squarely in the laps of those who already have access to healthcare and health education. Where homosexuality remains illegal—or where the broader social taboo against anal sex and sex between men continues (Kutner et al. 2020)—pleasure is just as meaningful and impactful on the lives of GBMSM, but far less likely to be embraced by policymakers. In a way, PrEP may function as a Trojan horse in these contexts, prioritised for the sake of HIV prevention and control but ultimately benefitting the additional aspects of sexual health we have discussed in this chapter. The trajectory by advocacy groups in countries that have embraced PrEP may point to a promising process. To the extent that the promotion of PrEP purely as HIV prevention lends strength to the voices of those GBMSM who experience enhanced sexual health, more holistically defined, these GBMSM may bear the fruit of not only survival but also promoting a discourse about the benefits of PrEP on reduced anxiety and enhanced sexual expression. The problem, of course, remains that even in countries where PrEP is more readily available, stigma associated with homosexuality continues to impede access as does stigmatising discourse about the right to sexual pleasure itself.

Acknowledgements Dr. Kutner's work was supported by the US National Institutes of Health through the National Institute of Mental Health grants K23MH124569 (PI: Bryan Kutner, PhD, MPH), T32MH19139 (PI: Theodorus Sandfort, PhD), and P30MH43520 (PI: Robert Remien, PhD).

References

An Roinn Sláinte/Department of Health. (2015). *National Sexual Health Strategy 2015–2020 and action plan 2015–2016*. Dublin: Department of Health for Ireland.

Aunon, F. M., Wagner, G. J., Maher, R., Khouri, D., Kaplan, R. L., & Mokhbat, J. (2015). An exploratory study of HIV risk behaviors and testing among male sex Workers in Beirut, Lebanon. *Social Work in Public Health, 30*(4), 373–384. https://doi.org/10.1080/19371918.2014.979274.

Bourne, A., Hammond, G., Hickson, F., Reid, D., Schmidt, A. J., Weatherburn, P., & Network, E. (2013). What constitutes the best sex life for gay and bisexual men? Implications for HIV prevention. *BMC Public Health, 13*(1), 1083. https://doi.org/10.1186/1471-2458-13-1083.

British HIV Association & British Association for Sexual Health. (2018). *BHIVA/BASHH guidelines on the use of HIV pre-exposure prophylaxis (PrEP)*. London: BHIV/BASHH.

Calabrese, S. K., & Underhill, K. (2015). How stigma surrounding the use of HIV Preexposure prophylaxis undermines prevention and pleasure: A call to destigmatize "Truvada whores". *American Journal of Public Health, 105*(10), 1960–1964. https://doi.org/10.2105/ajph.2015.302816.

Crosby, R. A., & Mena, L. (2017). Correlates of enhanced sexual pleasure from condom use: A study of young black men who have sex with men in the United States. *AIDS and Behavior, 21* (5), 1491–1496. https://doi.org/10.1007/s10461-016-1564-x.

Donovan, C., Mearns, C., McEwan, R., & Sugden, N. (1994). A review of the HIV-related sexual behaviour of gay men and men who have sex with men. *AIDS Care, 6*(5), 605–617. https://doi.org/10.1080/09540129408258674.

Eaton, L. A., Kalichman, S. C., Cain, D. N., Cherry, C., Stearns, H. L., Amaral, C. M., et al. (2007). Serosorting sexual partners and risk for HIV among men who have sex with men. *American Journal of Preventive Medicine, 33*(6), 479–485. https://doi.org/10.1016/j.amepre.2007.08.004.

Ekstrand, M. L. (1992). Safer sex maintenance among gay men. *AIDS, 6*(8), 875–878. https://doi.org/10.1097/00002030-199208000-00017.

Feustel, N. (Director) (2017). *PrEP17: The coming of age of PrEP* [film]. Georgetown Media (http://www.georgetownmedia.de/).

French, R. S., Bonell, C., Wellings, K., & Weatherburn, P. (2014). An exploratory review of HIV prevention mass media campaigns targeting men who have sex with men. *BMC Public Health, 14*(1), 616. https://doi.org/10.1186/1471-2458-14-616.

Frost, D. M., Stirratt, M. J., & Ouellette, S. C. (2008). Understanding why gay men seek HIV-seroconcordant partners: Intimacy and risk reduction motivations. *Culture, Health & Sexuality, 10*(5), 513–527.

Gamarel, K., & Golub, S. (2015). Intimacy motivations and pre-exposure prophylaxis (PrEP) adoption intentions among HIV-negative men who have sex with men (MSM) in romantic relationships. *Annals of Behavioral Medicine, 49*(2), 177–186. https://doi.org/10.1007/s12160-014-9646-3.

Giguere, R., Dolezal, C., Bauermeister, J. A., Frasca, T., Valladares, J., Febo, I., & Carballo-Diéguez, A. (2015). Influence of partner type on acceptability and likelihood of use of a rectal microbicide among young men who have sex with men in the United States and Puerto Rico. *Journal of Sex Research, 53*(6), 633–641. https://doi.org/10.1080/00224499.2014.1002127.

Girard, G. (2016). HIV risk and sense of community: French gay male discourses on barebacking. *Culture, Health & Sexuality, 18*(1), 15–29. https://doi.org/10.1080/13691058.2015.1063813.

Gold, R. S., & Rosenthal, D. A. (1998). Examining self-justifications for unsafe sex as a technique of AIDS education: The importance of personal relevance. *International Journal of STD & AIDS, 9*(4), 208–213. https://doi.org/10.1258/0956462981922052.

Golden, M. R., Stekler, J., Hughes, J. P., & Wood, R. W. (2008). HIV serosorting in men who have sex with men: Is it safe? *Journal of Acquired Immune Deficiency Syndrome, 49*(2), 212–218.

Grace, D., Jollimore, J., MacPherson, P., Strang, M. J. P., & Tan, D. H. S. (2018). The pre-exposure prophylaxis-stigma paradox: Learning from Canada's first wave of PrEP users. *AIDS Patient Care and STDs, 32*(1), 24–30. https://doi.org/10.1089/apc.2017.0153.

Gredig, D., Uggowitzer, F., Hassler, B., Weber, P., & Nideröst, S. (2016). Acceptability and willingness to use HIV pre-exposure prophylaxis among HIV-negative men who have sex with men in Switzerland. *AIDS Care, 28*(sup 1), 44–47. https://doi.org/10.1080/09540121.2016.1146212.

Gruskin, S., & Kismödi, E. (2020). A call for (renewed) commitment to sexual health, sexual rights, and sexual pleasure: A matter of health and Well-being. *American Journal of Public Health, 110* (2), 159–160. https://doi.org/10.2105/ajph.2019.305497.

Hartney, T., Westrop, S. J., Anderson, J., Brigstock-Barron, O., Hadley, A., Guthrie, K., & Connor, N. (2015). *Health promotion for sexual and reproductive health and HIV strategic action plan, 2016 to 2019*. London: Public Health England.

Holt, M., Lea, T., Bear, B., Halliday, D., Ellard, J., Murphy, D., et al. (2019). Trends in attitudes to and the use of HIV pre-exposure prophylaxis by Australian gay and bisexual men, 2011–2017: Implications for further implementation from a diffusion of innovations perspective. *AIDS and Behavior, 23*(7), 1939–1950. https://doi.org/10.1007/s10461-018-2368-y.

Holt, M., Lee, E., Lea, T., Bavinton, B., Broady, T., Mao, L., et al. (2020). HIV preexposure prophylaxis cascades to assess implementation in Australia: Results from repeated, national behavioral surveillance of gay and bisexual men, 2014–2018. *Journal of Acquired Immune Deficiency Syndromes, 83*(3), e16–e22. https://doi.org/10.1097/qai.0000000000002243.

Jaspal, R., & Nerlich, B. (2016). Polarised press reporting about HIV prevention: Social representations of pre-exposure prophylaxis in the UK press. *Health, 21*(5), 478–497. https://doi.org/10.1177/1363459316649763.

Keen, P., Hammoud, M. A., Bourne, A., Bavinton, B. R., Holt, M., Vaccher, S., et al. (2020). Use of HIV pre-exposure prophylaxis (PrEP) associated with lower HIV anxiety among gay and bisexual men in Australia who are at high risk of HIV infection: Results from the flux study. *Journal of Acquired Immune Deficiency Syndromes (1999), 83*(2), 119–125. https://doi.org/10.1097/qai.0000000000002232.

Kiguwa, P. (2015). 'I provide the pleasure, I control it': Sexual pleasure and 'bottom' identity constructs amongst gay youth in a stepping stones workshop. *Reproductive Health Matters, 23* (46), 117–126. https://doi.org/10.1016/j.rhm.2015.11.016.

Kippax, S., Noble, J., Prestage, G., Crawford, J. M., Campbell, D., Baxter, D., & Cooper, D. (1997). Sexual negotiation in the AIDS era: Negotiated safety revisited. *AIDS, 11*(2), 191–197.

Kutner, B. A., Simoni, J. M., King, K. M., Goodreau, S. M., Pala, A. N., Creegan, E., et al. (2020). Does stigma toward anal sexuality impede HIV prevention among men who have sex with men in the United States? A structural equation modeling assessment. *The Journal of Sexual Medicine, 17*(3), 477–490. https://doi.org/10.1016/j.jsxm.2019.12.006.

Landers, S., & Kapadia, F. (2020). The public health of pleasure: Going beyond disease prevention. *American Journal of Public Health, 110*(2), 140–141. https://doi.org/10.2105/ajph.2019. 305495.

Lorimer, K., Kidd, L., Lawrence, M., McPherson, K., Cayless, S., & Cornish, F. (2013). Systematic review of reviews of behavioural HIV prevention interventions among men who have sex with men. *AIDS Care, 25*(2), 133–150. https://doi.org/10.1080/09540121.2012.699672.

Love Lazers. (2015). *Who we are*. Retrieved May 13, 2020, from https://www.lovelazers.org/en/.

Mabire, X., Puppo, C., Morel, S., Mora, M., Castro, D., Chas, J., et al. (2019). Pleasure and PrEP: Pleasure-seeking plays a role in prevention choices and could Lead to PrEP initiation. *American Journal of Men's Health, 13*(1), 1–14. https://doi.org/10.1177/1557988319827396.

Manley, D. (2017). *Understanding and negotiating access to preventative sexual health care biotechnology in online communities: a thematic analysis of the Facebook group "PrEP Facts: rethinking HIV prevention and sex"*. Masters Thesis, Smith College, Northampton, MA.

Ministry of Health. (2015). *National Strategic Plan: Ending AIDS 2016–2030*. Putrajaya, Malaysia: Ministry of Health.

Ministry of Health & National AIDS & STI Control Programme. (2016). *Guidelines on use of antiretroviral drugs for treating and preventing HIV infection in Kenya*. Nairobi, Kenya: NASCOP.

Nath, R., Grennan, T., Parry, R., Baharuddin, F., Connell, J. P., Wong, J., & Grace, D. (2019). Knowledge and attitudes of syphilis and syphilis pre-exposure prophylaxis (PrEP) among men who have sex with men in Vancouver, Canada: A qualitative study. *BMJ Open, 9*(11), e031239. https://doi.org/10.1136/bmjopen-2019-031239.

Nutland, W. (2016). *The acceptability of pre exposure HIV prophylaxis among gay men in London*. DrPH thesis. London School of Hygiene & Tropical Medicine, London.

Pantalone, D. W., Holloway, I. W., Goldblatt, A. E. A., Gorman, K. R., Herbitter, C., & Grov, C. (2019). The impact of pre-exposure prophylaxis on sexual communication and sexual behavior of urban gay and bisexual men. *Archives of Sexual Behavior, 22*(151), 1–14. https://doi.org/10.1007/s10508-019-01478-z.

Parsons, J. T., Schrimshaw, E. W., Wolitski, R. J., Halkitis, P. N., Purcell, D. W., Hoff, C. C., & Gomez, C. A. (2005). Sexual harm reduction practices of HIV-seropositive gay and bisexual men: Serosorting, strategic positioning, and withdrawal before ejaculation. *AIDS, 19*(Suppl 1), S13–S25.

Philpot, S., Prestage, G., Holt, M., Haire, B., Maher, L., Hammoud, M., & Bourne, A. (2020). Gay and bisexual Men's perceptions of pre-exposure prophylaxis (PrEP) in a context of high accessibility: An Australian qualitative study. *AIDS and Behavior*, 1–12. https://doi.org/10.1007/s10461-020-02796-3.

PrEPster. (2020). *My PrEP story: Louis (part 1)*. Retrieved May 13, 2020, from https://prepster.info/2020/01/prep-story-louis-part-1/.

Queensland Department of Health. (2016). *Queensland sexual health strategy*. Brisbane: State Government of Queensland.

Rangel, J. C., & Adam, B. D. (2014). Everyday moral reasoning in the governmentality of HIV risk. *Sociology of Health & Illness, 36*(1), 60–74. https://doi.org/10.1111/1467-9566.12047.

Rhodes, T., & Cusick, L. (2000). Love and intimacy in relationship risk management: HIV positive people and their sexual partners. *Sociology of Health & Illness, 22*(1), 1–26.

Siegler, A. J., Rosenthal, E. M., Sullivan, P. S., Ahlschlager, L., Kelley, C. F., Mehta, C. C., et al. (2019). Double-blind, single-center, randomized three-way crossover trial of fitted, thin, and standard condoms for vaginal and anal sex: C-PLEASURE study protocol and baseline data. *JMIR Research Protocols, 8*(4), e12205. https://doi.org/10.2196/12205.

Simaleko, M. M., Longo, J. D. D., Police, S. M. C., & Piette, D. (2018). Attitude of men who have sex with men toward condom use in Bangui, Central African Republic (CAR). *Medecine et Sante Tropicales, 28*(4), 424–429. https://doi.org/10.1684/mst.2018.0857.

Smith, D. K., Herbst, J. H., Zhang, X., & Rose, C. E. (2015). Condom effectiveness for HIV prevention by consistency of use among men who have sex with men in the United States.

Journal of Acquired Immune Deficiency Syndromes (1999), 68(3), 337–344. https://doi.org/10.1097/qai.0000000000000461.

The Australasian Society of HIV, Viral Hepatitis and Sexual Health Medicine (ASHM). (2019). *PrEP Guidelines Update.* Sydney: ASHM.

Underhill, K. (2015). Intimacy, condom use, and pre-exposure prophylaxis (PReP) acceptability among men who have sex with men (MSM) in primary partnerships: A comment on Gamarel and Golub. *Annals of Behavioral Medicine: A Publication of the Society of Behavioral Medicine, 49*(2), 151–153. https://doi.org/10.1007/s12160-014-9651-6.

Van de Ven, P., Kippax, S., Crawford, J., Rawstorne, P., Prestage, G., Grulich, A., & Murphy, D. (2002). In a minority of gay men, sexual risk practice indicates strategic positioning for perceived risk reduction rather than unbridled sex. *AIDS Care, 14*(4), 471–480. https://doi.org/10.1080/09540120220133008.

Whitfield, T. H. F., Jones, S. S., Wachman, M., Grov, C., Parsons, J. T., & Rendina, H. J. (2019). The impact of pre-exposure prophylaxis (PrEP) use on sexual anxiety, satisfaction, and esteem among gay and bisexual men. *Journal of Sex Research, 56*(9), 1128–1135. https://doi.org/10.1080/00224499.2019.1572064.

WHO. (2006). *Defining sexual health: Report of a technical consultation on sexual health 28–31 January 2002.* Geneva: WHO.

WHO. (2016). *Consolidated guidelines on the use of antiretrovial drugs for treating and preventing HIV infection: Recommendations for a public health approach* (2nd ed.). Geneva: WHO.

WHO. (2019). *What's the 2+1+1? Event-driven oral pre-exposure prophylaxis to prevent HIV for men WHO have sex with men: Update to WHO's recommendation on oral PrEP.* Geneva: WHO.

Wohlfeiler, D., Hecht, J., Volk, J., Raymond, H. F., Kennedy, T., & McFarland, W. (2013). How can we improve online HIV and STD prevention for men who have sex with men? Perspectives of hook-up website owners, website users, and HIV/STD directors. *AIDS and Behavior, 17*(9), 3024–3033. https://doi.org/10.1007/s10461-012-0375-y.

Chapter 9
New Hierarchies of Desirability and Old Forms of Deviance Related to PrEP: Insights from the Canadian Experience

Adrian Guta, Peter A. Newman, and Ashley Lacombe-Duncan

9.1 Introduction

> Assemblages are passional, they are compositions of desire. Desire has nothing to do with a natural or spontaneous determination; there is no desire but assembling, assembled, desire. The rationality, the efficiency, of an assemblage does not exist without the passions the assemblage brings into play, without the desires that constitute it as much as it constitutes them (Deleuze and Guattari 1987, p. 399).

The current moment of the global HIV pandemic is characterised by continued transmission and stigma, but also a turn to bio-pharmacological and technological solutions that may realise the promise of an 'AIDS-free generation.' Despite decades of calls for investments in inexpensive upstream behavioural prevention options like education and free condoms, to expensive but needed structural interventions to reduce inequity and health disparities, the most sustained investments have been in bio-pharmacological and technological approaches to managing the epidemic. Among these are pharmaceutical treatments which can both treat *and* prevent HIV (including long-acting injectables), that promise to be easy to manage and absent the side-effects and challenges of earlier treatments and technologies. Technology-based approaches to managing the epidemic include smartphone applications that help promote adherence, diagnostic technologies for viral load monitoring, the use of geographic information technology combined with molecular sequencing to identify viral hotspots and risk clusters, and social media platforms that provide mediums to

A. Guta (✉)
School of Social Work, University of Windsor, Windsor, Canada
e-mail: aguta@uwindsor.ca

P. A. Newman
Factor-Inwentash Faculty of Social Work, University of Toronto, Toronto, Canada

A. Lacombe-Duncan
School of Social Work, University of Michigan, Ann Arbor, MI, USA

© Springer Nature Switzerland AG 2021   117
S. Bernays et al. (eds.), *Remaking HIV Prevention in the 21st Century*, Social
Aspects of HIV 5, https://doi.org/10.1007/978-3-030-69819-5_9

connect, disseminate, and educate (Guta et al. 2016a, b; McClelland et al. 2019). In recent years these technologies have been advanced alongside a resurgence of militaristic language in relation to HIV (Guta and Newman 2016). These new ways of engaging with HIV are said to be creating new social relations and ways of organising among those affected (Girard et al. 2019).

In what has been described in the United States as a 'High-Impact HIV Prevention' approach, HIV treatment and prevention have been combined in a single programmatic response 'using combinations of scientifically proven, cost-effective, and scalable interventions targeted to the right populations in the right geographic areas' (Centers for Disease Control and Prevention 2011). In this chapter, we focus on the targeted scale-up of HIV pre-exposure prophylaxis (PrEP), in which individuals deemed at high risk of acquiring HIV take the HIV medication Truvada (tenofovir and emtricitabine) daily, or intermittently, as directed by a physician, for prevention purposes. PrEP is marketed, as we will discuss in this chapter, as both desirable as a risk reduction strategy from an individual and public health standpoint, and, from an individual and community standpoint, for increasing sexual desire. The drug has been marketed to all those at risk, but with a predominant emphasis on gay, bisexual, and other men who have sex with men (GBMSM). Indeed, the World Health Organization (WHO) (2014, p. xix) was early to recommend PrEP for men who have sex with men 'as an additional HIV prevention choice within a comprehensive HIV prevention package.' As we have discussed elsewhere (Guta et al. 2016a), GBMSM are often defined by their sexuality and relationship to HIV, and as unable/unwilling to sublimate their desires – which ignores the complex social and structural determinants of HIV risk. Contrary to decades of messaging about the rational health-seeking neoliberal subject, health and risk are complex and multifaceted assemblages which require thoughtful and nuanced discussion (Fox 2011; Duff 2014).

In this chapter, we explore new (and old) forms of desire in the context of PrEP availability and their implications for the health and wellness of GBMSM. Through a 'new materialist' informed reading of data we have generated (interviews) and collected (health promotion campaigns), we explore the ways PrEP mediated risk-taking, health-seeking, and hierarchies of desirability are being produced, reproduced, and deployed, and to what ends. We reflect on the productive function of desire and the PrEP assemblage that includes people, affects, relations, pills, technologies, politics, spaces, and temporalities, and respond to calls to think beyond the biomedical framing of PrEP (Rosengarten and Michael 2010).

9.2   GBMSM, HIV, PrEP and the Canadian Context

The development, evaluation, efficacy, and implementation of PrEP globally have been well documented elsewhere (Cairns et al. 2016; Pinto et al. 2018). We offer a brief overview of realities for GBMSM, HIV and PrEP in Canada, where much of our scholarship is based. Canada is considered a global leader in LGBTQ rights with legal protections (workplace, housing, human rights), and was the fourth country globally to grant same-sex marriage rights (Tremblay 2019). The metropolitan centres of Vancouver, Toronto, and Montreal attract LGBTQ migrants from smaller communities within Canada and from around the world seeking safety and the ability to live and love freely (Kahn et al. 2017). Despite many positive gains and legal protections, Canadian GBMSM continue to experience complex social stressors related to homophobia, resultant mental health disparities, and structural barriers amid adverse social determinants of health that increase their HIV risk (Adam et al. 2017; Ferlatte et al. 2018).

There are an estimated 63,110 (plausible range 55,500–70,720) persons living with HIV in Canada, with GBMSM, African, Caribbean, and Black communities, and Indigenous peoples overrepresented (Public Health Agency of Canada 2016). The epidemic is localised among GBMSM, with estimates of over 50% of infections attributable to this category inclusive of GBMSM who inject drugs (Public Health Agency of Canada 2016). Increases in Canadian HIV cases in the past few years (Haddad et al. 2019) may be surprising considering Canada is the birthplace of 'seek-test-and-treat' initiatives (Vonn 2012) and 'treatment-as-prevention' (Nguyen et al. 2011), which served as the basis of the United Nations 90-90-90 strategy (Sidibé et al. 2016). However, despite being a leader in bio-behavioural initiatives, Canada also continues to aggressively criminalise HIV, which has negative implications for prevention and treatment efforts (Mykhalovskiy et al. 2020). PrEP scale-up also has been slower in Canada than in other jurisdictions (formally or through community-driven 'DIY' approaches, such as in England [Paparini et al. 2018]). Whereas the US Food and Drug Administration (FDA) approved the use of Truvada for HIV PrEP in 2012, Health Canada took until 2016 to issue PrEP approval (Canadian AIDS Treatment Information Exchange 2019), with substantial negative ramifications for persons at risk and for public health. In those intermittent years, only those who could afford it (and oftentimes those aware of US FDA approval) were being prescribed the drug 'off-label'.

In Canada, as elsewhere, PrEP was initially contentious. Concerns traversed PrEP stigma and shaming at the community level, in the queer and popular media, and from health care providers; apprehension about the levels of clinical engagement required (e.g., regular HIV and STI monitoring, and testing for kidney and liver function); and anxieties about 'risk compensation' in which GBMSM were expected to reduce or discontinue condom usage in the context of PrEP (Knight et al. 2016). Other concerns focused on the cost of the drug, the superordinate role of pharmaceutical companies, and ongoing gaps in treatment access for people living with HIV in Canada and beyond (Millett et al. 2012). PrEP coverage is now more accessible in Canada because of reduced costs from the manufacturer and increased national coverage through provincial drug plans and private insurance companies.

The initial debates about PrEP, especially at the community-level, often became narrowly focused and bifurcated – for or against PrEP? Is PrEP good or bad? Anti-stigma campaigns with #TruvadaWhore presented images of young GBMSM with pills on their tongues or holding their prescription bottles, in an attempt to reduce stigma. For some, this crystallised the idea that PrEP is about taking a pill to have sex; for others, it was a symbol of a new era of health and sexual liberation. Our aim is to think beyond these binaries and reductions and ask different kinds of questions about the social implications of PrEP. Moving beyond the driving focus on stigma as an organising (and sometimes sole) conceptual framework in the study of PrEP, we are interested in approaches that transcend biomedical and social science orthodoxies and rigid categorisations, and that invite new ways of thinking about health, research, and representation.

9.3   New Materialism, PrEP, and Assembling Desire

As a team, we share disciplinary training in social work and social psychology and conduct public health research using a range of methods and theoretical approaches (Newman et al. 2018; Lacombe-Duncan et al. 2021). We have written (together and separately) about the social and structural determinants of health, the lived realities of people living with and at risk of HIV (Lacombe-Duncan et al. 2020; Newman and Guta 2020), and about the governing effects of HIV prevention and treatment technologies (Guta et al. 2016b; Guta and Newman 2016; Guta and Murray 2019). In this chapter, we draw on new materialism's relational and 'flat' ontology which attempts to reconcile discourse and material realities, and when applied to the study of health considers the 'materiality of bodies as they engage with other material (natural and cultural) relations' (Fox 2015, p. 70). Our approach is informed by the contributions of both Michel Foucault and the team of Gilles Deleuze and Felix Guattari to make sense of the ever-growing complexity of health issues (Duff 2014). Drawing on Foucault, we remain attuned to modes of governance and the 'interrelatedness and entanglements of men [sic] and things, the natural and the artificial, the physical and the moral' (Lemke 2015, p. 5). This includes the continued impact of neoliberalism (Brown 2019) and the divestment, individualisation, and privatisation of health (Ayo 2012). Much has been written about the implications of neoliberal governance on sexual subjectivities and HIV interventions (Adam 2005). The health-seeking neoliberal actor is one who lives an evidence-based life, seeks health, and mitigates risk; but biomedical evidence and lived realities often conflict (Adam 2011; Guta et al. 2016b). Drawing on Deleuze and Guattari (1987), we move beyond fixed binaries to flows and possibilities and the productive function of desire, affects, and assemblages. When considering the sexuality-assemblage, a materialist approach moves beyond individual bodies to consider the broader fields in which sexuality and desire are produced and reproduced, and forms of resistance and *becoming* (Alldred and Fox 2015).

9.4   Methods (Talk, Text, and Visual Productions)

With these theoretical threads in mind, we turn to an analysis of key health promotion campaigns that promote a vision of PrEP, and empirical data about the lived realities of PrEP. We will discuss a few notable PrEP-related health promotion campaigns that have circulated in the USA and Canada in the past few years, which invoke messages about the relationship between PrEP, desire, and sexuality. Our selection of campaigns is strategic and partial, and we do not claim to provide a systematic review. Nor do we attempt to understand their motivations, though most are described as focused on reducing PrEP stigma and increasing access to PrEP. Additionally, we revisit data collected as part of our PrEP Choice study conducted in Toronto, Canada: we interviewed 29 GBMSM – 15 PrEP users and 14 non-users (at the time) (for details, see Lacombe-Duncan et al. 2021; Newman et al. 2018). These interviews were conducted during the period from immediately before to just after PrEP approval in Canada, when community debates were at their height (including on-line fora with active discussions of research, along with profiling of academics who raised concerns about PrEP implementation), and when PrEP health promotion campaigns were being introduced. Our interviews captured decision-making related to PrEP (choosing to initiate, resist, terminate), but also broader insights into the zeitgeist of the PrEP moment. The interviews, then and now, appear to be in dialogue with health promotion campaigns that appealed to the potentiality of PrEP, and especially desire (for intimacy, passion, and to end a perpetual state of sexual risk-related anxiety experienced by many GBMSM in relation to AIDS). We draw on our data in dialogue with notable PrEP campaigns to show the constellation of elements within the PrEP assemblage and to complicate the dominant narrative about PrEP as just a pill that reduces HIV infection risk. Finally, we recognise our role within the research-assemblage and how we have/are/will shape knowledge production in relation to PrEP (Fox and Alldred 2015).

9.5   Findings

Our research was conducted in an era marked by concerns from public health practitioners and researchers about PrEP leading to 'risk compensation,' and concerns primarily attributed to the so-called 'old guard' of the HIV movement, committed to established prevention technologies like condoms. The latter framed Truvada as a 'party drug' which will lead a to promiscuity (#TruvadaWhores); this is in stark contrast to radical invitations on guerrilla poster campaigns from a new generation of activists –to 'fuck raw' and be liberated on PrEP (Spieldenner 2016). Within this contentious milieu, we asked a seemingly simple series of questions to individual GBMSM about their motivations to take or not take PrEP.

We heard complex narratives from the GBMSM we spoke with that reflected neoliberal risk discourses where being in control was a central factor – for both PrEP users and non-users – but mediated by trust. For example, one of the most ardent non-PrEP users shared:

> I am the only person wholly responsible for my health and wellbeing, and I have always felt that way...ultimately it comes down to me and I can't imagine relinquishing an ounce of control or trust in someone who says they are taking a pill. Now, the hypocrisy of that statement is, you are trusting that your partner is not out having risky sex and bringing something home; but that's a risk I'm willing to take. (Non-user, P13)

In turn, one of the most fervent PrEP users said their decision to *start* PrEP was based on the inability to trust others:

> They've said they're negative, but are they negative? I started to read statistics like, 64-percent of new infections come from people that say that they're negative. My take on it all, basically, turned to well, PrEP is recommended by the CDC as at least 86-percent effective or more. Trusting somebody is proven to be zero-percent effective at preventing HIV. (PrEP user, P10)

All participants described themselves as responsible for their own actions, with many simultaneously rejecting, embracing, and resisting that responsibility. This ranged from participants who could be described as engaging in 'higher-risk' sex (e.g., condomless sex with multiple partners) and rejecting the idea of PrEP as an imposition, to those who saw themselves as 'empowered' to make the 'right' decision about their health and start taking PrEP. Empowerment is featured in many PrEP campaigns which draw on personal narratives of people who use PrEP and claim it has enabled them to 'take control' of their health (see for example PleasePrEPME.org). However, empowerment has been critiqued as a neoliberal strategy to 'responsibalize' individuals to make the 'right' decisions (framing those who 'fail' to make informed decisions as wilfully disempowered).

This neoliberal orientation to health-seeking and the *will to know* led many participants to immerse themselves in information about PrEP efficacy and demonstration trials happening around the world at the time, despite lacking formal scientific training (e.g., knowledge of clinical trial design). The same participant who was uncomfortable trusting sexual partners consumed the scientific evidence as well as reaching out to others who were already using PrEP:

> So, I started researching it and I am like a dog with a bone. I read every single study. I read every single clinical practice guideline that had been published. I went through tables of data and pulled out all the information and everything. I just kind of switched my tune. I started speaking to people that were on PrEP, as well, too. I think that was actually, potentially, the most important part of my journey. I just started to inform myself and ask some questions about whether it was actually a real thing or not. (PrEP user, P10)

For others, the science of PrEP was confusing. A participant shared that he followed the studies until he was comfortable with the results: 'I think the main concern was the effectiveness of it, like when I first researched it was like 42-percent effectiveness.' This caused him to read further about the flaws in that particular trial. 'So, doing a whole bunch of research, what is the actual effectiveness rate of it? I'm seeing 92-percent. I'm seeing 99-percent. I'm seeing 100-percent' (PrEP user, P22). Several PrEP users proudly described taking this evidence (printed research studies and reports) to their physicians and convincing them to prescribe PrEP off-label. For many of the non-users we heard from, no amount of risk or less-than-perfect efficacy was acceptable, even as some were regularly engaging in condomless sex. Among the PrEP users following clinical trials and guidance, some admitted to missing doses. The neoliberal health-seeking subject is alive and well, but how individuals interpret and translate the meaning of risk remains complicated.

9.6 Assemblages of Pills, Relations, Technology, Spaces, Affects, and Temporality

In this section, we discuss emergent and overlapping themes related to pills, technology, affects, relations, spaces, and temporality. As we moved to discussions about how PrEP fits into individuals' lives, the binary between user and non-user, and user as fixed status (e.g., continuous PrEP throughout one's sexually active years) became increasingly complicated. We heard from PrEP users who were not sure about why they were taking it and non-users who were considering it but were not ready or could not access it at the time. Some interviews started with an adamant rejection of PrEP ('it's not for me') and ended with participants openly questioning how they might feel in the future once PrEP becomes established ('maybe someday'). Early PrEP adopters reflected on whether they would continue using PrEP if they began a long-term relationship: 'I guess the question that I would be asking myself is, what would happen if I really get into a relationship; would that make me change my mind?' (PrEP user, P18). Several PrEP users took breaks during periods of low sexual activity, life changes, and illness. Some intended to start up again, and others were unsure. One participant who felt pressured into accepting a prescription following a doctor's visit explained: 'I kind of convinced myself and took it, but then I regretted it. I thought that I would start using it tomorrow, maybe next week, maybe the week after. And I think it's been like two weeks now and I haven't used it' (PrEP user, P29).

In these discussions, PrEP *as pill* emerged as an important theme, with many non-users averse to the idea of having to take a pill daily and what it might do to their body (within their internal system): 'I'm always worried about medication, what it does to you all the time, because I don't know what's in Truvada, I don't know what it does and what it affects, what cells or whatever. Like I said, I don't like taking prescriptions' (Non-user, P8). For others, the pill had the same connotations, but these concerns were outweighed by the preventative benefit they offered; and for others, the pill was easily integrated into an established health regimen of vitamins, protein powders, and medications. All but one of our participants lived and worked within Toronto's LGBTQ community and reported access to relatively affirming healthcare and queer-positive providers, many of whom knew about PrEP and were on it themselves. More than one participant described hearing about PrEP through physicians, not as healthcare providers, but as sexual partners. The decision to start

PrEP was often influenced by discussions with friends, social media, health promotion campaigns, scientific dissemination, and negotiating with sexual partners (e.g., 'will PrEP be part of our open relationship') and healthcare providers who were prescribing and overseeing ongoing clinical monitoring. There were discussions that took place in bathhouses: 'I met someone at [bathhouse] who said he was on PrEP before he told me his name, but after he began to try to fuck me bareback without a condom; and let's just say, I wasn't convinced in that circumstance' (Non-user, P17), bedrooms, dinner parties, nightclubs, doctor's offices, and virtually on sexual networking applications like Grindr as well as social media: 'I talk to everybody about this. I've shared some articles on my Facebook wall' (PrEP user, P24). For some, taking the pill was an act of liberation followed by the then ubiquitous PrEP selfie, with the pill resting on their tongue, to share on PrEP user forums. Further to being a source of information, and offering a space to 'come out' and build community, technologically-mediated fora created opportunities to sort between users and non-users: 'I have friends who want to take it because they have been rejected by guys on Grindr or Scruff because they won't have unprotected sex with them. They have said they want to go on it because they don't want to be rejected' (Non-user, P13).

9.7 Desire, Pleasure, Intimacy, and Transgression

In the 'sex that you want' campaign produced by the Toronto-based Gay Men's Sexual Health Alliance (www.thesexyouwant.ca), readers are told that sex is complicated because GBMSM encounter 'homophobia, transphobia, HIV stigma, and nasty attitudes about sex, gender, identity, and relationships'; and that 'shame and misunderstanding about sex and pleasure can make it hard to be honest with ourselves and others about the sex we're having and the sex we really want. And if we can't talk honestly about our desires, how can we make sure we're looking out for ourselves and for each other?' The site, which also includes PrEP resources, invites one to 'Ask yourself, what is the sex you want?'

The '#ItFeelsGood' campaign from AIDS Project Los Angeles combines subtle but sexually charged language with health affirming messages like '#ItFeelsGood...protecting myself against HIV with PrEP' (Dehlin et al. 2019). While acknowledging the range of possible answers, including those which emerged in our interviews with some men preferring condoms under certain circumstances, condomless sex is often constructed as the most desirable form of sexual expression for GBMSM (see Varghese 2019). Participants we spoke to echoed this language: '[PrEP] represents an opportunity for you to actually enjoy your sex life, have the sex that you want to have without the fear that it could kill you' (PrEP user, P10). PrEP offered the promise of pleasure and intimacy: 'Intimacy was another thing that I felt. I could feel closer to my partners and my partner, in general, without putting them at risk or putting myself at risk. It was a great feeling. It is a great feeling' (PrEP user, P24).

Subjected to the dominant neoliberal affective milieu in which fear, shame, and anxiety become embodied and repressive, many participants used PrEP to liberate themselves:

> I'm having the best sex I've ever had in my life. I'm taking lots of loads in my ass, I'm giving them. It's so much more intimate, and the only thing that's not there is the anxiety. I used to have guys over, there'd usually be a condom, but sometimes there wouldn't be; maybe they'd cream me, it'd be over, I'd be sitting on the couch, writing it down. This is the date. I'm going to have to keep this date in mind, because I might have seroconverted. That piece is gone. The anxiety has decreased so fucking much. It might as well be an anti-anxiety drug for me. (PrEP User, P11)

Another participant reflected on observing an erotic scene in a Berlin nightclub where people were having sex and using drugs (a common convergence of risk and pleasure [Bourne et al. 2015]), as an interested but risk-averse outsider and how PrEP could help him transgress:

> One of the very first things that came to my mind when I started PrEP, I said, I'm going to have this shield; metaphorically; I would see myself going back to Berlin, and fully enjoying what I saw. Because I said, okay, maybe now I can do everything that I saw there, and I can go crazy, and I can finally be part of that. That was the very first thought I had when I started using PrEP. In other words, having the freedom to experience something that has been prohibited while keeping myself negative. (PrEP user, P18)

We contrast these new forms of desire, freedom, and pleasure with the potential for new forms of exclusion and internal conflict. The following PrEP user expects a very high standard to have to use a condom: 'I just don't like having sex with condoms. So now I do look for people who don't want to have sex with condoms. I think that's one way to say it on my profile ["on PrEP"]. I'm like, are you okay with bareback? If they say, "yeah, you're on PrEP, cool", perfect! If no, it depends how hot they were. In general, yeah, I definitely have a 90-percent preference for no condoms' (Non-user, P25). We further contrast the talk of freedom with a PrEP user who felt he had lost control because of PrEP, and recounted having sex during a break from PrEP and feeling 'like not being on PrEP made it easier in the sense that there was no debate at all internal, I guess, about whether having unprotected sex was an option. I didn't think about it; there wasn't any pressure to have it unprotected. It was basically just, I'm putting a condom on and I'm going to fuck you now. It was easy and natural, and I had fun and I felt good about it – whereas with PrEP in the mix, there's kind of that debate, you know what I mean?' (PrEP user, P14). Finally, and most pointedly, a non-user questioned the logic and limits of pharmaceutically enabled intimacy: 'I think it puts us in a really gross position where it's like all gay people need to be medicated just to have the sex that we supposedly want. That feels gross to me. I just don't like it' (Non-user, P25).

One participant rejected the notion of freedom based on the anxieties and constraints that PrEP dispels, and discussed what they viewed as the additional burden of PrEP, the narrowing of pleasure, and the relationship to HIV:

> When I hear from people, "now that I'm on PrEP I can finally be free," was it the condom that was your oppressor? Was it the looming spectre of HIV constantly present, and this fear

that you had of "my god, this is the night where I contracted HIV?" *Or are you freeing yourself from something that. . .hasn't been articulated* (emphasis added), that will take a lot of grounded theory work to uncover? I read about the condom, being free from condoms, and having to always have this device around in order to have sex. You could not have sex unless you had that? People forget that there are all kinds of ways of getting sexual pleasure; but it's about penetrative sex all the time. PrEP does not free you from HIV. In fact, it ties you to HIV for perpetuity because you're trying to prevent it constantly. So, what are you actually free from? Now you've actually added something else to your routine. You've actually added a ball-and-chain. (Non-user, P02)

9.7.1 The Abject and Marginal

Throughout our interviews, there were subtle and overt allusions to undesirable and dangerous 'others' for whom PrEP (and sometimes condoms in addition) was necessary. Despite claims that PrEP is an equaliser that will bring HIV+/HIV-GBMSM together, PrEP users expressed strong preferences for sex with HIV-negative men, and some preferred sex with other men on PrEP, but would consider HIV-positive men if they had an undetectable viral load. That being on PrEP and the other partner being undetectable was a necessary condition for sex does not align with the science of U=U — as if the medicated/treated HIV subject is indelibly the infected or untrusted other. There were explicit concerns raised throughout the interviews about men who might have a high viral load and allusions to questionable *others*. Several participants referred to using condoms in certain contexts and with certain persons, but these were brief, fleeting, and were not picked up during our interviews at the expense of focusing on talk of sexual liberation. These were missed opportunities in the research process.

Looking back on our project, we have reflected on what was not captured in interviews conducted with primarily middle-class white men: who is desirable, who is more likely to have a high viral load, and who might be left behind in the PrEP revolution. As one participant explained: 'Yeah, I'm sure there's a huge class divide. I'm sure there's a huge race divide. I'm sure there's a lot of fucked up shit that comes out of this, and [it's] sickening. And, we already have shitty racism in the queer community as it is, and now we're going to have people even more not wanting to fuck people of colour because they're not on PrEP because they can't afford it.' (Non-user, P25). We consider the #PrEP4Love campaign that was disseminated across Chicago and generated 40,913,560 unique views across various social media platforms (Dehlin et al. 2019). We recognise the need to address racial PrEP disparities by increasing access but are concerned about how desire is mobilised in these campaigns that feature people of colour and tell them to 'catch desire' and 'transmit love' instead of HIV. We are troubled that to have the sex that you want for some people requires making themselves more desirable and less threatening through PrEP; that this does little to address racism while racialised health and HIV disparities continue to rage (especially in the USA, but also in Canada) is deeply concerning.

9.8   Conclusion

Our analysis of interview data and PrEP health promotion campaigns has attempted to complicate the PrEP binary that we encountered, and in part reproduced, through the PrEP Choice Project. We have attempted to redress this through writings that challenge both the PrEP binary and linearity imagined for PrEP users (learn about it, get on it, use it indefinitely) and reflect the complexity of decision-making along the prevention cascade (Lacombe-Duncan et al. 2021; Newman et al. 2018). In this chapter we engaged directly with questions of desire and pleasure and how they are part of a PrEP assemblage that includes pills, bodies, people, relationships, time, and space, and surfaced thoughtful perspectives from participants along the way. We continue to reflect on the kinds of freedom (and subjugation) PrEP has enabled and what remains lacking, which we, our participants, research, and health promotion campaigns struggle to articulate.

References

Adam, B. D. (2005). Constructing the neoliberal sexual actor: Responsibility and care of the self in the discourse of barebackers. *Culture, Health & Sexuality, 7*(4), 333–346. https://doi.org/10.1080/13691050500100773.

Adam, B. D. (2011). Epistemic fault lines in biomedical and social approaches to HIV prevention. *Journal of the International AIDS Society, 14*(2), S2. https://doi.org/10.1186/1758-2652-14-S2-S2.

Adam, B. D., Hart, T. A., Mohr, J., Coleman, T., & Vernon, J. (2017). HIV-related syndemic pathways and risk subjectivities among gay and bisexual men: A qualitative investigation. *Culture, Health & Sexuality, 19*(11), 1254–1267. https://doi.org/10.1080/13691058.2017.1309461.

Alldred, P., & Fox, N. J. (2015). The sexuality-assemblages of young men: A new materialist analysis. *Sexualities, 18*(8), 905–920. https://doi.org/10.1177/1363460715579132.

Ayo, N. (2012). Understanding health promotion in a neoliberal climate and the making of health conscious citizens. *Critical Public Health, 22*(1), 99–105. https://doi.org/10.1080/09581596.2010.520692.

Bourne, A., Reid, D., Hickson, F., Torres-Rueda, S., & Weatherburn, P. (2015). Illicit drug use in sexual settings ('chemsex') and HIV/STI transmission risk behaviour among gay men in South London: Findings from a qualitative study. *Sexually Transmitted Infections, 91*(8), 564–568. https://doi.org/10.1136/sextrans-2015-052052.

Brown, W. (2019). *In the ruins of neoliberalism: The rise of antidemocratic politics in the west.* New York: Columbia University Press.

Cairns, G. P., Race, K., & Goicochea, P. (2016). PrEP: Controversy, agency and ownership. *Journal of the International AIDS Society, 19*(7S6), 21120. https://doi.org/10.7448/ias.19.7.21120.

Canadian AIDS Treatment Information Exchange. (2019). *A history of HIV/AIDS.* Retrieved July 25, 2020, from https://www.catie.ca/en/world-aids-day/history.

Centers for Disease Control and Prevention. (2011). *High-impact HIV prevention: CDC's approach to reducing HIV infections in the United States.* Retrieved July 25, 2020, from http://www.cdc.gov/hiv/pdf/policies_NHPC_booklet.pdf.

Dehlin, J. M., Stillwagon, R., Pickett, J., Keene, L., & Schneider, J. A. (2019). #PrEP4Love: An evaluation of a sex-positive HIV prevention campaign. *JMIR Public Health and Surveillance, 5*(2), e12822–e12822. https://doi.org/10.2196/12822.

Deleuze, G., & Guattari, F. (1987). *A thousand plateaus: Capitalism and schizophrenia*. Minneapolis: University of Minnesota Press.

Duff, C. (2014). *Assemblages of health: Deleuze's empiricism and the ethology of life*. Dordrecht: Springer.

Ferlatte, O., Salway, T., Trussler, T., Oliffe, J. L., & Gilbert, M. (2018). Combining intersectionality and syndemic theory to advance understandings of health inequities among Canadian gay, bisexual and other men who have sex with men. *Critical Public Health, 28*(5), 509–521. https://doi.org/10.1080/09581596.2017.1380298.

Fox, N. J. (2011). The ill-health assemblage: Beyond the body-with-organs. *Health Sociology Review, 20*(4), 359–371. https://doi.org/10.5172/hesr.2011.20.4.359.

Fox, N. J. (2015). Health sociology from post-structuralism to the new materialisms. *Health, 20*(1), 62–74. https://doi.org/10.1177/1363459315615393.

Fox, N. J., & Alldred, P. (2015). Inside the research-assemblage: New materialism and the micropolitics of social inquiry. *Sociological Research Online, 20*(2), 122–140. https://doi.org/10.5153/sro.3578.

Girard, G., Patten, S., LeBlanc, M.-A., Adam, B. D., & Jackson, E. (2019). Is HIV prevention creating new biosocialities among gay men? Treatment as prevention and pre-exposure prophylaxis in Canada. *Sociology of Health & Illness, 41*(3), 484–501. https://doi.org/10.1111/1467-9566.12826.

Guta, A., & Murray, S. J. (2019). On the possibility of being governed otherwise: Exploring Foucault's legacy for critical social science studies in the field of HIV/AIDS. In E. Mykhalovskiy & V. Namaste (Eds.), *Thinking differently about HIV/AIDS: Contributions from critical social science* (pp. 39–71). Vancouver: UBC Press.

Guta, A., & Newman, P. A. (2016). Of HIV, kings, and cures: Troubling the apocryphal apothecary. *The American Journal of Bioethics, 16*(10), 25–27. https://doi.org/10.1080/15265161.2016.1214313.

Guta, A., Gagnon, M., Mannell, J., & French, M. (2016a). Gendering the HIV "treatment as prevention" paradigm: Surveillance, viral loads, and risky bodies. In E. van der Meulen & R. Heynen (Eds.), *Expanding the gaze: Gender and the politics of surveillance* (pp. 156–184). Toronto: University of Toronto Press.

Guta, A., Murray, S. J., & Gagnon, M. (2016b). HIV, viral suppression and new Technologies of Surveillance and Control. *Body & Society, 22*(2), 82–107. https://doi.org/10.1177/1357034x15624510.

Haddad, N., Robert, A., Weeks, A., Popovic, N., Siu, W., & Archibald, C. (2019). HIV in Canada-surveillance report, 2018. *Canada communicable disease report = Releve des maladies transmissibles au Canada, 45*(12), 304–312. https://doi.org/10.14745/ccdr.v45i12a01.

Kahn, S., Alessi, E., Woolner, L., Kim, H., & Olivieri, C. (2017). Promoting the wellbeing of lesbian, gay, bisexual and transgender forced migrants in Canada: Providers' perspectives. *Culture, Health & Sexuality, 19*(10), 1165–1179.

Knight, R., Small, W., Carson, A., & Shoveller, J. (2016). Complex and conflicting social norms: Implications for implementation of future HIV pre-exposure prophylaxis (PrEP) interventions in Vancouver, Canada. *PLOS One, 11*(1).

Lacombe-Duncan, A., Logie, C. H., Newman, P. A., Bauer, G. R., & Kazemi, M. (2020). A qualitative study of resilience among transgender women living with HIV in response to stigma in healthcare. *AIDS Care, 1*–6. https://doi.org/10.1080/09540121.2020.1728212.

Lacombe-Duncan, A., Guta, A., & Newman, P. (2021). Pre-exposure prophylaxis (PrEP) implementation for gay, bisexual and other men who have sex with men: Implications for social work practice. Health & Social Work, hlaa038, https://doi.org/10.1093/hsw/hlaa038

Lemke, T. (2015). New materialisms: Foucault and the 'government of things'. *Theory, Culture & Society, 32*(4), 3–25. https://doi.org/10.1177/0263276413519340.

McClelland, A., Guta, A., & Gagnon, M. (2019). The rise of molecular HIV surveillance: Implications on consent and criminalization. *Critical Public Health*, 1–7. https://doi.org/10.1080/09581596.2019.1582755.

Millett, G. A., Peterson, J. L., Flores, S. A., Hart, T. A., Jeffries, W. L., Wilson, P. A., et al. (2012). Comparisons of disparities and risks of HIV infection in black and other men who have sex with men in Canada, UK, and USA: A meta-analysis. *The Lancet, 380*(9839), 341–348. https://doi.org/10.1016/S0140-6736(12)60899-X.

Mykhalovskiy, E., Sanders, C., Hastings, C., & Bisaillon, L. (2020). Explicitly racialised and extraordinarily over-represented: Black immigrant men in 25 years of news reports on HIV non-disclosure criminal cases in Canada. *Culture, Health & Sexuality*. https://doi.org/10.1080/13691058.2020.1733095.

Newman, P. A., & Guta, A. (2020). How to have sex in an epidemic Redux: Reinforcing HIV prevention in the COVID-19 pandemic. *AIDS & Behaviour, 24*(8), 2260–2264. https://doi.org/10.1007/s10461-020-02940-z.

Newman, P. A., Guta, A., Lacombe-Duncan, A., & Tepjan, S. (2018). Clinical exigencies, psychosocial realities: Negotiating HIV pre-exposure prophylaxis beyond the cascade among gay, bisexual and other men who have sex with men in Canada. *Journal of the International AIDS Society, 21*(11), e25211. https://doi.org/10.1002/jia2.25211.

Nguyen, V.-K., Bajos, N., Dubois-Arber, F., O'Malley, J., & Pirkle, C. M. (2011). Remedicalizing an epidemic: From HIV treatment as prevention to HIV treatment is prevention. *AIDS, 25*(3), 291–293. https://doi.org/10.1097/QAD.0b013e3283402c3e.

Paparini, S., Nutland, W., Rhodes, T., Nguyen, V.-K., & Anderson, J. (2018). DIY HIV prevention: Formative qualitative research with men who have sex with men who source PrEP outside of clinical trials. *PLOS One, 13*(8), e0202830. https://doi.org/10.1371/journal.pone.0202830.

Pinto, R. M., Berringer, K. R., Melendez, R., & Mmeje, O. (2018). Improving PrEP implementation through multilevel interventions: A synthesis of the literature. *AIDS and Behavior, 22*(11), 3681–3691. https://doi.org/10.1007/s10461-018-2184-4.

Public Health Agency of Canada. (2016). Summary: Estimates of HIV incidence, *Prevelence and Canada's Progress of Meeting the 90-90-90 HIV Targets, 2016*. Retrieved July 25, 2020, from https://www.canada.ca/en/public-health/services/publications/diseases-conditions/summary-estimates-hiv-incidence-prevalence-canadas-progress-90-90-90.html.

Rosengarten, M., & Michael, M. (2010). HIV pre-exposure prophylaxis (PrEP) and the complexities of biomedical prevention: Ontological openness and the prevention assemblage. In M. Davis & C. Squire (Eds.), *HIV treatment and prevention Technologies in International Perspective* (pp. 167–183). London: Palgrave Macmillan.

Sidibé, M., Loures, L., & Samb, B. (2016). The UNAIDS 90-90-90 target: A clear choice for ending AIDS and for sustainable health and development. *Journal of the International AIDS Society, 19*(1), 21133–21133. https://doi.org/10.7448/IAS.19.1.21133.

Spieldenner, A. (2016). PrEP whores and HIV prevention: The queer communication of HIV pre-exposure prophylaxis (PrEP). *Journal of Homosexuality, 63*(12), 1685–1697. https://doi.org/10.1080/00918369.2016.1158012.

Tremblay, M. (2019). *Queering representation: LGBTQ people and electoral politics in Canada*. Vancouver: UBC Press.

Varghese, R. (2019). *Raw: PrEP, pedagogy, and the politics of barebacking*. Regina: University of Regina Press.

Vonn, M. (2012). British Columbia's 'seek and treat'strategy: A cautionary tale on privacy rights and informed consent for HIV testing. *HIV/AIDS Policy & Law Review, 16*(1), 4.

WHO. (2014). *Consolidated guidelines on HIV prevention, diagnosis, treatment and care for key populations* (9241507438). Retrieved July 25, 2020, from https://apps.who.int/iris/bitstream/handle/10665/128048/9789241507431_eng.pdf?sequence=1.

Chapter 10
Agency, Pleasure and Justice: A Public Health Ethics Perspective on the Use of PrEP by Gay and Other Homosexually-Active Men

Julien Brisson, Vardit Ravitsky, and Bryn Williams-Jones

10.1 Introduction

When in 2010 Truvada as pre-exposure prophylaxis (PrEP) was shown empirically to prevent HIV transmission (Grant et al. 2010), the field of public health became engaged in investigating the effects of this new biomedical tool for population health. As is common with the introduction of any new biomedical technology, there were mixed reactions. Some people were enthusiastic about the idea of a pill that could prevent HIV transmission (Feinberg 2012), while others were uneasy, believing that PrEP might lead individuals to abandon the use of condoms (Mansergh et al. 2012) or contribute to the growth of HIV drug-resistance (Wood 2012). The focus of much of this initial discussion was on HIV and other sexually transmitted infections (STIs), often neglecting the social dimensions of PrEP. With time, however, social scientists began to study this new biomedical technology, paying particular attention to the socio-cultural aspects of its development, implementation and uptake. Specifically, social scientists sought to understand how PrEP might bring about social change in terms of new and different biosocial relationships within gay communities (Girard et al. 2019).

One of the key contributions made by the social sciences has been the development of theoretical frameworks to enable the multi-faceted examination of biomedical innovation which, in the case of a new drug regimen such a PrEP, can foreground issues that might be overlooked by classic biomedical frameworks (Collin and David 2016). Yet, some social analyses of PrEP can also be problematic and these must also be examined critically. For example, some social scientists have argued that PrEP is a worrying form of medicalisation or pharmaceuticalisation of

J. Brisson (✉) · V. Ravitsky · B. Williams-Jones
Bioethics Program, Department of Social and Preventive Medicine, School of Public Health, University of Montreal, Montreal, Canada
e-mail: julien.brisson@umontreal.ca

© Springer Nature Switzerland AG 2021
S. Bernays et al. (eds.), *Remaking HIV Prevention in the 21st Century*, Social Aspects of HIV 5, https://doi.org/10.1007/978-3-030-69819-5_10

HIV prevention and sex (Giami and Perrey 2012; Gitome et al. 2014; Mc Manus and Mercado-Reyes 2016). The messages accompanying such an analysis can and should raise concerns about how the agency of PrEP users is framed, and the legitimate place of pleasure in sex.

In a previous paper (Brisson et al. 2019b), we argued for understanding PrEP as part of a safe sex ethics framework[1] for gay and other homosexually-active men. Our position there was anchored in a biomedical approach to public health ethics and sought to challenge some epidemiologically misinformed critiques of PrEP. For example, working from such a perspective, one could analyse the epidemiological cost-effectiveness of a public health intervention with a focus on lowering rates of incidence of disease on a population scale –respecting the ethical principal of beneficence by reference to a biomedical concern (e.g., HIV incidence). In parallel, however, a more social approach to public health ethics would pay greater attention to social issues in public health, not limiting itself to focusing on biomedical problems. For example, while some public health initiatives might help lower the incidence rates of disease within a population (in accordance with the ethical principal of beneficence), if these same initiatives result in increased stigmatisation towards historically marginalised communities then they might be unethical due to their non-respect for the ethical principles of nonmaleficence and justice. There can be friction therefore between biomedical and social approaches regarding how best to determine the most ethical action to take. This is notably the case with PrEP. While it might seem intuitive to endorse this new technology as a means to preventing HIV transmission (a biomedical problem of public health), when attending to social dimensions of PrEP such as advertisements targeting marginalised groups (a social problem of public health), ethical principles and values can come into conflict.

It is important to recognise that a public health ethics framework should extend beyond biomedical and/or epidemiological reasoning to explore ethical issues such as justice, stigmatisation and discrimination towards marginalised groups from a social perspective. Applying such a social perspective to PrEP and gay and other homosexually-active men is the goal of this chapter. We ground our position in a *social justice* approach that aligns with a reproductive justice framework (Luna and Luker 2013). The main argument we advance is that the agency of gay PrEP users, and the pleasure that may arise from using PrEP, should not be censored or diminished when analysing the pertinence of making PrEP more widely accessible. Instead of framing gay PrEP users as passive and disempowered agents of processes such as medicalisation and pharmaceuticalisation, we argue that they can and should be understood as active agents able to make autonomous and pragmatic decisions relating to sexual health. Following a similar logic to that articulated in reproductive

---

[1]The main ethical principles within this safe sex ethics framework are respect for autonomy and justice (Brisson et al. 2019b, pp. 54–55): *respect for autonomy* by acknowledging the right to engage in sex and to choose preventive measures; and *respect for justice* by paying attention to social context, in this case how the HIV epidemic principally affects already socially marginalised communities, hence creating the need to address issues related to justice.

justice frameworks advocating for women to have access to the contraceptive options of their choice, we argue that PrEP should be made readily available to gay men who wish to use it, without any moral judgment being attached to these choices.

We begin by reviewing some recent social science analyses of PrEP, showing why the way in which these represent gay PrEP users' agency is problematic. We then move to pleasure in sex, something that is often neglected or censored in discussions of PrEP—by policy makers for example—particularly as it relates to the question of PrEP users' agency. A final section focuses of issues of justice and uses the phenomenon of informal PrEP use to challenge some popular social science critiques.

10.2   Agency

Recent social analyses have viewed PrEP as a form of 'medicalization' of HIV prevention and sex (Giami and Perrey 2012; Gitome et al. 2014; Mc Manus and Mercado-Reyes 2016). Other theorisations have construed the process as 're-medicalization' (Syvertsen et al. 2014), 'biomedicalization' (Young et al. 2016), 'pharmaceuticalization' (Thomann 2018) or the exercise of 'pharmacopower' (Dean 2015; Schubert 2019). These concepts make distinct theoretical contributions to examining the social implications of PrEP. They have in common the presentation of PrEP users as the passive agents of a larger process: 'medicalization implies passivity on the part of the medicalized' (Rose 2007, p. 702). While these analyses do not always offer explicit critiques of PrEP, many of them do so. For example, the philosopher Paul Preciado (2015) uses the concept of pharmacopower to argue that the objective of Truvada as PrEP, similar to the contraceptive pill, is not to ameliorate the life of its user but rather to optimise their exploitation. More generally, the representation or 'framing' of key stakeholders plays a crucial role in public health ethics, especially when this involves marginalised communities (i.e., PrEP users). Our aim is to challenge the medicalisation framing of PrEP by examining the consequences it can have for the agency of PrEP users and their autonomy.

First, however, it is essential to situate the concept of medicalisation alongside interrelated concepts. Importantly, medicalisation is a 'term to designate issues that were not at one time but have become part of the province of medicine' (Rose 2007, p. 701). Over time, medical frameworks have come to be applied to a wide range of human conditions (Conrad 1992). As a result, previously social behaviours that do not necessarily involve disease or illness—e.g., sex and sexuality—have come to be included within the purview of medicine. The concept of medicalisation, as first introduced by Irving Zola (1972), embodies the idea 'of power [being exercised] over the bodies of unsuspecting target groups, most often patients' (Lock 2001, p. 481).

Biomedicalisation builds upon the notion of medicalisation to highlight the power of technoscience to transform biomedicine (Clarke et al. 2000).

Pharmaceuticalisation is, we suggest, an example of biomedicalisation, since it represents the idea of the 'transformation of human conditions, capabilities and capacities into opportunities for pharmaceutical intervention' (Williams et al. 2011, p. 711). Pharmacopower—which references biopolitics and the role of multinational industrial actors, i.e., 'Big Pharma'—has been defined by Paul Preciado as 'the miniaturization, internalization, and reflexive introversion (an inward coiling toward what is considered intimate, private space) of the surveillance and control mechanisms of the disciplinary sexopolitical regime' (2013, p. 79).

Within this theoretical framing of medical innovation, the user of 'medical' products (e.g., drugs, diagnostics, PrEP) is often represented as a passive agent; that is, as the submissive patient or victim of powerful social processes mobilised by (and in the interests of) multinational corporations, the medical profession, neoliberal decision makers and elected officials. Alternatively, if not a passive agent, users are understood to be using medical technologies (e.g., PrEP) as a direct consequence of, or in response to, larger social processes. For example, Matthew Thomann (2018) argues that PrEP is a pharmaceuticalisation of neoliberal risk subjectivity 'that pushes the individual to acknowledge their risk for HIV, take pre-emptive action, and become biomedically responsibilised' (p. 1004). Through such processes, and via powerful and subtle public health messaging, gay and other homosexually active men become 'biomedically self-governed', unconsciously internalising social and biomedical norms about 'appropriate behaviour'. PrEP thus becomes a 'reasonable' and even 'obligatory' response to HIV prevention, and any reason not to use PrEP becomes illegitimate (Young et al. 2016).

We dispute this 'false consciousness' type of argument (Wells 2017), because it unjustly frames gay men as disempowered actors with limited agency who are the victims of larger social processes. Instead, we argue that gay men using PrEP can and should be recognised as actively, consciously and pragmatically choosing to reduce the risk of HIV transmission, as they might do with condoms.

In this respect, it is important to recognise that condoms are also a biomedical tool. Their purpose is to prevent the transmission of HIV and other STIs, and to prevent pregnancy when applicable. Pharmacies and manufacturers (e.g., of condoms, lubricants, contraceptive pills) all over the world sell and profit from the sale of condoms, a market that is largely driven by heterosexual practices. Like PrEP, condoms therefore embody a form of (bio)medicalisation or pharmaceuticalisation of sexuality and HIV/STI prevention. In recent decades, public health promotion campaigns and safe sex education programmes in schools have encouraged individuals, from a young age, to become biomedically responsibilised/self-governed. Sex is often presented using a medical language focused on risk and prevention, and the condom is the key biomedical tool to implement this medicalisation of sex. For example, an individual purchasing a condom is invited to acknowledge their risk of contracting HIV or other STIs if they engage in unprotected sex; they can take pre-emptive action by putting on a condom before having sex, the same way that someone at risk of HIV takes PrEP to prevent HIV transmission. Both these uses of biomedical tools involve the calculation of medical risks in sex. Interestingly, social science analyses of condom use for HIV/STI prevention, as well as advocacy by health professionals and community activists for the use of condoms to address HIV and the simultaneous conceptualisation of sex in medical terms, are rarely framed as problematic. Why then is PrEP perceived as so radically different from condom use in HIV prevention with regards to the user's agency?

Clearly, PrEP and condoms are not equivalent biomedical tools; there are significant differences in the dynamics of their use. For example, PrEP requires a prescription, whereas condoms do not. PrEP requires medical surveillance (e.g., frequent HIV/STI testing) while condoms do not. In other words, PrEP entails greater interaction with health professionals and healthcare systems, which can lead to challenging power relations, for example if a doctor refuses to prescribe PrEP to a patient. In contrast, no physician involvement is needed to access condoms; they can be easily purchased in pharmacies or supermarkets in many countries and are often distributed free of charge by health workers.

10.3   Pleasure

As highlighted by Gabriel Girard (2016, p. 217), sexual pleasure and erotism have been surprisingly absent from public discussion about the use of, and access to, PrEP. This absence creates a critical problem, especially from a public health ethics perspective. Specifically, the pleasurable dimensions of PrEP use provide a strong argument for greater access by those who want to use this tool—for example, research by Mabire et al. (2019) underscores the importance of pleasure in sex for gay and other homosexually active men's decisions to use PrEP.

Historically, with the development of the HIV epidemic, the gay community advocated for the use of condoms as part of a safe sex ethics framework. The public health argument here was obvious since condoms offered a risk reduction strategy with which to diminish HIV transmission rates. It should never be forgotten 'that gay men all over the world—through conversation, discussion, and debate, and through the lived practices of sex—literally invented safe or safer sex, even before HIV had been isolated and identified' (Berkowitz 2003 as cited in Aggleton and Parker 2015, p. 1566). However, it is crucial to remember too the question of pleasure in sex was also central to the promotion of condoms. As Kane Race has argued, 'the history of HIV prevention may be understood as a series of struggles on the part of affected groups to elaborate bodily practices capable of mediating between pleasure and safety [where] health does not stand in opposition to pleasure' (2009, pp. 1–2). There was an important political dimension to arguing for gay men being able to continue to gain pleasure through sex in an epidemic that mostly affected socially marginalised communities. It is therefore peculiar that this overwhelmingly positive attitude towards sex did not persist with the introduction of PrEP, especially in gay communities, and as discussed by social scientists.

Looking at the early part of the history of the HIV epidemic, there was a certain unanimity within gay communities—and on the part of many scholars in the social sciences—in favour of advocating for the promotion of condoms as a biomedical means to address the epidemic (Lau et al. 1992; Junge 2002; Race 2003), and thus a tolerance for the medicalisation of sex. There was in addition the promotion of an ethic of non-judgementality towards people's sexual behaviour, even if this might be labelled as 'riskier'. For example, it would have been ethically unacceptable to shame an individual taking pleasure from having sex with different partners, while using condoms to mitigate the risk of HIV transmission.

In contrast, there was a parallel movement by socially conservative groups who were opposed to talking about condom use or pleasure in sex, most noticeable in debates about comprehensive sex education for young people and in the Catholic Church's stance against the use and promotion of condoms. For many social conservatives, taking pleasure in certain sexual acts (e.g., sex outside of heterosexual monogamous relationships) is necessarily immoral and thus should be condemned and even prohibited. There was also an openness to shaming and stigmatising discourses regarding sexual behaviour. Individuals who engaged in heterosexual sex outside marriage—or, worse still, sex between men—were framed as immoral and as being the cause of the AIDS (Kowalewski 1990; Campbell et al. 2011). Yet, it was precisely the medicalisation of HIV and AIDS that made it possible to challenge this stigmatisation. HIV transmission was explained through biology as opposed to a moral/religious framing and it was possible to curtail this risk through the promotion and use of a medical technology (i.e., through the medicalisation of sex).

With the introduction of PrEP and its uptake by gay and other homosexually-active men, there came renewed stigmatisation and moralisation, but this time from within the gay community itself. Popular expressions such as 'Truvada whore' or 'PrEP whore' provide examples of this (Calabrese and Underhill 2015; Spieldenner 2016; Pawson and Grov 2018). In using PrEP, there is the implication that one does not always use condoms when having sex, something that has been so important in the struggle against HIV, and thus a justification, for some, to stigmatise PrEP users as immoral (Dean 2015). This phenomenon of gay men shaming PrEP users (who themselves are predominantly gay men) embodies a radical shift of position on the subjects of sex and pleasure. Indeed, it reflects a discourse similar to that of socially conservative groups, for whom it is acceptable to shame the sexual practices of some while simultaneously ignoring the fact that biomedical interventions such as condoms and PrEP prevent HIV transmission.

From a public health ethics perspective, especially in the context of the ongoing global HIV epidemic, there is a serious problem when individuals are shamed for their sexual pleasures and practices, even more so when this shame involves the use of an HIV prevention tool. Generally speaking, 'in the HIV epidemic, slut shaming can be problematic, because it has a tendency to silence discussions about sex among gay men' (McDavitt and Mutchler 2014 in Spieldenner 2016, p. 1691). This is particularly true when it relates to the topic of pleasure in safe sexual behaviours, since at issue here is respect for individual choice, respect for groups (that are often marginalised), and justice in access to sexual health technologies.

10.4   Access to PrEP as a Justice Issue

When PrEP was first approved by the US Food and Drug Administration in 2012, it was reasonable to worry, from a biopolitical perspective, that there might be significant and undue pressure placed on high-risk and historically vulnerable groups (e.g., gay and bisexual men, sex workers, trans women) to take up and adhere to this new biomedical tool to prevent HIV transmission. Given PrEP's apparent efficacy, it would have been possible for governments and public health authorities around the world to accept this new HIV prevention tool, make it rapidly accessible to high risk populations, and even use moralising health promotion messages (e.g., that not using PrEP was irresponsible) to promote its use. This has not been the case.

As of 2020, PrEP is still largely inaccessible in many countries, and either cannot be formally prescribed or is too costly for most people to afford (UN 2017; Bekker et al. 2018; Hayes et al. 2019). In 2018, there were an estimated 381,580 PrEP users in 68 countries, with 59% of them in North America (Lancet HIV 2019b, p. e723). Yet, most people at high risk of HIV live outside of North America and are to be found in low and middle-income countries. In the USA, 'of the estimated 1.2 million people at risk of HIV, only around 250,000 people are using PrEP—most well educated, affluent, white gay men' (Lancet HIV 2019a, p. 483). In parallel, studies have shown that individuals from marginalised communities, such as Latinos (Page et al. 2017), trans people (Sevelius et al. 2016) and African American men and women in the Southern USA (Elopre et al. 2017) have difficulty accessing PrEP. While these examples come from the USA, in the majority of countries internationally marginalised communities are also excluded from access to PrEP.

The global health phenomenon of 'informal PrEP'—i.e., accessing antiretroviral drugs through informal channels (e.g., through the Internet or through friends) (Brisson et al. 2019a)—helps clarify the important justice issues regarding access. A clear parallel can be made here with women who get clandestine abortions because the medical procedure is illegal or because they lack the necessary financial resources in a context of private medicine. This latter issue has been effectively addressed by the reproductive justice movement, which began in the 1990s by women of colour in the USA in response to ongoing debates over reproductive health (Ross and Solinger 2017). Historically, feminist analyses had framed the discussion as one of access to contraceptives and abortion, i.e., being 'pro-choice'. But one problem with this framing was that it neglected to recognise women's ability to be capable of making choices in relation to their sexual and reproductive health. Reproductive justice advocates highlighted the structural factors, such as poverty and lack of access to healthcare services, that shaped—i.e., limited—the ability of many women to exercise their reproductive health rights, including ones as important as whether or not to have children (Smith 2005).

In terms of agency and pleasure in sex, the reproductive justice framework recognised the importance of advocating for women to be able to choose to engage in sex, to be able to enjoy sex and to have access to the necessary contraceptive tools to control their sexual and reproductive health. In 2017, 43% of pregnancies in developing countries were unplanned and '84% of these unintended pregnancies were in women who had an unmet need for modern contraception' (Bekker et al. 2018, p. 331). These statistics make it clear that lack of access to contraceptive tools and reproductive health services for women is a serious injustice and human rights issue. It is unjust that some women—particularly those belonging to marginalised groups—lack the same opportunities as others in terms of their reproductive health and rights. All women should have equal access to quality reproductive services, regardless of ethnicity, social class or socio-economic status.

Applying a reproductive justice framework to PrEP helps highlight ongoing and highly problematic geographic and class inequities around the world, of which the global health phenomenon of informal PrEP provides a telling illustration. The lack of accessibility to PrEP for most people around the world, except for the wealthy, arguably constitutes a much more serious concern than the threat of the possible social harms of PrEP (e.g., biopolitical surveillance, the medicalisation of sex) for gay men. Around the world, there are community groups, like PrEPster, PrEPara Salvador, and IwantPrEPNow, that advocate for greater accessibility to PrEP while simultaneously stressing the importance of acknowledging pleasure in sex and fighting PrEP-related stigma. These groups help demonstrate the applicability and pertinence of a reproductive justice framework for PrEP and gay men by underscoring how PrEP's inaccessibility foremost constitutes a justice issue.

10.5 Conclusion

Social scientific and ethical discussion of the introduction of new HIV prevention technologies is crucial, especially as these analyses allow us to explore and comment on the possible consequences (good and bad) of a new technology. Authors who have developed critical analyses of PrEP, such as those presented in this chapter, are often well-intentioned and wish to protect the wellbeing of PrEP users, who often belong to marginalised groups. It is understandable and important to take a critical stance in relation to the development of a new HIV prevention technology intended for individuals at high risk of HIV. Nonetheless, as we have argued, when analysing PrEP from a social position, it is crucial also not to overlook essential elements, such as the agency of potential and current gay and other homosexually active men PrEP users and the pleasurable elements that are related to the use of PrEP. Just as importantly, however, while PrEP use can be problematised, it is the worldwide inequity and inaccessibility of PrEP that constitutes a much more serious public health ethics issue.

Funding This work was supported by a doctoral research award to Julien Brisson from the Canadian Institutes of Health Research [grant number 201610GSD-385545-283387] in honour of Nelson Mandela.

References

Aggleton, P., & Parker, R. (2015). Moving beyond biomedicalization in the HIV response: Implications for community involvement and community leadership among men who have sex with men and transgender people. *American Journal of Public Health, 105*(8), 1552–1558.

Bekker, L. G., Alleyne, G., Baral, S., Cepeda, J., Daskalakis, D., Dowdy, D., et al. (2018). Advancing global health and strengthening the HIV response in the era of the sustainable development goals: The international AIDS society—Lancet commission. *The Lancet, 392* (10144), 312–358.

Berkowitz, R. (2003). *Stayin' alive: The invention of safe sex, a personal history.* Boulder: Westview.

Brisson, J., Ravitsky, V., & Williams-Jones, B. (2019a). Informal PrEP: An emerging need for nomenclature. *The Lancet Public Health, 4*(2), e83.

Brisson, J., Ravitsky, V., & Williams-Jones, B. (2019b). Towards an integration of PrEP into a safe sex ethics framework for men who have sex with men. *Public Health Ethics, 12*(1), 54–63.

Calabrese, S. K., & Underhill, K. (2015). How stigma surrounding the use of HIV preexposure prophylaxis undermines prevention and pleasure: A call to destigmatize "Truvada whores". *American Journal of Public Health, 105*(10), 1960–1964.

Campbell, C., Skovdal, M., & Gibbs, A. (2011). Creating social spaces to tackle AIDS-related stigma: Reviewing the role of church groups in sub-Saharan Africa. *AIDS & Behavior, 15*(6), 1204–1219.

Clarke, A. E., Fishman, J. R., Fosket, J. R., Mamo, L., & Shim, J. K. (2000). Technoscience and the new biomedicalization: Western roots, global rhizomes. *Sciences Sociales et Santé, 18*(2), 11–42.

Collin, J., & David, P. M. (2016). *Vers une pharmaceuticalisation de la société: le médicament comme objet social.* Québec: Presses de l'Université du Québec.

Conrad, P. (1992). Medicalization and social control. *Annual Review of Sociology, 18*, 209–232.

Dean, T. (2015). Mediated intimacies: Raw sex, Truvada, and the biopolitics of chemoprophylaxis. *Sexualities, 18*(1–2), 224–246.

Elopre, L., Kudroff, K., Westfall, A. O., Overton, E. T., & Mugavero, M. J. (2017). The right people, right places, and right practices: Disparities in PrEP access among African American men, women and MSM in the deep south. *Journal of Acquired Immune Deficiency Syndromes (1999), 74*(1), 56–59.

Feinberg, J. (2012). Truvada PrEP: Why I voted "yes". *Annals of Internal Medicine, 157*(7), 521–522.

Giami, A., & Perrey, C. (2012). Transformations in the medicalization of sex: HIV prevention between discipline and biopolitics. *Journal of Sex Research, 49*(4), 353–361.

Girard, G. (2016). "La pilule qui change tout?": Analyses des débats québécois autour de la prophylaxie préexposition du VIH. In J. Collin & P. M. David (Eds.), *Vers une pharmaceuticalisation de la société: le médicament comme objet social* (pp. 193–222). Québec: Presses de l'Université du Québec.

Girard, G., Patten, S., LeBlanc, M. A., Adam, B. D., & Jackson, E. (2019). Is HIV prevention creating new biosocialities among gay men? Treatment as prevention and pre-exposure prophylaxis in Canada. *Sociology of Health & Illness, 41*(3), 484–501.

Gitome, S., Njuguna, S., Kwena, Z., Ombati, E., Njoroge, B., & Bukusi, E. A. (2014). Perspective paper: Medicalization of HIV and the African response. *African Journal of Reproductive Health, 18*(3), 25–33.

Grant, R. M., Lama, J. R., Anderson, P. L., McMahan, V., Liu, A. Y., Vargas, L., et al. (2010). Preexposure chemoprophylaxis for HIV prevention in men who have sex with men. *New England Journal of Medicine, 363*(27), 2587–2599.

Hayes, R., Schmidt, A. J., Pharris, A., Azad, Y., Brown, A. E., Weatherburn, P., et al. (2019). Estimating the 'PrEP gap': How implementation and access to PrEP differ between countries in Europe and Central Asia in 2019. *Eurosurveillance, 24*(41), 1900598.

Junge, B. (2002). Bareback sex, risk, and eroticism: Anthropological themes (re)surfacing in the post-AIDS era. In E. Lewin & W. L. Leap (Eds.), *Out in theory the emergence of gay and lesbian anthropology* (pp. 186–221). Urbana & Chicago: University of Illinois Press.

Kowalewski, M. R. (1990). Religious constructions of the AIDS crisis. *Sociological Analysis, 51* (1), 91–96.

Lancet, H. I. V. (2019a). Are 2 million bottles of PrEP an empty gesture? *The Lancet HIV, 6*(8), PE483.

Lancet, H. I. V. (2019b). New PrEP formulation approved. . . but only for some. *The Lancet HIV, 6* (11), e723.

Lau, R. K. W., Jenkins, P., Caun, K., Forster, S. M., Weber, J. N., McManus, T. J., et al. (1992). Trends in sexual behaviour in a cohort of homosexual men: A 7-year prospective study. *International Journal of STD & AIDS, 3*(4), 267–272.

Lock, M. (2001). The tempering of medical anthropology: Troubling natural categories. *Medical Anthropology Quarterly, 15*(4), 478–492.

Luna, Z., & Luker, K. (2013). Reproductive justice. *Annual Review of Law and Social Science, 9*, 327–352.

Mabire, X., Puppo, C., Morel, S., Mora, M., Rojas Castro, D., Chas, J., et al. (2019). Pleasure and PrEP: Pleasure-seeking plays a role in prevention choices and could Lead to PrEP initiation. *American Journal of Men's Health, 13*(1), 1557988319827396.

Mansergh, G., Koblin, B. A., & Sullivan, P. S. (2012). Challenges for HIV pre-exposure prophylaxis among men who have sex with men in the United States. *PLoS Medicine, 9*(8), e1001286.

McManus, F., & Mercado-Reyes, A. (2016). Constructing publics, preventing diseases and medicalizing bodies: HIV, AIDS, and its visual cultures. *Sexualidad, Salud y Sociedad, 24*, 69–102.

McDavitt, B., & Mutchler, M. G. (2014). "Dude, you're such a slut!" barriers and facilitators of sexual communication among young gay men and their best friends. *Journal of Adolescent Research, 29*(4), 464–498.

Page, K. R., Martinez, O., Nieves-Lugo, K., Zea, M. C., Grieb, S. D., Yamanis, T. J., et al. (2017). Promoting pre-exposure prophylaxis to prevent HIV infections among sexual and gender minority Hispanics/Latinxs. *AIDS Education & Prevention, 29*(5), 389–400.

Pawson, M., & Grov, C. (2018). 'It's just an excuse to slut around': Gay and bisexual mens' constructions of HIV pre-exposure prophylaxis (Pr EP) as a social problem. *Sociology of Health & Illness, 40*(8), 1391–1403.

Preciado, B. (2013). *Testo Junkie: Sex, Drugs, and Biopolitics in the Pharmacopornographic Era*, (B. Benderson, Trans.). New York: Feminist Press.

Preciado, P. (2015, June 11). *Condoms chimiques. Libération.* https://www.liberation.fr/ chroniques/2015/06/11/condoms-chimiques_1327747

Race, K. D. (2003). Revaluation of risk among gay men. *AIDS Education & Prevention, 15*(4), 369–381.

Race, K. (2009). *Pleasure consuming medicine: The queer politics of drugs*. Durham, NC: Duke University Press.

Rose, N. (2007). Beyond medicalization. *The Lancet, 369*(9562), 700–702.

Ross, L., & Solinger, R. (2017). *Reproductive justice: An introduction*. Oakland: University of California Press.

Schubert, K. (2019). The democratic biopolitics of PrEP. In H. Gerhards & K. Braun (Eds.), *Biopolitiken–Regierungen des Lebens heute* (pp. 121–153). Wiesbaden: Springer VS.

Sevelius, J. M., Keatley, J., Calma, N., & Arnold, E. (2016). 'I am not a man': Trans-specific barriers and facilitators to PrEP acceptability among transgender women. *Global Public Health, 11*(7–8), 1060–1075.

Smith, A. (2005). Beyond pro-choice versus pro-life: Women of colour and reproductive justice. *The National Women's Studies Association Journal, 17*(1), 119–140.

Spieldenner, A. (2016). PrEP whores and HIV prevention: The queer communication of HIV pre-exposure prophylaxis (PrEP). *Journal of Homosexuality, 63*(12), 1685–1697.

Syvertsen, J. L., Bazzi, A. M. R., Scheibe, A., Adebajo, S., Strathdee, S. A., & Wechsberg, W. M. (2014). The promise and peril of pre-exposure prophylaxis (PrEP): Using social science to inform prep interventions among female sex workers. *African Journal of Reproductive Health, 18*(3), 74–83.

Thomann, M. (2018). On December 1, 2015, sex changes. Forever': Pre-exposure prophylaxis and the pharmaceuticalisation of the neoliberal sexual subject. *Global Public Health, 13*(8), 997–1006.

UN. (2017). *Ending AIDS. Progress towards the 90-90-90 targets.* Geneva: Joint United Nations Programme on HIV/AIDS.

Wells, S. (2017). Feminism, false consciousness, & consent: A third way. *Georgetown Journal of Gender and the Law, 18*(1), 251.

Williams, S. J., Martin, P., & Gabe, J. (2011). The pharmaceuticalisation of society? A framework for analysis. *Sociology of Health & Illness, 33*(5), 710–725.

Wood, L. V. (2012). Why I voted "no" to Truvada PrEP. *Annals of Internal Medicine, 157*(7), 519–520.

Young, I., Flowers, P., & McDaid, L. (2016). Can a pill prevent HIV? Negotiating the biomedicalisation of HIV prevention. *Sociology of Health & Illness, 38*(3), 411–425.

Zola, I. K. (1972). Medicine as an institution of social control. *The Sociological Review, 20*(4), 487–504.

Part III
Provision Politics and New Forms of Governmentality

Chapter 11
The Political Life of PrEP in England: An Ethnographic Account

Sara Paparini

11.1   Introduction

In April 2020, it was announced that the English National Health Service (NHS) would begin routine provision of pre-exposure prophylaxis (PrEP) for HIV. This happened approximately 6 years since the results of the English PROUD clinical trial were first made public in 2014 (McCormack et al. 2016). During these 6 years, PrEP was not available as a service on the English NHS, if not through alternative routes to access (see for example Paparini et al. 2018), including a public health trial (called IMPACT).

After the PROUD trial, implementation work that had been proceeding for around 18 months in what appeared to be the direction of a PrEP roll-out, was instead suddenly halted in March 2016, when NHS England announced that it would not commission PrEP. The reasons for NHS England's decision have since remained the subject of speculation and this paper, based on ethnographic research on the early emergence of PrEP in England, lays out the key debates and discourses articulated with regards to this 'NHS controversy'.

11.1.1   The Political Life of PrEP

NHS England's initial explanation for the decision on PrEP was that the 2012 restructure of the health and social care system in England had shifted responsibility for public health (including PrEP drugs for HIV prevention) directly to Local Authorities. This was an unexpected decision that, as we will see, was followed by

S. Paparini (✉)
Nuffield Department of Primary Care Health Sciences, University of Oxford, Oxford, UK
e-mail: sara.paparini@phc.ox.ac.uk

© Springer Nature Switzerland AG 2021   145
S. Bernays et al. (eds.), *Remaking HIV Prevention in the 21st Century*, Social
Aspects of HIV 5, https://doi.org/10.1007/978-3-030-69819-5_11

a remarkable response in press and media, a rise in PrEP activism, and a court case brought by the HIV charity the National AIDS Trust against NHS England. Although by no means the only drug-related controversy of this kind (see for example Charlton 2019), when compared to the favourable decisions about PrEP taken early on by other high-income countries (e.g. Australia, the USA, France and, even closer, Scotland), the position of NHS England on PrEP came nonetheless as a surprise.

So far, a number of international scholars have analysed PrEP as an example of a *biopolitical* intervention (Giami and Perrey 2012; Dean 2015; Young et al. 2016; Thomann 2018; Martinez-Lacabe 2019; Young et al. 2019). From these perspectives, PrEP produces a particular form of biopolitical subjects (the PrEP user) who display risk-aversion, self-governing and responsibility through the highly individualised use of a biomedical technology which also involves intensive, self-initiated and clinic-delivered surveillance (e.g. testing, counselling, behavioural reporting, therapeutic monitoring). This is linked to the observation that PrEP reinforces a re-medicalised 'turn' in HIV prevention as a clinic-centred, technocratic intervention which obfuscates, and may come at the expense of, broader collective responses to the epidemic (Nguyen et al. 2011; Kippax and Stephenson 2012; Cairns et al. 2016). Such approaches constitute some of the key building blocks towards a full understanding of the change in HIV prevention brought about by PrEP.

However, NHS England's decision in 2016 has also animated a *political* life of PrEP, by which I mean here a set of agonistic social interactions whose aim is to shape policy and affect the governmental distribution of resources (see Easton 1959). The NHS controversy has been politically productive in at least three ways. Firstly, by attracting media attention and galvanising a moral debate around PrEP provision. Secondly, by re-igniting a national PrEP activism which draws from the historical and international 'politics of recognition' in HIV. Thirdly, by making even more visible the politics of evidence in clinical research and, in the English case, how they are mobilised both in terms of remit (which part of the health system should pay for what), in legal debates, and in terms of cost-effectiveness.

I illustrate these three dimensions of the political life of PrEP by recounting a story of the NHS controversy from around the time of the PROUD trial through to the court case against NHS England (2012–2017). I wish to show how particular PrEP politics, in the English case, have emerged not only as a result of new techno-scientific discoveries, but, centrally, as a result of the health system's controversial response to their implementation.

11.2 Methods

This study is part of a larger anthropological group project called *Eradication*, which has been documenting the development of interventions aimed at ending the AIDS epidemic, such as PrEP and 'test-and-treat'. As a part of this project, between 2016 and 2018, I conducted an ethnographic study of the emergence of PrEP in England, using also my own archives and field notes from previous projects in academia and non-governmental organisations. Details of my fieldwork are shown in Table 11.1.

In this article, all quotes in inverted commas are direct quotes from texts, observations or oral interviews. Where not already in the public domain, all direct quotes are anonymous. The study was approved by the Ethics Committee of the Graduate Institute of International & Development Studies (Geneva) and of the London School of Hygiene & Tropical Medicine.

11.3 The NHS Controversy: A Story

11.3.1 Early Ambivalence

At a weekend workshop in Windsor in June 2013, clinical, academic and public health stakeholders gathered to take stock of 30 years of work in the HIV sector in the UK. Central to the meeting were discussions of the then recent reforms included in the Health and Social Care Act of 2012, in which the NHS in England (which operates separately to the NHS in Wales, Scotland and Northern Ireland) was tasked to pay for HIV treatment, Local Authorities would form local Health & Wellbeing boards to commission HIV prevention, and national HIV prevention funding would no longer be ring-fenced.

In this new and radically different landscape, PrEP appeared as (only) one of the main topics of the day. It was met with hope and concern in equal measures. The report from the Windsor meeting reads:

> There was some debate and difference of opinion as to whether and how PrEP should be used to prevent HIV spreading (. . .) There is clear evidence (. . .) that it should be regarded as an effective tool for treating this epidemic. However (. . .) PrEP is a complex technology and it is not just a matter of making it available (. . .) should we wait until proper scientific rigour has been applied? (Making Sense of HIV at 30 2013)

The meeting was taking place against the backdrop of community clashes about PrEP, mainly in the USA. The Director of the Los Angeles-based AIDSCare Health Foundation (AHF) had expressed strong criticism about PrEP as a 'party drug' (AHF 2016) and a profit-making venture, and lobbied against Gilead's submission to the Food and Drug Administration (FDA) for approval (AHF 2011; Tuller 2011). However, PrEP-ambivalent views were far from being mainstream. Indeed, the AHF position would be denounced by the gay press many times over the years as stigmatising gay men's choices (Lucas 2014; HIVPlusMag.com Contributor 2015) and key US media would question the origins of much resistance to PrEP (Glazek 2013).

Around this time, the evidence on PrEP's clinical efficacy was growing, particularly in the USA, and was being endorsed by gay communities in other countries

Table 11.1 Fieldwork and data collection

Method	Participants/Events	Quantity	Notes	Consent process
Individual interviews with stakeholders	Public health officials, HIV clinicians, members of PrEP trial teams, staff from community organisations, PrEP and HIV activists, and other academic researchers involved in PrEP studies.	22	All stakeholder interviews involved common questions about the early days of PrEP, the beginning of the PROUD study, and views on NHS England's position on PrEP. Interview guides were then refined as appropriate (e.g. how did researchers test their approach? How did policymakers view the translation of clinical evidence into policy? What were activists' main challenges around new HIV prevention technologies?).	A participant information sheet was distributed prior to our meetings and verbal consent was sought. Notes were taken during the interview and then returned to participants to check their accounts had been represented correctly. No compensation was offered for participation.
Key informants followed over time	PrEP activists	2	Informal conversations and exchanges were recorded in my field notes.	Same as above.
Focus group discussions	London-based MSM sourcing PrEP outside of clinical trials	20	A purposive sampling strategy was employed. The study was open to MSM (including trans men) over 18 years of age who had self-purchased, and self-administered PrEP in the past 12 months; and MSM who had purchased and used PrEP in the past 12 months but were not currently using PrEP. More details available in Paparini et al. (2018).	Consent to participate was given both verbally and in writing by participants in the focus groups. Focus group participants were given £30 to compensate for their time and for travel expenses.
Ethnographic observation	Twitter debates, and related media outputs, reports and journal articles; national and international HIV conferences; London PrEP mobilisation workshops; research meetings from fellow PrEP researchers (including clinic-based studies); activist arts and media events.	n/a	I recorded confidential notes of informal conversations with attendees, researchers, policymakers and industry representatives.	My position as a researcher was explained at the beginning of each interaction; all interactions have been kept anonymous.

such as in France (through the community-led IPERGAY trial in 2012) (Molina et al. 2015), Australia, The Netherlands and, eventually, in the UK too. Prior to the beginning of the PROUD trial, however, some UK stakeholders were still hesitant. Some clinicians in my study maintain, for example, that they were not sure at the time that the men most likely to adhere to PrEP would be those that PrEP would be most useful for.

Even when PROUD did start, recruitment was slow as community support for PrEP from gay and HIV organisations was still tenuous. In my interviews, community stakeholders recall worrying that a medical solution would take over years of community-based prevention, and that funding would go to more medical technologies and less to the 'traditional' health promotion needed to make them work. A few also mentioned that rushing into taking drugs was never a good idea and PrEP seemed like the 'mass-medication of gay men'.

11.3.2   'You Can't Argue with 86%': The PROUD Trial

In early 2013, PrEP was still seen somehow as a 'hard sell', and PROUD was portrayed as a pragmatic study that would settle some of the dispute about real PrEP usage in the UK (McCormack et al. 2016). After an unsuccessful larger bid, funding was pieced together for an initial pilot trial that would help '*circumvent*' concerns about costs and feasibility of a full trial. The pilot started in October 2012 to recruit 500 MSM, funded by the Medical Research Council Clinical Trials Unit and Public Health England, with routine NHS staff time and drugs donated by Gilead.

Notably, the trial was conceived of as a trial *for* MSM, to prove the usefulness of a new 'radical' intervention (McCormack et al. 2016) to overcome a long-standing problem in UK HIV epidemiology: the steady, persistent incidence of HIV, chiefly amongst gay and other MSM. And, in what many have described to me as an 'unexpected' turn of events, the trial recruited a group of MSM with extremely high HIV incidence. This meant that, since no transmission had occurred in the intervention arm, the trial had to be stopped earlier than planned to avoid men in the deferred arm (i.e. supposed to receive PrEP 12 months after men in the intervention arm) becoming HIV positive.

Many of those I have spoken with in 2017, referring to the effectiveness result of the study, use a common refrain: 'you can't argue with 86%'. This result finally turned the clinical and community tide around. The concurrent announcement of results in 2014 from both PROUD and the French IPERGAY trial were, according to a research clinician interviewee, 'shockingly influential' and a 'tipping point' was reached in the history of PrEP which shifted those views that the American iPrEx study alone (Grant et al. 2010) had not been able to.

11.3.3   The Erosion of HIV Prevention Funding

By 2015, then, the PROUD study had settled questions about whether PrEP 'works'. Yet the NGO and public health sectors had been in turmoil in the years during the study: since then, Local Authority spending on prevention had been dropping by around 15% each year, even more in some HIV high prevalence authorities. The government had withdrawn £200 m of the money it was due to Local Authorities in 2015–2016 for public health schemes (and is cutting another £331 m in 2020–2021) (Davies 2015).

As the austerity-driven political and economic climate worsened, justifying the cost of PrEP brought contention not only between communities, clinicians and the government, but within each of these networks, too. With HIV prevention funding under threat from the new government cuts and the reform of the NHS, would the NHS spending money on PrEP undermine existing measures (health promotion, condoms, testing, early treatment to make viral load undetectable)?

Informants recall how cost-effectiveness modelling at the time was a particularly sensitive political undertaking, as each scenario could be mobilised in favour or against PrEP, especially by public health commissioning bodies. The soon-to-be announced decision of the English NHS not to commission PrEP, however, would eventually turn the conversation around, and pivot the discussion not on whether PrEP made sense as a potential public health investment, but rather on the health service's responsibility of protecting, through the provision of PrEP, people otherwise deemed at inevitable risk of acquiring HIV.

11.3.4   The U-Turn

The rationale laid out in NHS England's announcement in March 2016 with regards to PrEP (non-)provision was ambivalent. On the one hand, it was framed in terms of legal remit: the reform of the health service had laid out that prevention is the responsibility of Local Authorities, hence the NHS *could not* commission a public health intervention. Importantly, the NHS *must not* set a precedent: it could not fund PrEP as this would have displaced funding for other 'specialised commissions' who, it would be argued, would also have a right to access preventative medicines:

> Including PrEP for consideration in competition with specialised commissioning treatments (. . .) could present risk of legal challenge from proponents of other 'candidate' treatments and interventions that could be displaced by PrEP if NHS England were to commission it (NHS England 2016).

On the other hand, whilst not debating the scientific value of PrEP, it questioned how definitive the PROUD results were:

> NHS England is keen to build on the excellent work to date and will be making available up to £2 m (. . .) to run a number of early implementer test sites (. . .) These will run over the next two years and will aim to test the 'real life' cost effectiveness and affordability of PrEP as part of an integrated HIV and STI prevention service (NHS England 2016).

The news didn't go down very well at all. Talks and process up to that point had always been based on NHS funding for PrEP: Truvada is a drug the NHS sources and provides as HIV treatment already and it was clear that Local Authorities could not afford a patented 'PrEP bill', even more given the latest budget cuts. Without NHS funding, PrEP would not happen.

Professor Sheena McCormack, PROUD PI, responded first to the suggestion that more evidence was needed:

> We strongly disagree with the inference that more 'real-life' evidence is required to assess the cost effectiveness and affordability of PrEP as part of an integrated service. This is exactly what PROUD has already established—and in the most astounding and scientifically robust way (NHS England 2016).

The argument over costs was met with counterargument about cost savings and legitimacy, as McCormack continued:

> PrEP is a powerful HIV prevention tool and avoids the need for NHS England specialist services to fund a lifetime of treatment...The risk of legal challenge is negligible compared to the benefits, which are financial for NHS England, and personal for the thousands of individuals destined to otherwise catch HIV (NHS England 2016).

According to community organisations, the financial offer of £2 million for new research was 'loose change found down the back of the sofa' (NAT 2016). A petition to 'make PrEP immediately available on the NHS' was launched, collecting over 13 thousand signatures (UK Government and Parliament 2016).

11.3.5 Politics of Recognition in Austerity

Some in my study speculated that NHS England's decision was a way to 'buy time' until Gilead's drug patents would expire, and PrEP could be sourced as a generic drug. But not everyone believed in financial or legal reasons for the decision not to pay for a PrEP routine service. For GMFA (a leading gay men's health charity) it was clear this was a 'let down' for gay men (Hodson 2016). Just a few days after the NHS England's announcement, the National AIDS Trust policy blog read:

> This fiasco will have serious human consequences in the many HIV transmissions which will take place (...) It epitomises the inability of our health system to value prevention. Perhaps also the failure of our health system to value equally the well-being of gay men (NAT 2016).

Doubts emerged as to whether NHS England's choice was based on a different question altogether: are gay men 'worth' all this investment? Especially against other specialised treatments? Many of the people I have spoken with think that this question, lurking in the pages of English tabloids at the time (see, for example, Platell 2015), weighed in favour of the decision not to fund PrEP.

United4PrEP—a coalition of HIV clinicians, charities and activists—called for a protest outside of the Department of Health in July 2016 (Siddons 2016). Reports of the protest had the familiar tone of early AIDS and treatment activism:

> The feeling among many protestors was that the decision [about PrEP] would not have been taken if HIV did not affect marginalised communities (...) "If this was an illness that disproportionately affected straight, white people" one protester argued, "we wouldn't be here today." (Siddons 2016).

The interpretation of NHS England's decision not to fund PrEP as a form of neglect of the health of minorities was an important development in the story of this controversy. The unexpected response from NHS England provoked an uproar about the state's exclusion of (particularly) gay men's health from its remit because, in McCormack's words, these men were otherwise 'destined to catch HIV'. Beyond signifying a breach of gay men's right to prevention options, in the midst of the controversy, PrEP was thus being reconfigured.

First, it was being reconfigured as the most effective way to avoid what was now increasingly framed as a highly likely, or inevitable, HIV diagnosis. For example, the very vocal message of PrEP activist Greg Owen, whose personal story of becoming HIV positive after failing to access PrEP has since been told many times in the media (Strudwick 2017). 'You either take ARVs before, or you take them after', one interviewee told me: the choice is between antiretrovirals for prevention of HIV, or for treatment of the HIV diagnosis that could not be prevented.

Second, PrEP increasingly represented the 'responsible choice'. This was to answer concerns that PrEP users may stop using condoms, and sexually transmitted infections (STI) rates would increase, with the counterargument that PrEP users are more likely to be those who are already not using condoms:

> Some people have portrayed PrEP use as irresponsible (...) But I think it's totally the opposite. It's an immensely responsible thing to do, particularly if you are one of those guys who doesn't consistently use condoms (Greenhalgh and Cookson 2017).

Finally, The NHS controversy amplified PrEP's profile in the media and galvanised community groups to endorse PrEP as a matter of principle and as a right for gay men. Framing PrEP as the best, most responsible choice for gay men decidedly cast NHS's England decision *not* to provide PrEP as a form of neglect.

Indeed, interest in 'DIY' ways of sourcing PrEP outside of clinical trials grew exponentially through the NHS controversy, as the end of the trial and lack of a PrEP roll-out left many without formal access to PrEP. Whereas in 2012 PROUD had opened to slow recruitment, by the end of 2016, a significant number of men were buying generic PrEP online by themselves (Paparini et al. 2018).

11.3.6 Future 'AIDS Victims' and the Treatment and Prevention Split

The notion of neglecting men 'otherwise destined to catch HIV' was most strikingly voiced in one of the judges' response to the court case brought against NHS England by the National AIDS Trust (NAT):

No one doubts that preventative medicine makes powerful sense. But one governmental body says it has no power to provide the service and the local authorities say that they have no money. The Claimant is caught between the two and *the potential victims of this disagreement are those who will contract HIV/AIDS* but who would not were the preventative policy to be fully implemented. (National Aids Trust v NHS England 2016, High Court Ruling. 4. My emphasis.)

NAT, a well-established HIV policy organisation, resorted to legal action because the NHS' decision appeared as a 'total closure' and no other policy route seemed possible. NAT's central supporting arguments were based on clinical evidence to a great degree. In all effects, and for the purpose of commissioning and responsibility, PrEP was argued to be the same as other forms of antiretroviral treatment as prevention, particularly post-exposure prophylaxis (PEP), already routinely provided by the NHS.

The courts' decision (in the High Court and in the Court of Appeal) provided legal basis to some very important claims: that PrEP is a form of *treatment* (as it works after transmission has occurred to avoid viral replication); that specialised commissioning includes treatment (which includes prevention); and that the NHS could work concurrently with Local Authorities on matters of public health.

At the appeal that followed, the Court of Appeal judges commented especially on the separation of prevention from care in the NHS reform:

Sadly, it seems to follow that bureaucratic squabbles about apportionment of responsibility will be the inevitable consequence of the Lansley [Health Care Act 2012] reforms. (National Aids Trust v NHS England 2016, 46, Appeal)

Some of the participants in my study have commented, in confidence, that the court case was indeed something that the NHS welcomed, possibly even actively sought, as a way to resolve the ambiguities of the 2012 Health and Social Care reform. Yet, the rocky road of PrEP in England did not end with the courts' decision. There was no immediate reversal of the U-turn and, and it wasn't until the spring of 2020 that the English NHS would start providing PrEP services.

11.4   Discussion and Conclusion

What I have presented so far is my partial view of the story. Aspects of it, such as the initial resistances to PrEP from some community groups, echo the broader readings of PrEP in social science literature as an instance of biomedicalisation of prevention. The difficulties encountered in implementing PrEP as such a new (and expensive) prevention technology can perhaps, however, be read also in an additional light.

The English controversy touched upon three important dimensions of the political life of PrEP. Firstly, specific constructions of risk and responsibility have been pitted against one another in the *moral domain* of PrEP, as an intervention mainly aimed at

MSM. In this domain, PrEP users (potential, imagined, actual) have been configured both as epitomes of the responsible and self-caring individual or—on the contrary—as reckless individuals uninterested in condoms and careless about STIs other than HIV (Holt 2015; Jaspal and Nerlich 2017; Williamson et al. 2019). This was the domain, for example, of progressive *versus* conservative UK media, but also the moral grounds delineated by participants in a number of qualitative studies looking at ideas about PrEP in the UK (and other contexts in the global North, such as the USA) (Young et al. 2014; Jaspal and Nerlich 2017; Pawson and Grov 2018; Williamson et al. 2019). PrEP has thus re-introduced important issues of moral value that have characterised previous HIV responses and fuelled national and international political engagement by (largely) gay men pushing back against claims that PrEP would increase sexual risk-taking and 'promiscuity'.

Secondly, pro-PrEP media and community publications, activists' and clinicians' collaborations in documentaries, events, conferences, and in some social science literature are evidence of the remarkable capacity of different communities to mobilise (once again) around HIV-related issues. Debates in this domain touch upon three current key interpretations of PrEP: first, PrEP as sexual liberation or revolution (freeing sex from the spectre of HIV and affording new pleasures and intimacies, especially in otherwise marginalised sexual spaces and across the HIV positive/negative sero-divide) (Grace et al. 2018; Martinez-Lacabe 2019); second, PrEP as a collaborative community and scientific triumph (a magic bullet that can eliminate HIV, a second antiretroviral revolution after the historical discoveries of effective HIV treatment); and, third, PrEP as an explicit commitment (embodied in the possibility of national PrEP programmes) to the health of sexual minorities (particularly gay and transgender) in the form of a new investment in HIV prevention, hence a form of inclusive health citizenship (Paparini et al. 2018).

Thirdly, the NHS controversy, culminating in a court case in which clinical evidence was used strategically, has shown how issues of remit between prevention and treatment are truly tangled in the English health system as a result of government reform. Moreover, linked questions of cost-effectiveness have highlighted the broader politics of evidence—in this case the ways in which clinical trials are designed and used to portray the 'real-world' impact of pharmaceutical interventions—from debates around 'risk compensation' (whether PrEP users will change their sexual practices and prevention strategies in ways that will alter the epidemiological landscape), to the mechanics of PrEP provision (e.g. feasibility, acceptability, service design, uptake, user adherence). Immediate examples of these are cost-effectiveness models and what they index (Paparini et al. 2019), but PrEP commissioning papers or clinical guidelines all offer evidence of these various tensions and the assumptions and values that guide public health policy.

The PrEP controversy thus makes visible the NHS as a complex, 'multivalent' network of actors (Roy 2017, p. 14) which is, concurrently, a site of co-production of potentially profitable knowledge (clinical evidence) and of political and moral values (state-citizen interactions). In creating a barrier in this case, NHS England has thus further highlighted questions about PrEP as an example of the broader tensions between private interests (such as those of pharmaceutical companies) and public health.

Controversy, as an analytical device, creates a space in which 'the deliberations as to what constitutes evidence, and the social contingencies of science-based actions' (Rhodes et al. 2018, p. 260) may become more explicit. For example, in debates about PrEP commissioning and cost-effectiveness, any assumptions about who is 'at risk enough' to benefit from PrEP, who should be eligible and targeted, how many should be treated to see an epidemiological shift (and a return on investment) were incrementally built on the logics (e.g. about HIV incidence or adherence) pertaining to clinical research in the PROUD trial.

The epidemiological and biomedical apparatus that supports the development of new interventions such as PrEP is thus broadly situated in public research (for PROUD as well as for the iPrEx and IPERGAY trials). Furthermore, it is only through a long-established network of collaborations between activists, clinicians and an extensive infrastructure of public health surveillance, that something like a *risk citizenship*, a constituency of future PrEP users, patients-in-waiting who would benefit from PrEP (or be harmed by its absence), could emerge. These same citizens have been agitating *for* PrEP and *against* the NHS since 2016.

The emergence of the use of pharmaceuticals for public health prevention thus alter the relationship between particular forms of clinical and epidemiological research (in this case, a PrEP randomised-controlled trial), and their relationships to health policy. The interruption in this relationship that the NHS controversy represents has made evident the ways which moral, political and material tensions can create new constituencies that are at once co-produced *and* excluded by the state. The emergence of PrEP as a biomedical prevention technology has been mired in polarised international discussions between clinicians, PrEP users, activists, researchers, drug manufacturers and policymakers for the last decade or so. I have highlighted here different moral and political domains of significant debate.

PrEP, perhaps more than previous HIV prevention strategies, both reveals and extends the important nexus between science, politics, and profit. In deciding to refuse and delay PrEP provision, the English NHS has opened up PrEP for analysis in new ways. By having to justify its position, by enlivening public debate, and by sparking substantial community responses, the NHS controversy has revealed some of the complex inner workings of the political life of HIV prevention technologies.

Funding and Acknowledgements   The study was funded by the European Research Council ERC CoG 617930, with additional funding from the Independent Social Research Foundation. I would like to thank all the people who agreed to have discussions with me during this study. I wish to thank the editors of this volume for their help. I would also like to thank Vinh-Kim Nguyen, Julie Castro, Ryan Whitacre, Christophe Broqua, Lucille Gallardo, Christopher Zraunig, Lesley Doyal, Hakan Seckinelgin, Thomas L. and Aileen Clarke for ideas and comments on different drafts of this paper.

References

AHF. (2011, December 16). *AHF slams Gilead "HIV prevention pill" FDA application*. Retrieved May 21, 2020, from https://www.aidshealth.org/2011/12/ahf-slams-gilead-hiv-prevention-pill-fda-application/.

AHF. (2016, January 8). *Gilead premieres HIV PrEP party drug ad*. Retrieved May 21, 2020, from https://www.aidshealth.org/2016/01/gilead-premieres-hiv-prep-party-drug-ad/.

Cairns, G. P., Race, K., & Goicochea, P. (2016). PrEP: Controversy, agency and ownership. *Journal of the International AIDS Society, 19*(7 (Suppl 6)). https://doi.org/10.7448/ias.19.7.21120.

Charlton, V. (2019). NICE and fair? Health technology assessment policy under the UK's National Institute for health and care excellence, 1999–2018. *Health Care Analysis*, 1–35. https://doi.org/10.1007/s10728-019-00381-x.

Davies, A. (2015, June 16). *£200m cuts to public health: The situation is getting serious*. Retrieved May 21, 2020, from https://www.nuffieldtrust.org.uk/news-item/200m-cuts-to-public-health-the-situation-is-getting-serious.

Dean, T. J. S. (2015). Mediated intimacies: Raw sex, Truvada, and the biopolitics of chemoprophylaxis. *Sexualities, 18*(1–2), 224–246.

Easton, D. (1959). Political anthropology. *Biennial Review of Anthropology, 1*, 210–262. Retrieved January 30, 2020, from www.jstor.org/stable/2949205.

Giami, A., & Perrey, C. (2012). Transformations in the medicalization of sex: HIV prevention between discipline and biopolitics. *Journal of Sex Research, 49*(4), 353–361. https://doi.org/10.1080/00224499.2012.665510.

Glazek, C. (2013, September 30). Why is no one on the first treatment to prevent H.I.V.? *New Yorker*. Retrieved May 21, 2020, from https://www.newyorker.com/tech/annals-of-technology/why-is-no-one-on-the-first-treatment-to-prevent-h-i-v.

Grace, D., Jollimore, J., MacPherson, P., Strang, M. J. P., & Tan, D. H. S. (2018). The pre-exposure prophylaxis-stigma paradox: Learning from Canada's first wave of PrEP users. *AIDS Patient Care and STDs, 32*(1), 24–30. https://doi.org/10.1089/apc.2017.0153.

Grant, R. M., Lama, J. R., Anderson, P. L., McMahan, V., Liu, A. Y., Vargas, L., et al. (2010). Preexposure chemoprophylaxis for HIV prevention in men who have sex with men. *The New England Journal of Medicine, 363*(27), 2587–2599.

Greenhalgh, H., & Cookson, C. (2017, January 4). The 'final nail in the coffin' for aids? *The Financial Times*. Retrieved May 21, 2020, from https://www.ft.com/content/24fc5ba6-c912-11e6-9043-7e34c07b46ef.

HIVPlusMag.com Contributor. (2015, June 24). *Op-Ed: 10 worst offenses of AIDS healthcare Foundation's Michael Weinstein*. Retrieved May 21, 2020, from https://www.hivplusmag.com/opinion/2015/06/24/op-ed-10-worst-offenses-aids-healthcare-foundations-michael-weinstein.

Hodson, M., (2016, March 24). *It's time for PrEP to be made available for those who need it*. Retrieved May 21, 2020, from https://www.gmfa.org.uk/blog/its-time-for-prep-to-be-made-available-for-those-who-need-it.

Holt, M. (2015). Configuring the users of new HIV-prevention technologies: The case of HIV pre-exposure prophylaxis. *Culture, Health & Sexuality, 17*(4), 428–439.

Jaspal, R., & Nerlich, B. (2017). Polarised press reporting about HIV prevention: Social representations of pre-exposure prophylaxis in the UK press. *Health (London, England), 21*(5), 478–497. https://doi.org/10.1177/1363459316649763.

Kippax, S., & Stephenson, N. (2012). Beyond the distinction between biomedical and social dimensions of HIV prevention through the lens of a social public health. *American Journal of Public Health, 102*(5), 789–799. https://doi.org/10.2105/AJPH.2011.300594.

Lucas, M. (2014, April 14). *Op-Ed: The danger in calling PrEP a "party drug"*. Retrieved May 21, 2020, from https://www.out.com/news-opinion/2014/04/14/op-ed-danger-calling-prep-party-drug.

Making Sense Making Sense of HIV at 30. (2013, June 12–14). *The achievements and challenges of thirty years of AIDS activism. A Cumberland Lodge residential conference summary report.* Retrieved May 21, 2020, from https://www.cumberlandlodge.ac.uk/read-watch-listen/making-sense-hiv-30-achievements-and-challenges-thirty-years-aids-activism.

Martinez-Lacabe, A. (2019). The non-positive antiretroviral gay body: The biomedicalisation of gay sex in England. *Culture, Health & Sexuality, 21*(10), 1117–1130. https://doi.org/10.1080/13691058.2018.1539772.

McCormack, S., Dunn, D. T., Desai, M., Dolling, D. I., Gafos, M., Gilson, R., et al. (2016). Pre-exposure prophylaxis to prevent the acquisition of HIV-1 infection (PROUD): Effectiveness results from the pilot phase of a pragmatic open-label randomised trial. *The Lancet, 387*(10013), 53–60. https://doi.org/10.1016/s0140-6736(15)00056-2.

Molina, J.-M., Capitant, C., Spire, B., Pialoux, G., Cotte, L., Charreau, I., et al. (2015). On-demand Preexposure prophylaxis in men at high risk for HIV-1 infection. *New England Journal of Medicine, 373*(23), 2237–2246. https://doi.org/10.1056/NEJMoa1506273.

NAT. (2016, March 22). *PrEP – What went wrong? What should happen? NAT Blog.* Retrieved May 21, 2020, from https://www.nat.org.uk/blog/prep-what-went-wrong-what-should-happen.

National AIDS Trust v NHS Commissioning Board. (2016) *EWHC 2005 (Admin).* Retrieved May 21, 2020, from https://www.judiciary.uk/judgments/national-aids-trust-v-nhs-england/.

Nguyen, V.-K., Bajos, N., Dubois-Arber, F., O'Malley, J., & Pirkle, C. M. (2011). Remedicalizing an epidemic: From HIV treatment as prevention to HIV treatment is prevention. *AIDS, 25*(3), 291–293. https://doi.org/10.1097/QAD.0b013e3283402c3e.

NHS England. (2016, March 21). *News: Update on commissioning and provision of pre exposure prophylaxis (PREP) for HIV prevention.* Retrieved May 21, 2020, from https://www.england.nhs.uk/2016/03/prep/.

Paparini, S., Nutland, W., Rhodes, T., Nguyen, V.-K., & Anderson, J. (2018). DIY HIV prevention: Formative qualitative research with men who have sex with men who source PrEP outside of clinical trials. *PLoS One, 13*(8), e0202830.

Paparini, S., Whitacre, R., & Nguyen, V.-K. (2019). *Modelling risk behaviours? The influence of behavioural risk variables in calculations of the cost-effectiveness of oral PrEP in the UK and US.* AIDS impact 14th international conference, London, United Kingdom, 29–31 July 2019.

Pawson, M., & Grov, C. (2018). 'It's just an excuse to slut around': Gay and bisexual mens' constructions of HIV pre-exposure prophylaxis (PrEP) as a social problem. *Sociology of Health & Illness, 40*(8), 1391–1403. https://doi.org/10.1111/1467-9566.12765.

Platell, A. (2015, February 28). Platell's people: Why should WE pay for gays to have unsafe sex? *Daily Mail.* Retrieved May 21, 2020, from https://www.dailymail.co.uk/debate/article-2973020/PLATELL-S-PEOPLE-pay-gays-unsafe-sex.html.

Rhodes, T., Lancaster, K., Harris, M., & Treloar, C. (2018). Evidence-making controversies: The case of hepatitis C treatment and the promise of viral elimination. *Critical Public Health, 29*(3), 260–273. https://doi.org/10.1080/09581596.2018.1459475.

Roy, V. (2017). *The Financialization of a Cure: A Political Economy of Biomedical Innovation, Pricing, and Public Health* (doctoral thesis). University of Cambridge. https://doi.org/10.17863/CAM.13671.

Siddons, E. (2016, July 8). Protesting for life-saving HIV drugs. *i-D.* Retrieved January 21, 2020, from http://i-d.vice.com/en_gb/article/protesting-for-life-saving-hiv-drugs.

Strudwick, P. (2017, February 25). Meet the man who stopped thousands of people becoming HIV-positive. *Buzzfeed News.* Retrieved May 21, 2020, from https://www.buzzfeed.com/patrickstrudwick/meet-the-man-who-stopped-thousands-of-people-becoming-hiv-po.

Thomann, M. (2018). On December 1, 2015, sex changes. Forever': Pre-exposure prophylaxis and the pharmaceuticalisation of the neoliberal sexual subject. *Global Public Health, 13*(8), 997–1006. https://doi.org/10.1080/17441692.2018.1427275.

Tuller, D. (2011, October 10). Questions on tactic to prevent H.I.V. *New York Times.* Retrieved May 21, 2020, from https://www.nytimes.com/2011/10/11/health/11hiv.html.

UK Government and Parliament. (2016). *Petition: Make pre-exposure prophylaxis (prep) immediately available on the NHS*. Retrieved May 21, 2020, from https://petition.parliament.uk/archived/petitions/113891.

Williamson, I., Papaloukas, P., Jaspal, R., & Lond, B. (2019). 'There's this glorious pill': Gay and bisexual men in the English midlands navigate risk responsibility and pre-exposure prophylaxis. *Critical Public Health, 29*(5), 560–571. https://doi.org/10.1080/09581596.2018.1497143.

Young, I., Flowers, P., & McDaid, L. M. (2014). Barriers to uptake and use of pre-exposure prophylaxis (PrEP) among communities most affected by HIV in the UK: Findings from a qualitative study in Scotland. *BMJ Open, 4*(11), e005717. https://doi.org/10.1136/bmjopen-2014-005717.

Young, I., Flowers, P., & McDaid, L. (2016). Can a pill prevent HIV? Negotiating the biomedicalisation of HIV prevention. *Sociology of Health & Illness, 38*(3), 411–425. https://doi.org/10.1111/1467-9566.12372.

Young, I., Davis, M., Flowers, P., & McDaid, L. M. (2019). Navigating HIV citizenship: Identities, risks and biological citizenship in the treatment as prevention era. *Health, Risk & Society, 21*(1–2), 1–16.

Chapter 12
Implementation Science or 'Show' Trial? England's PrEP Impact Study

Catherine Dodds

12.1 Introduction

The efficacy and effectiveness of Pre-Exposure Prophylaxis (PrEP) was first established globally through successive randomised (Grant et al. 2010; Molina et al. 2015) and non-randomised trials (McCormack et al. 2016) focussed primarily on its capacity to reduce the risk of sexual transmission among men who have sex with men (MSM). Alongside the development of HIV Treatment as Prevention over the past two decades, this work has underpinned a triumphal global narrative about how preventive uses of HIV antiretroviral treatments would mean new HIV infections would soon be a thing of the past. However, just as we witnessed with the introduction of HIV antiretroviral treatment in the 1990s, evidence that PrEP worked did not mean that accessible services would be implemented to reach all those in need.

This chapter focuses on how PrEP policy in England has played out vis-à-vis the launch of England's PrEP Impact trial in 2017 as the world's 'largest single PrEP implementation trial'. It purportedly aimed to address 'significant outstanding implementation questions that should be answered prior to using PrEP in a sustained way on a substantial scale in England' (NHS England 2016). These included: understanding how many sexual health clinic attendees need PrEP, willingness to take it, and duration—in order to inform an orderly roll-out of PrEP services in England (Public Health England and Chelsea and Westminster Hospital NHS Foundation Trust 2020). On paper, the PrEP Impact Trial existed in order to provide answers about how to best provide PrEP through England's health service, by filling an apparent gap between existing scientific knowledge and practical application.

C. Dodds (✉)
School for Policy Studies, University of Bristol, Bristol, UK
e-mail: catherine.dodds@bristol.ac.uk

© Springer Nature Switzerland AG 2021
S. Bernays et al. (eds.), *Remaking HIV Prevention in the 21st Century*, Social Aspects of HIV 5, https://doi.org/10.1007/978-3-030-69819-5_12

Behind the scenes, however, there were other reasons for the initiation of the Impact trial: the trial rhetoric offered an expedient, low cost solution to a political deadlock. This chapter offers first-hand insights into these backstage processes, revealing how the questionable motives of the PrEP Impact trial have resulted in troubling contradictions throughout its progress, which themselves create challenging implications for future PrEP policy in England.

12.2 Trials and Tribulations

Social scientists of medicine have pointed to profound challenges arising from a knowledge hierarchy that has prioritised the randomised control trial (RCT) as the pinnacle of acceptable health evidence-making (Wahlberg and McGoey 2007; Deaton and Cartwright 2018). This critique argues that the persistence of RCTs as the 'gold standard' of knowledge creation fails to recognise the ways in which strictly standardised conditions silence the complex social dynamics within which all health technologies are ultimately embedded. HIV provides exemplary evidence to support this critique, given the widely demonstrated inadequacy of focussing disproportionately on the outcomes of experimental research regimes to address an epidemic defined by its complex and particularised social, political, moral and economic disparities (Fassin 2007; Kingori and Sariola 2015; Kippax and Stephenson 2016; Camlin and Seeley 2018). This body of work closely examines how 'evidence' and its mode of production (Rhodes and Lancaster 2019) often becomes entrenched in systems designed to protect and benefit the interests of those organising the trial, at the cost of producing meaningful learning outcomes. As such, the HIV response has been profoundly impacted by biomedicalisation that renders the 'social issues (both carried and revealed by AIDS) practically inexpressible' (Fassin 2007, p. 189).

In response to these critiques of knowledge production, the emergent field of *implementation science* might appear to be a remedy. Implementation research is meant to examine how new interventions or technologies that proved efficacious in the controlled setting of the RCT might be made effective in 'real world' contexts. 'The basic intent of implementation research is to understand not only what is and isn't working, but how and why implementation is going right or wrong, and testing approaches to improve it' (Peters et al. 2013). This kind of approach is meant to pick up on contextual cues (including process issues, but also social inhibitors) which can then be acted upon in real time through pragmatic research design. Therefore, good implementation research is intended to be reliant upon open and iterative learning with rich data collected from stakeholders and users across the life of the project with regard not only to medical technologies, but also the messier processes and procedures of access and activation which are impacted by social interaction, diverse cultures of expectation and exchange, systems of meaning and structures of inequality.

However, the PrEP Impact Trial was not designed in a way that could enable it to promote this sort of advance through iterative learning. Perhaps this is because practitioners of implementation science can find it difficult to escape the habits of power and control that are embedded in the scientific knowledge hierarchy. In addition, these habits may have become entrenched as the trial practitioners sought to obliviate the trial's own genesis, given it was hastily developed to resolve a financial impasse between key health policy agencies. It could also be the case that the trial was simply a means of rationing access to the costly medicines being used for PrEP (at a time when they were still under patent), while funding for sexual health services across England simultaneously faced serious decline (Nagington and Sandset 2020). In examining these possibilities, this study provides evidence that the PrEP Impact trial was less an implementation trial and more of a 'show trial', a term traditionally associated with criminal or political trials that are arranged to satisfy public demands or purge opposition, rather than to achieve its nominal purpose.

12.3 Methods

Using my longstanding network of professional HIV contacts in England, I generated an opportunistic (and subsequently snowballed) list of key stakeholders to invite for interview between May and August 2019 near the mid-point of the Impact trial (see Table 12.1). I knew many across years of working relationships, including membership of United4PrEP—an activist coalition demanding government provision of PrEP. I am therefore embedded in the processes that I am analysing.

The invitation to take part was emailed by a research administrator, and included information explaining the aim of undertaking a policy analysis of the Impact's political and social context. Those who agreed to take part included: key PrEP activists, some of whom had paid roles connected to PrEP activism and others who did not (including those representing women, people in the sex work industry and Black African heterosexuals); senior staff in national and local HIV

Table 12.1 Roles of potential and actual study participants

Role description	Invited ($n=$)	Interviewed ($n=$)
Clinician/IMPACT trialist	4	1
Community activist/organiser/HIV organisation (paid and unpaid)	12	9
Participating clinic staff	2	1
Public Health England (PHE) staff	4	0
Local authority staff/elected council member	7	2
NHS England (NHSE) staff	2	0
Other	2	0
Total	33	13

organisations; and Local Authority commissioners of sexual health services. Many study participants were members of the trial's Community Advisory Board, alongside one member of the trial's Programme Oversight Board. Trial clinicians and PHE/NHSE staff were invited to take part but almost universally declined, saying things like: 'Sharing personal views at this point could place me in a conflicted position.' In addition, as fieldwork got underway, tensions had been reignited between NHSE and Local Authorities regarding proposals to expand the trial, making it a 'sensitive time' according to a further invitee. While interviews with more clinical and health infrastructure stakeholders may have provided wider perspectives, the data from this sample offer sharp, front-line insights into the drivers and responses to PrEP policy in England unavailable elsewhere. Although it is important to acknowledge the limited account afforded by these data, the acute reticence among particular groups to engage in the study indicates why investigating this trial in light of its political and social contexts (rather than from a hegemonic, scientific perspective) is essential. The matter of anonymisation was initially left open so that participants could exercise a choice to be named—however, as it turned out, very few wanted to be named, so the decision has been taken to anonymise all quotes. This study was granted ethical approval by the School for Policy Studies' Ethics Committee at the University of Bristol.

12.4   Why Was a 'Show' Trial Needed?

Following the earliest efficacy studies that showed PrEP worked, a wide array of volunteer PrEP activists self-organised, finding unique ways to disseminate unbiased information and to strategically build demand for public provision. These efforts were particularly notable among those working in sex industries, within networks of gay men, and among others with a particular stake in preventing HIV. A working group on PrEP had already been established by the National Health Service in England (NHSE) as early as September 2014 to work out costings and service design in anticipation of the results from the PROUD trial. So the focus of all of these volunteer efforts from many quarters was to provide information and support to help meet an interim gap in reliable information sources, to sustain support for public provision, and to support those who were already privately buying PrEP online.[1]

There was therefore a universal expectation among all stakeholders that national roll-out would take place as soon as England's own PROUD trial had concluded. However, on 21 March 2016 NHSE made a surprise announcement that commissioning PrEP was outside its powers. They argued that because the 2012 Health and Social Care Act had conferred responsibility on England's 343 elected Local

---

[1]Notable organisations involved nationally and internationally include: Porn4Prep, I Want PrEP Now, Prepster, ActUp London, Sophia Forum and United4PrEP.

Authorities (comprising boroughs, counties and municipalities) for public health services, NHSE said they were not in a legal position to take responsibility for PrEP provision. This policy backdrop set the stage for a serious impasse between Local Authorities and NHSE over who was responsible for considering provision of these costly medicines which remained under patent, and their associated clinical services—for the purposes of HIV prevention. It was a conflict that once again enabled a space for divergent accounts of morality to be debated in public, academic and policy narratives, frequently playing on supposed uncertainties in the PrEP evidence base (Sandset and Wieringa 2019).

The National AIDS Trust took NHSE to court, and NHSE's refusal to consider PrEP funding was overturned on appeal (Azad et al. 2018). However, this 'victory' was rapidly followed by defeat when, in late 2016, NHSE's annual review of treatments needing specialised commissioning did not approve PrEP. Thus, despite widespread clinical and community agreement that PrEP would play an important role in HIV prevention in England, the funding impasse remained. The PrEP Impact trial emerged as means of temporarily resolving uncertainty about whether any publicly funded PrEP could be accessed by those who needed it. Participants in my research overwhelmingly and independently identified that the trial was primarily set up to enable the legal use of generic formulations of medications (tenofovir and emtricitabine) rather than patented Truvada, thereby reducing PrEP's costs.

> [the decision to run the Impact study was driven by] the impact of budget. And it was the expedient way to deliver this innovation, umm. . .within a budget they could manage. Doing it under the umbrella of a research project allowed them to use generic drugs, which obviously is a fraction of the price of the real PrEP, and therefore allowed them to enrol a much larger number than they could have done for the budget they felt they could manage. (HIV clinician) #11

> If they were going to call it a trial, then they were able to use generic drugs instead of branded drugs. (Member of staff in local HIV organisation) #4

> The kind-of activist discussion was: "If it's a trial you can get generic drugs and what we need is access, and if this is the offer on the table then we should take it". (PrEP advocate) #7

Having been widely understood from the outset as the only opportunity of getting anyone on to publicly-funded PrEP in the near future, most stakeholders from the HIV sector said they and their colleagues had initially regarded their role in sustaining the pretence of this 'show trial' as a fair trade off for PrEP access. This open secret was said to have been widely acknowledged among those in PrEP activist networks who had closely followed events.

> Nobody really wanted a trial, and nobody could really see—actually, no, that's not true. Some people could see there will be some benefit in terms of the objectives of the trial, but to be frank, it was a just a vehicle: to enable as many people as possible to access PrEP in the quickest possible way. (Member of staff in national HIV organisation) #8

When asked what they felt the ultimate outcome or legacy of the Impact Trial was likely to be, half of all participants felt that the single gain provided by the study was that it had been the only strategy for enabling tens of thousands of people in England to get PrEP without having to pay for it privately.

> I think undoubtedly it will have stopped hundreds of people sero-converting, in spite of all of its problems and it has got PrEP to lots of folk. Is it good enough? No. But I think that's its legacy, other than that I can't really think of [its legacy] to tell you the truth. (Member of staff in local HIV organisation) #9

However, despite several respondents acknowledging their initial attraction to this short-term solution, many described how their perspective on the value of this expedient solution had changed as the trial progressed. At the half-way stage of the Impact trial, when our interviews were taking place, many said they were no longer able to keep up the pretence that this was a real trial, because the duplicity had pushed them towards burnout. These participants said they felt increasingly debased by the particular performance required by the trial narrative as a study to support and inform future roll-out, when the reality was that it had only ever been a managerialist mechanism designed to mitigate costs.

> We have for the longest time been colluding with each other that we need this trial for these reasons and the reasons really are about finance. It's that kind of disingenuous, dishonest process that has absolutely worn me down. (Sexual health commissioner for a Local Authority) #12

Those most directly involved in trial governance described being surprised by the 'rules of engagement' during formal trial meetings, including unspoken hierarchies of power which aimed to silence those who might pull back the curtain between the trial's front-stage and back-stage.

> One of my key questions [during official trial meetings] has always been what does he or she think? Does he or she know that this is a crock of shit? Could we have that conversation privately? I've come to realise we can never have it publicly. (Member of staff in national HIV organisation) #5

While most continued to adhere to 'rules' governing what should and should not be publicly expressed about the true nature of the trial, three interviewees (each involved in different ways) said they had openly critiqued the trial's façade. In each case, these individuals mentioned the personal costs of raising their concerns within and beyond the trial's own structures. While the conclusions of this chapter emphasise structural and population-level implications of this trial, the personal and intrapersonal toll for advocates and others working closely in and around PrEP Impact was at times considerable. Most of the stakeholders interviewed for this study had been closely involved in England's HIV landscape for a number of years, so they are not strangers to the political realities of compromise and pragmatism. However, most described the Impact trial as a particularly troubling and exhausting conflict zone which served to further alienate those who hold different understandings of what constitutes valuable 'evidence' from one another, while simultaneously driving wedges between stakeholder groups, organisations and individuals.

12.5 The Trial as an Expression of Power

As one would expect of a clinical trial, governance and oversight were held centrally by those in PrEP Impact's uppermost structures (including the trial team and senior figures in Public Health England and NHSE who chaired the Programme Oversight Board—or POB—which managed the trial's externally-facing narrative). Framed as an 'implementation trial' to help answer real world questions of uptake and access in order to test and inform future service design, around half of interviewees pointed out that the inflexibility of the trial structure meant that no space was created for iterative learning. It appears that the sanctity of following prescribed process, inherited from practices common in RCTs rather than implementation studies, seriously inflected this project. Stakeholders described how their recommendations to: better promote Impact to diverse audiences, help simplify patient management, support the sharing of live information about clinic spaces, monitor the impact of PrEP on the mental health and wellbeing of diverse users, and to better support the user experience, were ignored. Community stakeholders reported gaining the impression from the outset that their suggestions were regarded as meddlesome and irrelevant. Some reflected on other implementation studies where the relationships between triallists and their stakeholders were more engaging, ongoing and meaningful, with inbuilt opportunities to implement iterative learning throughout a trial's progress.

> [The trial leads] could have had community representation, and they chose to keep that separate as a Community Advisory Board [CAB]. (HIV clinician) #11

While this interviewee said that the trial team had tried to engage with community stakeholders, all other interviewees who sat on the trial's CAB consistently described it as a distinctly arms-length mechanism for disseminating updates from the centre. Some felt the CAB was a site for playing out community disputes, and had become consumed by 'busy-work'—rather than having their diverse forms of expertise meaningfully valued and incorporated. It remains unclear the extent to which the POB might have played a role in establishing these patterns, and to what extent it functioned on a different premise to the trial team.

A prevalent theme from the majority of interviewees was that those leading the trial sought to enforce the concept of *data integrity* as a disciplining tool, arguing that all trial outcomes would be tainted if strict adherence to the protocol was spoiled.[2] The argument that strict control of data flow was essential to maintain its integrity was, according to many, a key means through which the trial committee centralised its power by restricting access to meaningful interim data. What they described instead was Impact's own failure to function as an implementation trial, because it had disabled its own capacity to learn iteratively, study its own processes and procedures, adapt accordingly and study the ensuing effects. By the half-point

---

[2]A few of those interviewed did note that a change in the clinical leadership part way through the study had brought some renewed opportunity for dialogue.

stage of the trial, information about the demographic features of trial participants remained strictly confidential and cynicism was widespread among almost all of those interviewed. A high proportion of participants expressed considerable concern that it would only be at the end of the trial that it would become apparent how few people other than men who have sex with men (MSM) had been enrolled (with concerns about limited diversity even among this group), meaning the trial had curtailed its own capacity to learn what might have been done differently in order to understand and best meet the diverse needs of potential PrEP users.

Most interviewees drew links between controls on data-sharing and the trial protocol's stated intent not to promote PrEP, but instead to use a non-interventionist trial design that assessed and offered PrEP to eligible individuals already attending sexual health clinics. As a result—they argued—marginalised MSM, Black African migrant men and women, trans people, and workers in the sex industry remained at increased HIV risk because of their experience of barriers in accessing traditional sexual health services. There was concern that because many were not tuned in to the social media channels of most PrEP activism, it was even less likely that marginalised people would find out about PrEP—even despite the considerable efforts of dedicated volunteer sex workers, women and trans people who sought to help overcome these types of obstacles. Ultimately, what concerned these interviewees was that the 'show trial' would ultimately broaden those same gaps because of the trial team's determination to only enable access for existing users of sexual health services, while simultaneously not supporting any form of promotion.

> We need to understand what Black-African women need to uptake this, so we need to build that into the trial, it wasn't about that. It was like, "All communities that are at risk will understand their risk in the same way". (PrEP advocate) #2

Despite early assurances of 'ringfenced' trial allocations for groups at high risk of HIV beyond MSM, at the trial half-way point participants broadly agreed that the ringfencing strategy had failed, and that this was in part because the trial did not allocate funds for campaigns to support the promotion of information about PrEP or for trial recruitment.

> For those other communities we needed some investment and that wasn't done, that's a huge failing of the trial. (PrEP advocate) #2

Outside of the trial, Public Health England subsequently funded a few community groups to provide PrEP awareness interventions for targeted populations through its HIV Prevention Innovation Fund. Some other community organisations provided information about PrEP and the Impact trial from their own resources. However, stakeholders made it clear that these piecemeal arrangements did not amount to anything like the required national coordination or scale to ensure that news of PrEP's availability through the trial might reach a sufficiently diverse range of people in need in ways that would help ensure that the sample it gained could adequately and fully inform future services across England. Despite repeating their concerns at successive CAB meetings, stakeholders were deeply concerned that the sharing of trial evidence that had been promised was subsequently sequestered. This meant that collective learning would be delayed until the formal publication of results, long after such lessons could pragmatically be implemented into service plans.

> Is PrEP reaching the people that need it now, is it reaching people in their diversity? No. Is this trial going to lead to routine commissioning? Not necessarily. Is it gonna lead to equitable access? Almost certainly not, because they are I think going to conclude from this trial that some people just don't need or want PrEP. (PrEP advocate) #7

Ultimately, most stakeholders expressed frustration that despite the time and energy they had committed to supporting and enabling the Impact trial, they had come to realise it had been organised as a means of rationing PrEP demand via the trial's highly managerialist structures. At the outset, maximum trial allocations were dispensed to each of the 139 clinic sites, and 20% of the trial's 10,000 spaces were ringfenced for members of high-risk groups beyond MSM. Early demand was predictably strongest in urban locations with high MSM density, and as trial sites started to open in late 2017 some allocations filled rapidly. A new section of the trial website was quickly developed with the intention of directing (primarily MSM) users to clinics that still had available spaces for different user groups. In the summer of 2018, the 'non MSM' ringfence was dropped from 20% to 10% due to purportedly low demand among those who were not cis-gendered men who have sex with men. Some asserted that the posture of restraint about trial recruitment and promotion was a purposeful tactic to rein in spending not only for the trial itself, but as a means of rationing demand for the commissioned service that might follow.

> Places for getting homosexual men [were getting] filled up so then the solution was to say, "Well we overestimated the number of women that might use PrEP". No you didn't because you didn't estimate, you just came up with a number. It was never an estimate and it was never calculated properly. (PrEP advocate) #7

There was a real concern that this focus on demand management had not only pitted people against one another within the HIV sector, but among communities in need.

> I know there were people who are involved in the process who are quite annoyed. If a gay man who is really genuinely at risk goes somewhere and it's full. And then you say, "oh, we have 1000 places reserved for Blacks". And when they are not accepted, they are thinking, "it's not right. It's not right". I honestly think that inadvertently, they are really making people feel very bad. (Member of staff at a local HIV organisation) #4

A tiered set of inequalities had emerged, described by the participant above, with well-informed gay and bisexual men facing increasingly unpredictable access to trial places, accompanied by vanishingly low figures for more diverse men who have sex with men, and people having heterosexual sex. With so much ongoing change, community organisations and potential PrEP users they were supporting were increasingly unclear which clinics were accepting what categories of people into their remaining trial places.

Despite the strict expectations attached to the confidentiality of all trial data, it was notable during these interviews just how frequently some details and figures appeared to have leaked out among those on the CAB and those playing a role in other trial committees. However, such figures could never be formally acknowledged or built into future planning, they essentially only held 'hearsay' status.

> You know, only four percent of these places have been taken up by non-MSM people, and that's really crazy! (Member of staff at a local HIV organisation) #4

There was a lot of discontent about the inequalities of access that had become apparent through these informal knowledge networks.

> I think still a lot of people will have misunderstood it as a medical study [ie. RCT with placebo]. That inherently will have put so many communities off, particularly communities that often feel like they are not cared for and won't be cared for if the medical study is wrong. Particularly Black communities and even a lot of sex worker communities can feel like they'll all just be the lab rats. (PrEP advocate) #13.

> It was a trial that was designed for and about gay men, and particular gay men. (PrEP advocate) #7

This concern therefore added to many participants' disquiet about the ways in which the PrEP Impact trial had further entrenched existing bias in HIV prevention services towards urban, middle class white gay men who tend to disproportionately use the sexual health clinics through which the trial exclusively operated. During our interviews, participants had begun to predict how the failure to recruit and learn about PrEP needs amongst diverse populations would directly imprint itself onto future service design, built primarily around 'ideal users' who are already routinely attending sexual health services (Holt 2015; Young et al. 2020).

Adding to the complexity of this 'show trial' was NHSE's announcement that they would support additional medication costs that could enable the trial to expand first to 13,000 in June 2018, and then to 26,000 places in the spring of 2019 (NHS England n.d.). The latter announcement to double the trial size created significant conflicts with Local Authorities who carry responsibilities for running all of the sexual health clinics where the Impact trial was sited. Most balked at the match-funding needed to support the additional clinical caseloads and follow-on screening that would accompany trial expansion. Uneven and protracted negotiations ensued, with many local commissioners arguing that they could not afford the costs within a context of extensive funding cuts driven by a national politics of austerity. These conflicts were reported widely in the gay, local and national press, further compounding confusion about trial places for those who might want to enrol. Then, in the midst of the fieldwork for this study, on 5 July 2019, the NHS National Director of Special Commissioning released a letter via Twitter that said he was 'asking the trial researchers to support open ended additional places where any clinic and their local authority commissioner would like them' (Stewart 2019). Therefore, not only were the earlier attempts to ration trial places widely regarded as causing divisions and entrenching inequalities among those most impacted by HIV, but these calls for expansion then became a site for open conflict to be played out between NHSE and Local Authorities. These developments also raised questions about the inherent contradictions built into Impact's trial structure. Each time the NHSE made an unexpected announcement supporting trial expansion, this further deepened the rifts which had opened between these large institutional players. The vastly different working cultures between the highly centralised structures represented by Public Health England and the National Health Service, contrasted with hundreds of Local Authorities run by publicly-elected representatives came sharply into focus through the way the Impact trial had been managed.

> So privately [among local authority commissioners] for example, there is lots of, "We can never trust NHS England again". [. . .] there's been an ugly fraught process, but that will be its legacy. (Sexual health commissioner for a Local Authority) #12

This same individual described the impossible position in which they had been placed, being expected to gain approval for even more of their Local Authority's funds to support clinical provision for further trial expansion, while still having no access to interim trial data.

> I've got to take this back to a whole range of people and sell it, so throw me a fish for Christ's sake! Throw me something that can help me sell this back at base. (Sexual health commissioner for a Local Authority) #12

All participants expressed frustration about the continual conflicts between NHS and Local Authorities on responsibilities for additional running costs as the trial progressed and grew. The 'show trial' had been constructed in order to overcome conflicts about who would pay for PrEP but became the new location where that disagreement played out. Many participants took the view that the Impact trial was unable to resolve weaknesses caused by longer term disinvestment in sexual health service provision and HIV prevention, and that it could not be expected to resolve broader infrastructure challenges. The 'show' trial was devised as a means of squaring the circle, finding what appeared to be an ingenious way to keep down the costs of high-priced patent protected medicine by gaining legal access to generics instead. However, its carefully rationed access served to further entrench the structural determinants of health, which for many interviewees had become a more relevant issue than attempting to maintain the 'show' trial's façade.

> The Impact trial will finish with some limited data that will help us in our future planning and it's not going to solve the rest of the problems that still exist because of political and economic and cultural disinvestment in our sexual health services. (PrEP advocate) #1

> The reason why a lot of London clinics have not taken up the new places is because of capacity. So they don't have capacity in terms of seeing more patients. So I think that will be a kind of big impact. I think that, in terms of the trial itself, I think that one of the challenges they have is that they don't want to acknowledge some of the challenges they are facing. (Clinic staff member) #3

Some participants reflected on the way that these wider frustrations were ultimately directed into disputes over the machinations of the trial itself with the fall-out of these conflicts resonating across the sector. They described how this situation had dramatically increased internal competition between actors for funds, attention and recognition, thereby deflecting attention away from the under-resourced structures in which in which all actors were situated. All of this was understood to have resulted from careful PrEP rationing which had been crafted as part of the trial design. As a result of these combined factors, few of those interviewed expressed any confidence that the Impact trial could meet its goal of meaningfully shaping how England could deliver PrEP in the future.

> Interviewer: What kind of legacy will we end up with as a result of the Impact trial?
> Participant: In terms of what will we know?
> Interviewer: Sure.
> Participant: What will we know that we don't know now?
> Interviewer: Yes.
> Participant: I don't know, because it's difficult to… [long pause]… I'm really struggling with that question, I'm afraid, I really am.
> Interviewer: That's fine.
> Participant: I'm not sure how to answer that because there are still so many questions.
> (Sexual health commissioner in a Local Authority) #14

Most tended to agree with this sentiment, because in their view, Impact had neither pursued meaningful questions that would provide the answers that Local Authorities required for service design, nor had it shared any of what it had learned. In addition to this, along the way the trial's managerialist control functions had helped to sow discontent, distrust and conflict between groups were meant to be working towards the joint goal of HIV prevention.

12.6   The Impact Study and PrEP's Future in England

The PrEP Impact trial was framed as an implementation study but stakeholder accounts demonstrate the ways in which it is best regarded as a 'show' trial—concocted not as a genuine implementation study but an inherently flawed attempt to bypass conflicts between national and local government actors. While this compromise solution did enable access to generic PrEP for thousands who would have either had to pay for it privately or do without, even that element of the trial's success is mitigated by a range of associated harms.

Rather than celebrating the trial's 'gains', the majority of interviewees felt exhausted and personally complicit with a trial infrastructure that had actually served to deepen conflict and distrust between the very agencies who would need to co-commission the PrEP services of the future (NHSE alongside hundreds of Local Authorities), and also between some voluntary organisation actors. Furthermore, the vast majority of participants expressed profound concern that the implementation trial had actively functioned as a mechanism of healthcare rationing (Nagington and Sandset 2020), creating an expansion of barriers to PrEP's accessibility among the socially and economically marginalised. This trial was structured in ways that disabled many in need from learning about or receiving PrEP. The costs of the inequalities fostered by and woven into the fabric of PrEP provision in England through the Impact trial are inestimable. The feature of the trial that is most culpable for this state of affairs was its ongoing attachment to a hierarchy of evidence-making that prioritised process and 'purity' over functional outcomes.

Central to the stated outcomes of Impact was that it was meant to inform good commissioning practice when PrEP services were finally rolled out. To this end, in June 2018 the trial's Programme Oversight Board established a Short Term PrEP Commissioning Planning Group which was tasked with devising a set of recommendations for future PrEP Commissioning in England. These would be informed by trial outcomes and interim learning gained up to that point and shared for dissemination among key stakeholders. However, the report developed by that group was never allowed into the public domain. In July 2020, England's Department of Health and Social Care released budget and commissioning directions for Local Authorities to implement PrEP services in October 2020. The Short Term PrEP Commissioning Planning Group's report and recommendations, commissioned by the Impact oversight board and completed in 2018, remained unpublished until the end of October 2020—too late to be of use to planners.

With Local Authority sexual health commissioners expected to pull together a PrEP service in the 4 months between the release of commissioning directions and the conclusion of the Impact trial, there was no further sharing of insight from those holding the trial data during this short planning period. This is perhaps one of the most potent demonstrations of this trial's particular performance of the making of evidence from before the start of the trial to beyond its finish (Rhodes and Lancaster 2019). Rather than working in collaboration to share information that will benefit the design of immanent service, the evidence always remained in the hands of the actors closest to the centre of this show. Presumably that evidence will be packaged and prepared for future academic publication in esteemed scientific journals, but this does not meet the practical needs of planner and implementers who are rapidly having to design England's new PrEP service, with no functional insights to glean from the Impact trial. The only thing that has been made clear to current planners is that state-funded PrEP will still only be accessible to those already using sexual health clinics for the forseeable future. As with other 'show' trials, the final conclusions of the PrEP Impact trial will contain few surprises, and once all the final reports are written there is small chance of anything being done to address the way this trial has further entrenched structural injustices and inequalities in England's PrEP provision.

References

Azad, Y., Gold, D., & Smithson, K. (2018). *Going to law for prep: A case study from England* (poster). Presented at the international AIDS conference, National AIDS Trust, Amsterdam.

Camlin, C. S., & Seeley, J. (2018). Qualitative research on community experiences in large HIV research trials: What have we learned? *Journal of the International AIDS Society, 21*(S7), e25173. https://doi.org/10.1002/jia2.25173.

Deaton, A., & Cartwright, N. (2018). Understanding and misunderstanding randomized controlled trials. *Social Science & Medicine, 210*, 2–21. https://doi.org/10.1016/j.socscimed.2017.12.005.

Fassin, D. (2007). *When bodies remember: Experiences and politics of AIDS in South Africa.* Berkeley and Los Angeles: University of California Press.

Grant, R.M., Lama, J.R., Anderson, P.L., McMahan, V., Liu, A.Y., Vargas, L. et al. for the iPrEx study group. (2010). Preexposure chemoprophylaxis for HIV prevention in men who have sex with men. *New England Journal of Medicine, 363*(27), 2587–2599. https://doi.org/10.1056/NEJMoa1011205

Holt, M. (2015). Configuring the users of new HIV-prevention technologies: The case of HIV pre-exposure prophylaxis. *Culture, Health & Sexuality, 17*(4), 428–439.

Kingori, P., & Sariola, S. (2015). Museum of failed HIV research. *Anthropology & Medicine, 22*(3), 213–216. https://doi.org/10.1080/13648470.2015.1079302.

Kippax, S., & Stephenson, N. (2016). *Socialising the biomedical turn in HIV prevention*. London and New York: Anthem Press.

McCormack, S., Dunn, D. T., Desai, M., Dolling, D. I., Gafos, M., Gilson, R., et al. (2016). Pre-exposure prophylaxis to prevent the acquisition of HIV-1 infection (PROUD): Effectiveness results from the pilot phase of a pragmatic open-label randomised trial. *The Lancet, 387*(10013), 53–60. https://doi.org/10.1016/S0140-6736(15)00056-2.

Molina, J-M., Capitant, C., Spire, B., Pialoux, G., Cotte, L., Charreau, I., et al. for the ANRS IPERGAY Study Group. (2015). On-demand Preexposure prophylaxis in men at high risk for HIV-1 infection. *New England Journal of Medicine, 373*, 2237–2246.

Nagington, M., & Sandset, T. (2020). Putting the NHS England on trial: Uncertainty-as-power, evidence and the controversy of PrEP in England. *Medical Humanities*. https://doi.org/10.1136/medhum-2019-011780.

NHS England. (2016). *NHS England announces major extension of national HIV prevention programme with Public Health England and funding for ten new specialised treatments* [press release]. Retrieved August 21, 2020 www.england.nhs.uk/2016/12/hiv-prevention-pregramme/.

NHS England. (n.d.). *PrEP trial updates*. Retrieved July 13, 2020, from https://www.england.nhs.uk/commissioning/spec-services/npc-crg/blood-and-infection-group-f/f03/prep-trial-updates/.

Peters, D. H., Tran, N. T., Adam, T., & Alliance for Health Policy and Systems Research, World Health Organization (Eds.). (2013). *Implementation research in health: A practical guide*. Geneva: WHO.

Public Health England & Chelsea and Westminster Hospital NHS Foundation Trust. (2020). *PrEP impact trial: Trial protocol v6*.

Rhodes, T., & Lancaster, K. (2019). Evidence-making interventions in health: A conceptual framing. *Social Science and Medicine, 238*, 112488. https://doi.org/10.1016/j.socscimed.2019.112488.

Sandset, T., & Wieringa, S. (2019). Impure policies: Controversy in HIV prevention and the making of evidence. *Critical Policy Studies*. https://doi.org/10.1080/19460171.2019.1661865.

Stewart, J. (2019, July 5). *Letter to NAT, THT and prepster on PrEP access*. [Twitter] @NHSEngland. Retrieved August 19, 2020, from https://twitter.com/NHSEngland/status/1147170453586247680.

Wahlberg, A., & McGoey, L. (2007). An elusive evidence base: The construction and governance of randomized controlled trials. *BioSocieties, 2*, 1–10. https://doi.org/10.1017/S1745855207005017.

Young, I., Boydell, N., Patterson, C., Hilton, S., & McDaid, L. (2020). Configuring the PrEP user: Framing pre-exposure prophylaxix in UK newsprint 2012–2016. *Culture, Health & Sexuality*. https://doi.org/10.1080/13691058.2020.1729420.

Chapter 13
The Stigma Struggles of Biomedical Progress: Understanding Community Engagement with PrEP by People Who Use Drugs

Andy Guise

13.1 PrEP as Revolution or Ongoing Struggle in HIV Prevention?

"'The revolution is not an apple that falls when it is ripe. You have to make it fall" [quoting Che Guevara]. . .Welcome to the PrEP revolution!' (Baeten and McCormack 2016)

'One of the concerns is that well. . . like. . . we've given people PrEP so we don't need to give them access to any other harm reduction support' (Person who uses drugs, North America, cited in INPUD 2015)

Pre-exposure prophylaxis for HIV (PrEP) is generating widespread excitement as part of a new wave of biomedically focused HIV prevention. Evidence from PrEP trials show substantial reductions in HIV risk (Baeten et al. 2012; McCormack et al. 2016) and observational evidence suggests significant falls in HIV incidence in places like London following widespread PrEP access (O'Halloran et al. 2019). From such evidence comes talk of a 'PrEP revolution' in HIV prevention (Baeten and McCormack 2016). There are, however, marked differences emerging in access to, and experiences of, PrEP (Calabrese et al. 2017; Golub 2018). Whilst some communities have high access and use, others—such as some people who use drugs—do not (Ayala et al. 2017; McFarland et al. 2019). Indeed, for some communities the prospect of PrEP raises concern, rather than talk of a revolution (INPUD 2015).

Such concerns about PrEP are wide-ranging, although a focus is PrEP representing a 'medicalisation' of HIV prevention and narrow pursuit of biomedical strategies that negate social concerns (Nguyen et al. 2011; INPUD 2015). Such a narrow biomedical focus is in tension with how successful HIV prevention is negotiated by communities, and that biomedical technologies are themselves always

A. Guise (✉)
Faculty of Life Sciences & Medicine, King's College, London, UK
e-mail: andrew.guise@kcl.ac.uk

© Springer Nature Switzerland AG 2021
S. Bernays et al. (eds.), *Remaking HIV Prevention in the 21st Century*, Social Aspects of HIV 5, https://doi.org/10.1007/978-3-030-69819-5_13

negotiated into practice within particular social worlds (Kippax and Stephenson 2012; Kippax et al. 2013). There is potential that PrEP, and other biomedical technologies, could 'silence' the negotiation of HIV. To some, this 'silence' is a virtue of PrEP: it could, in theory, allow individuals to control HIV prevention, rather than, for example, negotiating condom use with a sexual partner. Such a 'silencing' of the social complexity of HIV is also possible at a macro level. Introducing PrEP could, some fear, silence the need for action on the social determinants of HIV. Communities of people who use drugs have raised concerns at how pursuit of PrEP could curtail action on the limited access to evidence-based HIV prevention interventions such as needle and syringe exchange or opioid therapies (Degenhardt et al. 2014; INPUD 2015).

Whilst some communities express concern, other communities are deeply engaged in radically negotiating PrEP access. One important case study is PrEPster in the UK, where community-based activists enabled private PrEP supplies, petitioned the English National Health Service (NHS), shaped a new PrEP trial, and fostered PrEP access through 'sex positive' messaging (PrEPster 2020). It is perhaps in the context of England and for particular groups of gay men and other men who have sex with men where reference—in the opening quote—to Che Guevara and talk of a revolution is apt. Community engagement is then not necessarily marginalised for PrEP, despite concerns over medicalisation.

There is no singular community of people affected by HIV however; the needs, experiences and resources of, for example, gay men and other men who have sex with men in London, UK have overlaps with, and divergences from, other communities. A significant contrast to the PrEPster experience is the controversy surrounding a PrEP trial for people who use drugs in Bangkok, Thailand and opposition to it from local activists. PrEP within the trial was offered within a 'standard of care', which in the Thai context did not assume needle and syringe exchange programming (NSP) or ongoing access to HIV care, reflecting the broader health system and a criminalisation attached to drug use in Thailand (Alcorn 2005; Jintarkanon et al. 2005; Hayashi et al. 2013; Thai Drug Users Network et al. 2013). This trial design was seen by activists to break ethical norms for research and to adapt to a criminalising context for people who use drugs (Jintarkanon et al. 2005) where government policy led to the unexplained killing of thousands of people (Human Rights Watch 2004). From this opposition to PrEP by activists and people who use drugs we can start to see how PrEP is not always a revolution, but its introduction instead meshes with on-going struggles for rights, citizenship and harm reduction services.

A question then emerges of why there are very different community responses to PrEP: of extremes of revolutionary change, and as on-going struggle? Experiences of gay men in London and people who use drugs in Bangkok offer a contrast that warrants consideration. Social scientists have suggested PrEP will be useful to some people, some of the time, in some places (Auerbach and Hoppe 2015). Policy and strategy have also long emphasised the need for HIV prevention to respond to specific needs and experiences of key populations (Ayala et al. 2017; Joint United Nations Programme on HIV/AIDS (UNAIDS) 2019). It follows, therefore, that we might well expect to see some communities experiencing PrEP—and other biomedical advances—as a revolution in how we respond to HIV, whilst others not. Despite this agreed principle of varying needs and experiences, these differing experiences of PrEP have not been critically scrutinised, nor has policy and strategy adapted to them. PrEP is instead principally promoted with little engagement with concerns, beyond framing such issues as 'barriers' that should be 'overcome' (e.g. Allen et al. 2020); that PrEP is universally appropriate is assumed. A fuller debate on HIV prevention needs to understand whether and how novel biomedical interventions, including PrEP, might be realised in particular contexts.

This chapter explores these diverging experiences of PrEP revolution and struggle with a specific focus on the experiences of people who use drugs. Through situating these experiences within their social and historical context, and comparing to past eras of biomedical advance, the chapter aims to help conceptualise the community negotiation of PrEP and biomedical advance framed by analyses of stigma and structural violence (Epstein 1996; Parker and Aggleton 2003; Farmer 2004; Kippax and Stephenson 2012). The chapter first explores the context for PrEP-related concern for some people who use drugs, through situating how PrEP is being negotiated within contexts of 'structural violence'. Second, the chapter outlines a framework for understanding the introduction of new biomedical technologies like PrEP as bound up in broader and longer-running 'stigma struggles'; from this perspective community negotiation and contest of PrEP is one struggle enmeshed in longer-running struggles against stigma. The third section explores how the processes and institutions of biomedical science that drive PrEP help create and exacerbate these stigma struggles. Through this discussion, a core theme is developed of how for many people who use drugs, PrEP is necessarily subordinate to broader progress on the social determinants of health and the stigma and discrimination that limit this. By locating analysis of PrEP within the stigma surrounding it, and understanding the struggles against stigma, the chapter concludes with reflections on how stigma can be resisted.

13.2   Understanding Concerns: Negotiating PrEP Amidst Structural Violence

Reflecting PrEP's recent emergence, there is as yet little evidence for how people who use drugs are negotiating and experiencing PrEP in practice. A recent global consultation led by the International Network of People who Use Drugs (INPUD 2015) reported enthusiasm from some, but also concerns: that PrEP wasn't feasible or ethical considering other deficiencies in HIV prevention and care, that it might be a substitute for other harm reduction strategies constrained by the prevailing criminalisation of drugs, and that PrEP heralds a re-medicalisation of HIV that will undermine action on the social determinants of HIV (INPUD 2015; Guise et al. 2016).

Available studies published since the INPUD consultation, mainly in settings such as the USA and Canada, echo the consultation themes. Studies report limited knowledge of PrEP amongst people who use drugs and varying levels of interest; some people report enthusiasm, others less or none (Bazzi et al. 2018; McFarland et al. 2019; Sherman et al. 2019; Allen et al. 2020). These studies also point to how there are a range of structural barriers to the uptake of PrEP: social exclusion, criminalisation, and limits on health care access and harm reduction services (Biello et al. 2018).

There is also, as yet, little indication of high-profile community led organisation by people who use drugs to enable PrEP (in comparison to PrEPSter in the UK, for example). Furthermore, networks of people who use drugs are not placing clear priority on PrEP. A review of resources and online campaigns by networks of people who use drugs would suggest they have not prioritised PrEP access in recent advocacy (see websites of International Network of People who Use Drugs, European Network of People who Use Drugs, Asian Network of People who Use Drugs, International Harm Reduction Association accessed August 2020).

Understanding concerns about PrEP, or a lack of priority of it, is aided by considering the contexts of structural violence faced by many people who use drugs (Farmer 2004): structural violence being the indirect and invisible forms of violence that result from a particular social order (Farmer 2004; DeVerteuil 2015). This structural violence is expressed through long-running societal stigma against drug use that combines with multiple forms of power and domination to exclude and oppress, particularly through the criminalisation of drug use and how people are denied access to various resources, of harm reduction services, health care, housing, employment and social position (Bourgois 1998, 2000). PrEP is being introduced within these social orders, and so constraining PrEP access and raising the possibility of PrEP deepening the effects of structural violence; e.g. as in the INPUD consultation, of providing PrEP being a logic for not providing NSP.

Whilst recognising how contexts of structural violence currently constrain many people who use drugs, we also need to consider whether PrEP uptake will continue to be constrained by structural violence? Or might PrEP have the potential to combat or mitigate it? Exploring these questions follows the suggestion, as above, that PrEP could mitigate the HIV stigma that currently limits other prevention modalities (Auerbach and Hoppe 2015). Other potentials have emerged as PrEP challenges prevailing understandings of sex and sexuality for gay men and other men who have sex with men, with PrEP providing another route through which people can think of sex without a condom, and so focus on the potential for pleasure rather than risk (and stigma) associated with sex (Calabrese and Underhill 2015). Caution is, however, needed: whilst there has been some destigmatisation of condomless sex, there is also an emergence of new stigmatised identities, such as the 'truvada whore' (Auerbach and Hoppe 2015; Calabrese and Underhill 2015; Golub 2018).

Holding that potential and caution in mind, could PrEP challenge or mitigate prevailing structural barriers and stigma for people who use drugs? Could PrEP foster new ways of thinking about drug use, as, for example, pleasurable rather than as deviant and criminal? The emergence of these new potential identities and norms—both stigmatising and non—we should explore in their context, and understand their links to other cultural and political shifts. For example, the popularity of PrEP use and how that links to evolving norms of sexuality for some gay men and men who have sex with men reflect long-running shifts: shifts in gay rights we might link to broader changes and shifts in public attitudes as well as legal regimes, as seen in rising public support and legislation for gay marriage in some settings (Grace et al. 2018). The potential for PrEP to mobilise other meanings is then tied to broader cultural and political shifts. In contexts of drug use we might then consider how stigma shifting would require change in, for example, the 'war on drugs'. Some punitive approaches towards drug use are shifting, particularly with regard to the use of cannabis, and government policy towards drug use is shifting in specific settings, such as south east Asia (Jha 2019). However, despite long-running advocacy pressure from health and drug use advocates to end the war on drugs, these forms of stigma are persistent and enduring. There is little sense in most settings of large-scale change that PrEP might catalyse or extend, even if this could still emerge.

PrEP has also been remarkable for the ways in which some communities have sourced their own supply and created distribution networks. Could PrEP be taken on and controlled by individuals and groups of people who use drugs and made to work despite prevailing criminalisation and marginalisation? Private PrEP markets may be emerging, reflecting economic resources available to some, and dependent on particular legal environments. That communities of people who use drugs might, and likely are, sourcing and providing PrEP needs to be understood within the—little told—histories of how needle and syringe provision, and wider secondary distribution, were led and established by communities themselves (Friedman et al. 2007), and how unsanctioned supervised injecting sites have emerged in highly criminalised environments (Davidson et al. 2018). However, such community-led initiatives are frequently covert, given the particular criminalising environments in which they emerge. There are also potential points of contrast with PrEP, which limit these community initiatives as future models: such community driven efforts are frequently 'low-tech' and don't need clinical monitoring or other supervision (e.g. needle and syringe programmes), or rely on community expertise rather than extensive material resources (e.g. supervised injection). A closer parallel to PrEP might instead be efforts to increase access to naloxone as a response to opioid overdose: naloxone access can be constrained by a range of administrative and legal issues (Davis and Carr 2020), which could mirror how formal health systems may be reluctant for people who use drugs to lead their own community focused supply and monitoring of PrEP, but which might prove successful. Whilst such a process seems more feasible, this too reinforces the notion of how any negotiation of PrEP, like naloxone, is ultimately constrained by overarching structural limits from a health system, and its political contours. PrEP then for many people who use drugs seems likely to be controlled by the same institutions and structures that are shaped· by criminalisation and marginalisation, rather than by individuals and communities.

The introduction of PrEP and concerns about it amongst some people who use drugs can be understood for how it is being negotiated in contexts of structural violence that are defined by stigma and limits on material security and health care access. This brief review suggests there is only limited potential for a negotiation of structural violence to create access to PrEP for people who use drugs. Instead, PrEP access for many people who use drugs is potentially inseparable from overlapping concerns of stigma and criminalisation, and battles to support the availability of harm reduction and action on the social determinants of health (INPUD 2015).

13.3   The Stigma Struggles of Biomedical Progress

Identifying the structural violence that shapes the experiences of many people who use drugs is central to understanding concerns and potential opposition to PrEP. And yet many communities face or have faced varying degrees of structural violence: consider the history of struggle for gay rights in the UK that preceded todays supposed PrEP 'revolution', or the ongoing persecution of many gay men in settings as varied as Poland (Human Rights Watch 2020). Structural violence is not unique to any one community, especially given a historical perspective. An understanding of diverging community responses then needs further analysis, and particular engagement with the specifics of context and history. Here, the chapter develops a framework for this analysis, building on prior study of community engagement and activism through the HIV epidemic, and focusing on how PrEP becomes part of long-running 'stigma struggles'.

The differing potentials for PrEP engagement can be illuminated through comparison to past eras of biomedical advance in HIV. In particular, the activism that shaped the development of ART in the 1990s and enabled radical structural change in how drugs were developed and made available (Epstein 1996). The community mobilisation across the global north and south that drove access to ART, and its development, has become a core part of the history of HIV. Groups of people living with or affected by HIV organised and engaged in a range of ways with the dominant political, bureaucratic and scientific institutions governing the early HIV response and forced substantial change through the 1980s and 1990s (Epstein 1996; France 2016). These changes included forcing attention to the ignored issues of HIV and AIDS, pressuring for financial resources for drug development, and campaigning on how drugs were developed and evaluated. These efforts bear comparison to today's situation with PrEP: of some communities deeply engaged in negotiating access to biomedical innovation, whilst others have very different access and engagement.

For Epstein, activist engagement with ART through the 1980s and 90s was contingent on the resources, or 'capitals', available to particular communities (Epstein 1996). Epstein builds on Bourdieu's analysis of capitals: the resources people can use, which is dependent on their position in society. Some communities—particularly those identifying as white and gay in the USA and Western Europe—were often highly educated (cultural capital) and had health care access (material or economic capital). 'Getting drugs into bodies' was therefore a primary goal for people with this experience and resources. For others, including for many people who use drugs, HIV drug access was only part of an equation that also required action on poverty, health care access and multiple forms of stigma (Epstein 1996). A prioritisation of ART by all communities was not possible amidst a lack of other 'capitals' denied through structural violence (Epstein 1996).

Epstein's analysis resonates with the diverging responses to PrEP described above, for how different communities—gay men in London, people who use drugs in Bangkok—might have access to different capitals, and so potentials for engagement in PrEP. And yet we can expand and reorientate Epstein's approach to deepen understanding. The power of Epstein's approach is to relate ART engagement and activism to other social structures. We can continue this logic and decentre biomedical progress, whether ART or PrEP. Stigma is then not just context for negotiating biomedical progress, but can be understood as an overarching and longer-running struggle within which biomedical progress is set. PrEP then becomes enmeshed in much longer-running struggles against stigma and for rights and citizenship.

The notion of 'stigma struggles' derives from recent scholarship by Tyler (Tyler and Slater 2018; Tyler 2020), and is defined here as long-running community driven mobilisation against stigma and discrimination. Tyler builds on analyses of stigma that have sought to focus on the forms of power that shape who is stigmatised and marginalised, that in turn reflect a critical re-reading of scholarship of stigma that has often focused on individual level analyses (Link and Phelan 2001; Parker and Aggleton 2003). Tyler continues this approach (Tyler and Slater 2018; Tyler 2020) and explores various struggles for rights and freedom—e.g. the US civil rights movement—that have defined how stigma has been produced and used to generate and manage inequalities (Tyler 2020). Core to this approach is to take a long-running historical perspective on how stigma emerges, and in particular how these forms of power are resisted by communities (ibid).

Attention to 'stigma struggles' brings together an analytical focus on structures of power with attention to long-running forms of resistance to stigma (Tyler 2018) and with the existing literatures that have theorised community action in the context of HIV (Epstein 1996) and how community agency has been integral to challenging and mitigating structural violence (Friedman et al. 2007). The frame of stigma struggles is then useful for understanding diverging potential for community engagement with PrEP, and other biomedical advances. The local negotiations of PrEP we are seeing are then a contest over PrEP and related meanings and identities and the resources brought to these (Epstein 1996), but are also—and at the same time—part of a long-running contest over stigma and the structural expression of power that limit the capitals and resources communities have that limit other necessary battles.

To return to the Bangkok trial to explore this: the controversy reflected debates around the ethics of the trial, vis a vis PrEP being offered within a 'standard of care', which in the Thai context did not assume NSP or ongoing access to HIV care (Alcorn 2005; Jintarkanon et al. 2005; Hayashi et al. 2013; Thai Drug Users Network et al. 2013). The Thai controversy over the PrEP trial has many elements: pre-existing harm reduction services, the ethical norms of trials, how such methodologies should relate to context, and this in contexts of suspicion over the motives of pharmaceutical companies. Here, a specific concern about PrEP is also an opposition to stigma, criminalisation and limits on harm reduction that has deep roots; debates about PrEP are not in isolation. The novel technology of PrEP is just one point of focus for longer-running debates and struggles against stigma and discrimination led by groups of people who use drugs. Broader structural forces and capitals shape the engagement with PrEP (Epstein 1996), but the engagement with PrEP also tells us about these other longer-running struggles for rights, services and freedom (Tyler 2020).

Understanding PrEP—and other biomedical advances—as situated within these longer-running stigma struggles (such as those effecting changes in social acceptance of gay men in several countries of the global north) brings a useful framing to understand why something apparently so revolutionary for some can be experienced very differently for others, whilst also emphasising both structural limits and community agency. It is useful then to see PrEP, and other products of biomedical progress, as something more than an object to be stigmatised or limited by stigma, and instead as something embedded in longer-running stigma struggles for rights and freedoms. Understanding PrEP and its implementation and use is then a context specific and historical question, but not one that many public health or scientific authorities are currently engaging with.

13.4   Erasing History? Science and Stigma Struggles

The analysis so far has sought to decentre biomedical progress in how we think about certain communities engaging with and negotiating technologies such as PrEP (and before that, ART). Whilst biomedicine might be usefully decentred in considering community needs and interests, biomedicine and the science involved in it are nonetheless central to understanding the particular nature of the stigma in the struggles described. As the history of HIV shows, biomedical advance and the work and methods of science have been frequently challenged by communities affected by HIV (Epstein 1996; Chan 2015; France 2016). The ongoing conduct of science is also central to the PrEP contests described above: the Impact trial of PrEP in England established in the wake of court findings that the NHS was unreasonably limiting PrEP access can be seen to function as a tool to ration PrEP access, rather than answering a scientific question (Nagington and Sandset 2020); the methodologies of the Bangkok trial and what is ethical conduct again illustrating this central role for science in the contests seen. Biomedical innovation and particular processes and institutions of science themselves buttress and deepen the stigma that communities are confronting. A particular feature of science is how it can remove a consideration of history: the erasure of history is an enabling condition for structural violence (Farmer 2004) and so the stigma struggles we describe here.

Returning to Epstein, the terrain of science has symbolic power to define credibility (Epstein 1996), and through this provoke, negate or support the stigma struggles communities are involved in. The early HIV activist battles were founded on efforts to develop this credibility within scientific institutions in charge of HIV biomedical research (Epstein 1996). Such processes of science determining symbolic capital and enacting symbolic violence are evident also in relation to PrEP. The conduct and discourses of science create particular dominant understandings of PrEP and people associated with it, that are then taken as 'natural', with particular negative consequences. For example, early doubts over PrEP efficacy led to concerns of 'risk compensation', and more recent targeting of PrEP at groups considered to be 'at high risk' that has generated its own dynamics that stigmatise PrEP (Golub 2018).

The specific discourse of 'evidence-based policy' also has effects. Scientific discourse inadvertently reinforces stigma towards people who use drugs by focusing the framing onto specific issues, which don't necessarily align with the priorities of people who use drugs. PrEP is promoted based on what is a problematic discourse of effect: a small number of RCTs, which show a lower reduction in HIV risk for people who use drugs (Choopanya et al. 2013) is widely repeated. That PrEP is then widely framed as 'effective' carries symbolic weight that is then used to target potential users of PrEP for 'adherence' and 'correct and consistent use', rather than other questions about contexts of criminalisation, as we return to below. This discourse of effect then structures consequent second order research questions of 'implementation science' and 'knowledge translation' that assume a universal evidence base (Rhodes et al. 2016). The emphasis of these questions and studies is then on whether people can adhere, or 'use PrEP consistently and correctly', and what interventions will support adherence. The narrow framing of these implementation science questions creates a silence on social and historical factors in analysis, this despite long calls for social perspectives to be integrated in efforts to achieve comprehensive HIV prevention (Kippax 2012; Auerbach and Hoppe 2015). Here then, the symbolic power of particular scientific discourses to elevate some questions and frameworks for thinking as authoritative and consequential, and others—promoted by community organisations—that might ask different questions of PrEP are not. As above, the negotiation of PrEP by many networks and groups of people who use drugs aims to locate PrEP within long-running challenges of access to, and funding of, harm reduction or the criminalisation of drug use (INPUD 2015). That these frameworks for analysis sought by communities do not figure centrally in dominant scientific discourse is then the basis through which other authorities—e.g. government, police forces—can deprioritise action on stigma and criminalisation, and so deepen stigma struggles.

A core focus for future action are then the analytical frameworks that dominate and figure centrally within the stigma struggles around PrEP. Discourses of evidence-based policy need to adopt more expansive conceptual framing that is attentive to history; as with the questions asked in trials and the development of trial methodologies through the era of HIV treatment development (Epstein 1996). Such a conceptual framing then needs to attend to that sought by communities, of locating PrEP within questions of stigma, criminalisation and harm reduction access. Debates about PrEP and communities of people who use drugs, especially in Bangkok, also provide more insight into how relationships with science might be more productive: of contest and dissent. As others have noted, a pursuit of solidarity in the response to HIV may be limiting dissent that could generate productive new insights (Aggleton and Parker 2015). An intolerance of dissent also elides with a tokenistic stance towards the involvement of affected communities, and their general under-resourcing; community representatives are invited to the table, but their differing questions and priorities are not engaged with. Whilst efforts to involve affected communities—e.g. inclusion of people who use drugs in study design, development and implementation should continue or be sought—we might also imagine new institutions through which dissent can be aired and responded to, that current routines for community engagement don't necessarily foster.

13.5 PrEP as an Ongoing Stigma Struggle

Whilst PrEP might figure as revolution for some, it is most useful, as argued in this chapter, that we understand PrEP as being enmeshed in long-running stigma struggles; the stage or outcome of these struggles is what determines the particular response any community might make to this novel intervention. From this, we might then need to imagine very different HIV prevention strategies, and advocacy in support of them, with respect to whether PrEP is appropriate and desirable for all, or if it is, when and how. Conceptualising and then responding to these different potentials for engagement, and how they are tied to the resources and contexts for specific communities, is a challenge for a HIV policy community attuned to univer-sal notions of human rights, solidarity and equality (Aggleton and Parker 2015). A continuing challenge is how to enable distinct responses tailored to particular community needs that can allow for cautious or delayed responses to technological innovation that also maintains progress on broader struggles against stigma and for rights and citizenship. Following an analysis of stigma struggles we could suggest that policy and strategy recognise the primacy of stigma and its historical roots. Stigma here not merely as introductory preamble or vaguely defined context for an intervention, but clearly conceptualised. A stigma struggles analysis decentres biomedical technology and progress, but also underscores the core role for biomed-ical frameworks in this struggle: to develop frameworks for research and analysis of PrEP that can test and explore efficacy in a context bound way that relates to the experiences of people that might need it; these frameworks and methods are needed to replace those that assume an ahistorical setting and 'other' with little understood needs. The scientific institutions driving PrEP, like those in a previous era of biomedical progress before, can also engage more with the needs of communities, in a myriad of ways already promoted in terms of resourcing, respect and adapting processes, but especially in understanding that the struggles led by particular com-munities are a form of engagement with PrEP. Community organisations and networks of people who use drugs are faced with a challenging negotiation; how best to embrace the multiple meanings and potentials for PrEP whilst working for the social change that is necessary to confront the stigma that defines the longer running struggles for many.

References

Aggleton, P., & Parker, R. (2015). Moving beyond biomedicalization in the HIV response: Implications for community involvement and community leadership among men who have sex with men and transgender people. *American Journal of Public Health, 105*(8), 1552–1558. https://doi.org/10.2105/AJPH.2015.302614.

Alcorn, K. (2005). Thai tenofovir trial runs into trouble after ethics protests from drug users. *NAM aidsmap.* Retrieved March 9, 2020, from https://www.aidsmap.com/news/mar-2005/thai-tenofovir-trial-runs-trouble-after-ethics-protests-drug-users.

Allen, S. T., O'Rourke, A., White, R. H., Smith, K. C., Weir, B., Lucas, G. M., Sherman, S., & Grieb, S. M. (2020). Barriers and facilitators to PrEP use among people who inject drugs in rural Appalachia: A qualitative study. *AIDS and Behavior, 24*(6), 1942–1950. https://doi.org/10.1007/s10461-019-02767-3.

Auerbach, J. D., & Hoppe, T. A. (2015). Beyond "getting drugs into bodies": Social science perspectives on pre-exposure prophylaxis for HIV. *Journal of the International AIDS Society, 18*(Supplement 3), 19983.

Ayala, G., Chang, J., Matheson, R., Sprague, L., & Thomas, R. M. (2017). *Reconsidering primary prevention of HIV: New steps forward in the global response.* New York: The Global Forum on MSM & HIV.

Baeten, J., & McCormack, S. (2016). Welcome to the preexposure prophylaxis revolution. *Current Opinion in HIV and AIDS, 11*(1), 1–2.

Baeten, J. M., Donnell, D., Ndase, P., Mugo, N. R., Campbell, J. D., Wangisi, J., et al. (2012). Antiretroviral prophylaxis for HIV prevention in heterosexual men and women. *New England Journal of Medicine, 367*(5), 399–410. https://doi.org/10.1056/NEJMoa1108524.

Bazzi, A. R., Biancarelli, D. L., Childs, E., Drainoni, M.-L., Edeza, A., Salhaney, P., et al. (2018). Limited knowledge and mixed interest in pre-exposure prophylaxis for HIV prevention among people who inject drugs. *AIDS Patient Care and STDs, 32*(12), 529–537. https://doi.org/10.1089/apc.2018.0126.

Biello, K. B., Bazzi, A. R., Mimiaga, M. J., Biancarelli, D. L., Edeza, A., Salhaney, P., et al. (2018). Perspectives on HIV pre-exposure prophylaxis (PrEP) utilization and related intervention needs among people who inject drugs. *Harm Reduction Journal, 15*(1), 55. https://doi.org/10.1186/s12954-018-0263-5.

Bourgois, P. (1998). The moral economies of homeless heroin addicts: Confronting ethnography, HIV risk, and everyday violence in San Francisco shooting encampments. *Substance Use & Misuse, 33*, 2323–2351.

Bourgois, P. (2000). Disciplining addictions: The biopolitics of methadone and heroin in the United States. *Culture, Medicine and Psychiatry, 24*, 165–195.

Calabrese, S. K., & Underhill, K. (2015). How stigma surrounding the use of HIV Preexposure prophylaxis undermines prevention and pleasure: A call to destigmatize "Truvada whores". *American Journal of Public Health, 105*(10), 1960–1964. https://doi.org/10.2105/AJPH.2015.302816.

Calabrese, S. K., Krakower, D. S., & Mayer, K. H. (2017). Integrating HIV Preexposure prophylaxis (PrEP) into routine preventive health care to avoid exacerbating disparities. *American Journal of Public Health, 107*(12), 1883–1889. https://doi.org/10.2105/AJPH.2017.304061.

Chan, J. (2015). *Politics in the corridors of dying. AIDS activism and global health governance.* Baltimore: Johns Hopkins University Press.

Choopanya, K., Martin, M., Suntharasamai, P., Sangkum, U., Mock, P. A., Leethochawalit, M., et al. (2013). Antiretroviral prophylaxis for HIV infection in injecting drug users in Bangkok, Thailand (the Bangkok Tenofovir study): A randomised, double-blind, placebo-controlled phase 3 trial. *The Lancet, 381*(9883), 2083–2090.

Davidson, P. J., Lopez, A. M., & Kral, A. H. (2018). Using drugs in un/safe spaces: Impact of perceived illegality on an underground supervised injecting facility in the United States. *International Journal of Drug Policy, 53*, 37–44. https://doi.org/10.1016/j.drugpo.2017.12.005.

Davis, C. S., & Carr, D. (2020). Over the counter naloxone needed to save lives in the United States. *Preventive Medicine, 130*, 105932.

Degenhardt, L., Mathers, B. M., Wirtz, A. L., Wolfe, D., Kamarulzaman, A., Carrieri, M. P., et al. (2014). What has been achieved in HIV prevention, treatment and care for people who inject drugs, 2010–2012? A review of the six highest burden countries. *International Journal of Drug Policy, 25*(1), 53–60. https://doi.org/10.1016/j.drugpo.2013.08.004.

DeVerteuil, G. (2015). Conceptualizing violence for health and medical geography. *Social Science & Medicine, 133*, 216–222.

Epstein, S. (1996). *Impure Science*. Los Angeles: University of California Press.

Farmer, P. (2004). An anthropology of structural violence. *Current Anthropology, 45*(3), 305–325.

France, D. (2016). *How to survive a plague. The story of how activists and scientists tamed AIDS*. London: Picador.

Friedman, S. R., de Jong, W., Rossi, D., Touzé, G., Rockwell, R., Des Jarlais, D. C., & Elovich, R. (2007). Harm reduction theory: Users' culture, micro-social indigenous harm reduction, and the self-organization and outside-organizing of users' groups. *International Journal of Drug Policy, 18*(2), 107–117. https://doi.org/10.1016/j.drugpo.2006.11.006.

Golub, S. A. (2018). PrEP stigma: Implicit and explicit drivers of disparity. *Current HIV/AIDS Reports, 15*(2), 190–197. https://doi.org/10.1007/s11904-018-0385-0.

Grace, D., Jollimore, J., MacPherson, P., Strang, M. J. P., & Tan, D. H. S. (2018). The pre-exposure prophylaxis-stigma paradox: Learning from Canada's first wave of PrEP users. *AIDS Patient Care and STDs, 32*(1), 24–30. https://doi.org/10.1089/apc.2017.0153.

Guise, A., Albers, E. R., & Strathdee, S. A. (2016). 'PrEP is not ready for our community, and our community is not ready for PrEP': Pre-exposure prophylaxis for HIV for people who inject drugs and limits to the HIV prevention response. *Addiction, 112*(4), 572–578. https://doi.org/10.1111/add.13437.

Hayashi, K., Small, W., Csete, J., Hattirat, S., & Kerr, T. (2013). Experiences with policing among people who inject drugs in Bangkok, Thailand: A qualitative study. *PLoS Medicine/Public Library of Science, 10*(12), e1001570; discussion e1001570. https://doi.org/10.1371/journal.pmed.1001570.

Human Rights Watch. (2004). *Thailand—Not enough graves: The war on drugs, HIV/AIDS, and violations of human rights*. New York: Human Rights Watch. Retrieved August 17, 2020, from http://www.hrw.org/reports/2004/thailand0704/thailand0704.pdf.

Human Rights Watch. (2020). *Poland: Crackdown on LGBT activists*. Retrieved August 18, 2020, from https://www.hrw.org/news/2020/08/07/poland-crackdown-lgbt-activists.

INPUD. (2015). *Pre-exposure prophylaxis (PrEP) for people who inject drugs: Community voices on pros, cons, and concerns*. London: International Network of People who Use Drugs.

Jha, P. (2019). *Why Malaysia's new proposal could change Southeast Asia's drugs debate. The diplomat*. Retrieved August 17, 2020, from https://thediplomat.com/2019/07/why-malaysias-new-proposal-could-change-southeast-asias-drugs-debate/.

Jintarkanon, S., Nakapiew, S., Tienudom, N., Suwannawong, P., & Wilson, D. (2005). Unethical clinical trials in Thailand: A community response. *The Lancet, 365*(9471), 1617–1618. https://doi.org/10.1016/S0140-6736(05)66501-4.

Kippax, S. (2012). Effective HIV prevention: The indispensable role of social science. *Journal of the International AIDS Society, 15*(2), 17357.

Kippax, S., & Stephenson, N. (2012). Beyond the distinction between biomedical and social dimensions of HIV prevention through the Lens of a social public health. *American Journal of Public Health, 102*(5), 789–799. https://doi.org/10.2105/AJPH.2011.300594.

Kippax, S., Stephenson, N., Parker, R. G., & Aggleton, P. (2013). Between individual agency and structure in HIV prevention: Understanding the middle ground of social practice. *American Journal of Public Health, 103*(8), 1367–1375. https://doi.org/10.2105/AJPH.2013.301301.

Link, B., & Phelan, J. (2001). Conceptualising stigma. *Annual Review of Sociology, 27*, 363–385.

McCormack, S., Dunn, D. T., Desai, M., Dolling, D. I., Gafos, M., Gilson, R., et al. (2016). Pre-exposure prophylaxis to prevent the acquisition of HIV-1 infection (PROUD): Effectiveness results from the pilot phase of a pragmatic open-label randomised trial. *The Lancet, 387*(10013), 53–60. https://doi.org/10.1016/S0140-6736(15)00056-2.

McFarland, W., Lin, J., Santos, G.-M., Arayasirikul, S., Raymond, H. F., & Wilson, E. (2019). Low PrEP awareness and use among people who inject drugs, San Francisco, 2018. *AIDS and Behavior, 24*, 1290–1293. https://doi.org/10.1007/s10461-019-02682-7.

Nagington, M., & Sandset, T. (2020). Putting the NHS England on trial: Uncertainty-as-power, evidence and the controversy of PrEP in England. *Medical Humanities.* https://doi.org/10.1136/medhum-2019-011780.

Nguyen, V.-K., Bajos, N., Dubois-Arber, F., O'Malley, J., & Pirkle, C. M. (2011). Remedicalizing an epidemic: From HIV treatment as prevention to HIV treatment is prevention. *AIDS, 25*(3), 291–293.

O'Halloran, C., Sun, S., Nash, S., Brown, A., Croxford, S., Connor, N., et al. (2019). *HIV in the United Kingdom: Towards zero 2030.* London: Public Health England.

Parker, R., & Aggleton, P. (2003). HIV and AIDS related stigma and discrimination: A conceptual framework and implications for action. *Social Science and Medicine, 57*, 13–24.

PrEPster. (2020). *About.* Retrieved March 9, 2020, from https://prepster.info/about/.

Rhodes, T., Closson, E. F., Paparini, S., Guise, A., & Strathdee, S. (2016). Towards "evidence-making intervention" approaches in the social science of implementation science: The making of methadone in East Africa. *International Journal of Drug Policy, 30*, 17–26. https://doi.org/10.1016/j.drugpo.2016.01.002.

Sherman, S. G., Schneider, K. E., Park, J. N., Allen, S. T., Hunt, D., Chaulk, C. P., & Weir, B. W. (2019). PrEP awareness, eligibility, and interest among people who inject drugs in Baltimore, Maryland. *Drug and Alcohol Dependence, 195*, 148–155. https://doi.org/10.1016/j.drugalcdep.2018.08.014.

Thai Drug Users Network (TDN), Thai AIDS Treatment Action Group (TTAG), and Treatment Action Group (TAG). (2013). *U.S. centers for disease control and prevention (CDC) sponsored HIV preexposure prophylaxis (PrEP) trial among thai injection drug users marred by lack of response to community concerns [Press release].* Available at https://www.treatmentactiongroup.org/statement/u-s-centers-for-disease-control-and-prevention-cdc-sponsored-hiv-preexposure-prophylaxis-prep-trial-among-thai-injection-drug-users-marred-by-lack-of-response-to-community-concerns/ Accessed 9 March 2020.

Tyler, I. (2018). Resituating Erving Goffman: From stigma power to black power. *The Sociological Review, 66*(4), 744–765. https://doi.org/10.1177/0038026118777450.

Tyler, I. (2020). *Stigma, the machinery of inequality.* London: Zed Books.

Tyler, I., & Slater, T. (2018). Rethinking the sociology of stigma. *The Sociological Review, 66*(4), 721–743. https://doi.org/10.1177/0038026118777425.

UNAIDS. (2019). *Global AIDS update: Communities at the Centre.* Geneva: UNAIDS.

Chapter 14
How the Science of HIV Treatment-as-Prevention Restructured PEPFAR's Strategy: The Case for Scaling up ART in 'Epidemic Control' Countries

Ryan Whitacre

14.1 Introduction

Over the past decade, the clinical logics of HIV treatment as prevention (TasP) have transformed the global response to the epidemic. While clinical knowledge about the efficacy of TasP dates back to the turn of the twenty-first century when investigators first demonstrated that antiretroviral therapy (ART) could greatly reduce the chances of onward viral transmission (Cohen 2000; Quinn et al. 2000), in more recent years epidemiological modelling studies provided evidence that TasP could have population-level effects on HIV incidence and HIV-related mortality (Granich et al. 2009; Cambiano et al. 2010; Cohen 2010). On the heels of these findings, health organisations have launched ambitious strategies to change the course of the HIV epidemic. Strategies for creating an 'AIDS-free generation' began to be announced in 2010 (UNAIDS 2010) and have continued for several years.[1] For example, in 2010, the Joint United Nations Programme on HIV/AIDS (UNAIDS) outlined a vision for 'getting to zero' including zero new HIV infections, zero AIDS-related deaths and zero discrimination (UNAIDS 2010). In 2011, the US President's Emergency Plan for AIDS Relief (PEPFAR) also began to devise a new strategy to 'control' the HIV epidemic (PEPFAR 2012).

One of the earliest signs PEPFAR was crafting this strategy appeared in the organisation's annual report to US Congress, when PEPFAR leadership declared a commitment to 'saving lives by moving science into programs through smart investments' (PEPFAR 2012, p. 1). Guided by recent 'breakthroughs' in HIV

---

[1]For a detailed account of the rise of 'end of AIDS' rhetoric and strategies, see Kenworthy et al. 2018.

R. Whitacre (✉)
Anthropology and Global Health, Graduate Institute of International and Development Studies, Geneva, Switzerland
e-mail: ryan.whitacre@graduateinstitute.ch

© The Author(s) 2021
S. Bernays et al. (eds.), *Remaking HIV Prevention in the 21st Century*, Social Aspects of HIV 5, https://doi.org/10.1007/978-3-030-69819-5_14

science, PEPFAR would harness 'the power of evidence-based interventions to dramatically drive down the rate of new infections and save more lives' (PEPFAR 2012, p. 1). Later that same year, PEPFAR published a 'blueprint' for 'Creating an AIDS-Free Generation.' And by 2013 PEPFAR had officially launched its new strategic initiative to achieve 'epidemic control' in all recipient countries and regions (PEPFAR 2014b).

In 2014, UNAIDS updated its vision to 'end AIDS'. To achieve this ambitious goal, UNAIDS recommended a massive scale-up of HIV testing and expansion of access to ART, and set specific targets for achievement, including to ensure: 90% of people living with HIV know their status; 90% of them are on effective treatment; and 90% of people on effective treatment have an undetectable viral load. If '90-90-90' could be achieved by 2020, UNAIDS contended, we would see the 'end of AIDS' by 2030 (UNAIDS 2014).

Evidence that TasP could have population-level effects justified the new global agenda and the use of a new set of health metrics for monitoring performance. Whereas PEPFAR had previously measured programme reach by the number of people receiving clinical services, including HIV testing, counselling, condoms and ART, after the clinical logics of TasP were adopted, these organisations adjusted their metrics for impact to focus on reductions in HIV viral load among people living with HIV (PLWH), the number of new HIV cases averted, and HIV-related mortality. Drawing on the clinical science associated with TasP, PEPFAR's new strategy aimed to lower the number of people who acquire HIV below the number of people with HIV who die annually. By realising these two related aims, disease surveillance experts within the organisation suggested PEPFAR could effectively achieve 'epidemic control'.

To support the goals of the strategy, PEPFAR also began to update methods for monitoring the impact on the epidemic through a new set of health metrics, which track mortality among people living with HIV and population-wide HIV incidence. In the following years, PEPFAR analysed data in recipient countries to monitor the impact of this new strategy, and represented the outcomes in its annual report to Congress. By 2017, the organisation had identified a subset of 13 recipient countries that demonstrated potential to meet the identified targets. While maintaining its broad approach to control the epidemic in all recipient countries and regions, the organisation announced a new initiative to 'accelerate' epidemic control in this select group of 13 countries, which showed promise to achieve the goals of the strategy (2017b).

PEPFAR's new strategy has been influenced by larger transformations in global public health, including the rise of 'evidence-based medicine' (EBM). Since the turn of the twenty-first century, evidence-based medicine has increasingly influenced global public health and the imperative to generate evidence has transformed the world of health provision and care into a space of calculation and accountability (Adams 2016). Models for health forecasting have obscured the political and economic factors influencing health through several layers of statistical abstraction (Erikson 2016). Programmes to improve basic health care, which have historically defined the contributions of international development agencies have been overshadowed by biomedical interventions (Lock and Nguyen 2018), which can be more easily measured, even though these measures tend to be abstract, and in some cases, divorced from any meaningful evidence of impact (Wendland 2016). The consequences of this turn towards the biomedical approaches to care have manifested themselves in under-developed health systems (Pfeiffer 2013), where getting 'good numbers' has become a requirement for successful governance and increased aid (Oni-Orisan 2016). Just as EBM has transformed the logics and practices of this globalising field, TasP has reshaped the global agenda to 'end AIDS' and contributed to the ongoing biomedicalisation of the epidemic (Nguyen et al. 2011).

PEPFAR's strategic approach has also been influenced by political factors, including US Congressional oversight and a recent change in the budgetary approval process. The United States Congress first authorised the establishment of PEPFAR through the Leadership Act, and dedicated $15 billion to 'lead' the global response to the HIV/AIDS epidemic around the world (Hyde 2003). In 2008, Congress reauthorised PEPFAR (through the Lantos-Hyde Act) and increased its budget for bilateral aid to $48 billion (Biden 2008). However, in more recent years, Congress has not reauthorised a predetermined budget amount. While continuing to support PEPFAR's ongoing operations, Congress has required PEPFAR to implement a flexible budget structure, which would be reviewed annually. This change in budgetary oversight coincided with PEPFAR's new strategic approach to the global epidemic, and may have intensified reporting on programme performance. Therefore, the push for evidence-based interventions must also be examined within the context of an ongoing era of increasing austerity, and greater demands for accountability (Basu et al. 2017; Whitacre 2020).

Against this background, this chapter examines how the clinical logics of TasP structured PEPFAR's latest strategic initiative to achieve 'epidemic control' including the organisation's decisions for allocating funds to specific programmes and a subset of recipient countries, based on a set of metrics for evaluating performance. The findings draw from analysis of publicly available documents and data sets produced by PEPFAR, including the organisation's annual reports to the US Congress (PEPFAR 2005–2019), strategic updates (PEPFAR 2005, 2009a, 2013a, 2017b), and data sets on planned spending (PEPFAR 2020b). At the time of writing, strategic updates and annual reports were available online (US Department of State 2020) for all years of operations (PEPFAR 2004–2019) and planned spending data was available for all but the two most recent years (PEPFAR 2004–2017). In my analysis of this data set I traced broad trends in PEPFAR's planned spending, including by programme area and recipient countries, and changes in the use of health metrics after the strategy for achieving epidemic control was initiated.[2] To understand longitudinal trends in epidemic control countries, I also reviewed the

---

[2]The author has published the full analysed data set of PEPFAR's planned spending in 'epidemic control' countries for years 2004–2017. DOI: https://doi.org/10.5281/zenodo.4323072

epidemiological data provided by PEPFAR in supplementary tables included in annual reports, and plotted health outcomes by country over time.

Based on this research it is possible to observe how the clinical logics of TasP structured PEPFAR's latest strategic initiative to achieve 'epidemic control' including the organisation's metrics for evaluating performance, and decisions for allocating funds to specific programmes and countries. Supported by evidence from modelling studies that TasP could have population-level effects, 'epidemic control' was conceptualised as an 'evidence-based' solution that could be consistently measured and reported on. However, after several years of working toward the goals of this new biomedical approach to the epidemic, PEPFAR has not demonstrated its benefits over previous strategies. The organisation has not even demonstrated the ability to measure impact. The only clear effects of the new strategy are evident in the organisation's budget, including increased spending on treatment and decreased spending on other program areas, including care, govenrnance and systems, and management and operations, as well as decreased spending on countries not designated as priorities under the new strategy. The budget clearly shows programmes and countries that could not produce the right kinds of evidence to meet the goals of epidemic control have been systematically under-funded since the initiative began.

By highlighting this shift in PEPFAR's strategic approach, I do not intend to undermine the historical or contemporary importance of the organisation. PEPFAR has made undeniable contributions to the global response to the HIV epidemic. However, I do aim to tease out the strangeness of the particular set of metrics used to measure programme success, probe the reasons for using these metrics for bilateral assistance, or any such health programme, and call attention to the way this set of metrics has emerged in concert with evidence-based medicine, and the biomedical prevention of HIV.

14.2   Measuring Impact: From Providing Clinical Services to Projecting Health Outcomes

The clinical logics of TasP have reshaped PEPFAR's methods for tracking programme performance and measuring impact. Since its establishment, PEPFAR has utilised many key indicators to measure its own impact.[3] In the earliest years of PEPFAR's operations (2004–2008), the majority of indicators counted the number of clients receiving HIV care services from sponsored programmes (PEPFAR 2007b). These indicators monitored the number of HIV testing and counselling services, mothers and newborns who know their HIV status, prevention services for orphans and vulnerable children, and patients receiving ART, newly per year and

---

[3]Information about indicators is available for download in the 'Additional Data' section of PEPFAR's website, listed under the 'Historical Data' tab: https://data.pepfar.gov/additionalData

ongoing. When the organisation updated its strategy in 2009, PEPFAR started to measure the number of patients who were retained in HIV care for at least 12 months, and the number who agreed to voluntary male medical circumcision (VMMC) (PEPFAR 2009b, pp. 61–64). In 2011, PEFAR added more indicators to its annual report to measure the scale of services provided and number of patients receiving HIV care, including those who received treatment for tuberculosis (TB) in addition to HIV (PEPFAR 2013b, pp. 75–77, 184). In 2013 and again in 2015, the organisation added yet more indicators: one counted the number of people living with HIV who were pregnant and on ART (PEPFAR 2013b, pp. 44–47); and a second measured the number of clients who maintained a suppressed HIV viral load for at least 12 months (PEPFAR 2015b).

Over this history PEPFAR expanded the scope and number of indicators it used to measure its own impact, including by tracking services offered for the biomedical prevention of HIV. By documenting the number of services provided as a result of US bilateral aid, PEPFAR could demonstrate how the USA was 'leading' the global response to the epidemic in low- and middle-income countries (LMICs). As PEPFAR added new indicators to its audit structure, the organisation could make further claims to its own impact while generating evidence about performance. But ultimately, these many indicators could only demonstrate the ways in which bilateral aid had facilitated the provision of HIV care services, as opposed to health outcomes.

After PEPFAR introduced the strategy to achieve epidemic control in 2013 the organisation started reporting health outcomes associated with TasP and related biomedical methods of HIV prevention in its annual report to Congress, including the number of new HIV cases averted and lives saved (PEPFAR 2014a). PEPFAR's leadership also began to make clear statements about the importance of this new method of measurement. For example, in the executive summary of the annual report leadership proclaimed, 'saving lives is the ultimate metric of success' (PEPFAR 2012, p. 1). However, PEPFAR had not collected data to support the use of these new metrics. To make claims about progress toward achieving the stated goals, PEPFAR leveraged data sets from UNAIDS, which were generated through a wide range of sampling methods, and used to estimate incidence of HIV and HIV-related mortality across entire populations (UNAIDS 2019).

PEPFAR's claims about progress toward achieving or accelerating 'epidemic control' present troubling issues, given this significant difference between the data PEPFAR collected from aid recipients and the metrics the organisation reported to Congress. UNAIDS data were based on country-level estimates, and therefore, not specific to hospitals or clinics that received funding from PEPFAR. The measures were also not proportional to the presence of US bilateral aid in the country. Since the majority of funding for HIV care and services originated from domestic sources (UNAIDS 2018), the impact of any of PEPFAR's programmes could have only been abstractly correlated to the country-level health outcomes reported by UNAIDS. Furthermore, to represent progress toward epidemic control, PEPFAR reported estimates of health outcomes from a single year—either one or 2 years previous—and thus did not represent impact over time. Nevertheless, PEPFAR published single-year, country-level estimates in its annual report to Congress to suggest its

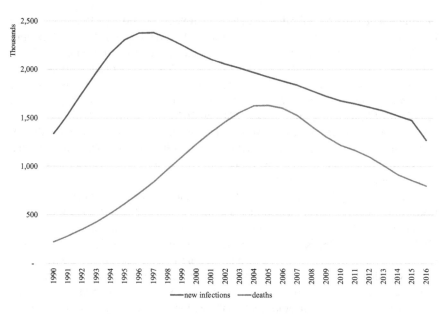

Fig. 14.1 Progress toward epidemic control in all PEPFAR countries (1990–2016)

programmes had discrete impact in specific countries that received bilateral aid from the USA.

Even if one were to bracket the limitations of this data and its uses, PEPFAR's claims about progress toward 'epidemic control' would be limited. For all countries receiving PEPFAR support, the ratio between new HIV cases and HIV-related deaths has not improved over the history of PEPFAR's existence. In fact, according to the UNAIDS data PEPFAR relied on to make claims about these metrics, the divide between new infections and deaths has widened over the organisation's history (Fig. 14.1). There were roughly 340,000 more new HIV infections than HIV-related deaths in 2004 (1.97 million new infections and 1.63 HIV-related deaths), and 470,000 more new infections than HIV-related deaths in 2016 (1.27 million infections vs. 0.8 million deaths).

The remaining distance between new infections and deaths complicates the picture of PEPFAR's progress toward epidemic control. On the one hand, it shows a glaring shortcoming of the strategy, which was not acknowledged in the annual report to Congress, but instead is tucked away in supplemental tables and buried within audit documents that number near 1000 pages. On the other hand, the gap between new infections and deaths could have been understood as the central ambition of the strategy. While the data demonstrate there has been no progress toward achieving the stated goals of 'epidemic control' across the entire group of PEPFAR's recipient countries, HIV incidence and HIV-related mortality have both decreased substantially over this same timeline, and the push to decrease incidence below mortality would be the ultimate mark of success. In any case, PEPFAR has not represented progress toward the metrics of epidemic control in aggregate (as shown

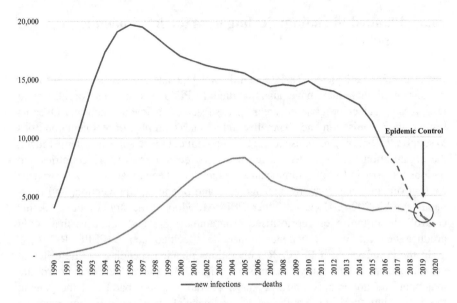

Fig. 14.2 Swaziland—Pathway to reaching epidemic control

in Fig. 14.1). Instead, the organisation has published individual charts for countries that have demonstrated progress toward realising the goals of epidemic control.

One chart representing progress toward epidemic control appeared in the 2017 strategic update (PEPFAR 2017b). It highlighted PEPFAR's impact on the epidemic in a single country: Swaziland (Fig. 14.2). According to data from 2016, the last available year data were available from UNAIDS, there had been no significant progress toward meeting the goals of the new strategy in Swaziland. In this sense, it mirrored the figure for all of PEPFAR's recipient countries. However, in this chart PEPFAR also projected possible future health outcomes to demonstrate what achieving 'epidemic control' would look like. By leveraging these broad epidemiological estimates, PEPFAR constructed a hypothetical future in which success would be realised. Of course, without current data this hypothetical 'future' could not be validated.

The clinical logics of TasP have guided PEPFAR's use of a new set of health metrics, and allowed the organisation to make claims about its potential impact on the epidemic through estimates of population-wide health outcomes. These metrics were divorced from any data PEPFAR collects from recipient countries, and only very loosely connected to the organisation's impact by a string of abstract correlations based on the very presence of US bilateral aid for HIV. Yet, PEPFAR has used these data to represent the impact of its programmes on the epidemic.

14.3   Planned Spending: Scaling up ART in 'Epidemic Control' Countries

Just as the clinical logics of TasP have influenced the use of a new set of metrics for measuring impact, they have also justified PEPFAR's decisions for allocating resources to select programme areas in a subset of recipient countries. Over its history, the organisation had channelled aid to a large number of recipient countries to support the ongoing response to the HIV epidemic. In fact, since its establishment, the organisation has expanded its reach to provide resources to 42 countries and regions for work in five programme areas, which have been broadly characterised as: care, governance and systems, management and operations, prevention, and treatment (amfAR 2020). However, when PEPFAR adopted the strategy of 'epidemic control' the organisation reprioritised programme areas and countries that could produce the right kinds of evidence to meet the specified metrics (PEPFAR 2013a).

In the initial years of PEPFAR's operations planned spending on the different programme areas was relatively consistent (Fig. 14.3). The budget for antiretroviral treatment and governance and systems, for example, both paralleled the general trend of rising spending. Shortly after the financial crisis of 2008, however, the budget for all programme areas plateaued, and planned spending for treatment dropped to levels approximately equivalent to prevention. However, since the implementation of PEPFAR's most recent strategic initiative, spending on treatment has greatly outpaced spending on other programme areas. In fact, since 2013, spending on treatment has increased by nearly 150% meanwhile planned spending

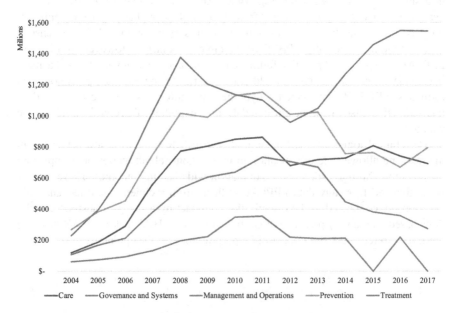

Fig. 14.3 PEPFAR's planned spending by programme area, 2004–2017

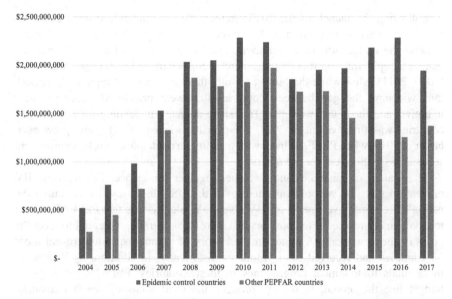

Fig. 14.4 PEPFAR's planned spending in 'epidemic control' countries vs. other recipient countries, 2004–2017

for governance and systems has been significantly reduced, and the budget for management and operations has been gutted.

There has been a similar trend in PEPFAR's planned spending in specific countries. Under the most recent initiative to 'accelerate epidemic control' PEPFAR announced it would prioritise countries that had the greatest potential to achieve epidemic control by 2020. With this announcement, the organisation suggested it would shift resource commitments from 42 countries and regions across the globe to 12 countries in sub-Saharan Africa in addition to Haiti.[4] While the prioritisation of these countries suggested a significant transition in resource allocation, upon review of the organisation's budget, it is clear that PEPFAR has historically given more aid to this subset of 13 countries over the history of its existence (Fig. 14.4). In fact, the planned spending differential between these 13 countries and all others began in 2004, the very first year of reported spending when this subset of countries collectively received just over $500 million, whereas the rest of the countries and regions given PEPFAR funds collectively received approximately half of that amount— $270 million. This spending differential has been maintained year-over-year for every year of PEPFAR's history, reaching a peak in 2010 when PEPFAR earmarked $2.3 billion for these 13 countries, and set aside approximately $500 million less ($1.8 billion) for all others.

---

[4]The list of countries chosen to 'accelerate epidemic control' includes: Botswana, Côte d'Ivoire, Haiti, Kenya, Lesotho, Malawi, Namibia, Rwanda, Swaziland, Tanzania, Uganda, Zambia, and Zimbabwe.

Following the launch of the 2013 strategy, the 13 epidemic control countries continued receiving disproportionately more funding than other recipients, but not because the budget for these countries grew to unprecedented levels. Instead the budget for epidemic control countries merely returned to the levels of previous years (2010, 2011). Meanwhile the budget for all other countries and regions decreased, thus widening the gap between countries that were prioritised under the new initiative, and those that were not. This steep decrease in funding for non-priority countries was first evident in 2014, however it widened in 2015, and grew even larger in 2016, when PEPFAR increased spending in epidemic control countries, and set aside $1 billion less for the others.

The strategy of epidemic control stitched together the science of biomedical HIV prevention with the geopolitical interests of the USA in a way that obscured the nation's declining investments in HIV abroad. While it is true that PEPFAR started to devote more resources to countries that were demonstrating potential to meet the goals of the new strategy, trends in the history of planned spending reveal these 13 countries had received more resources historically. In addition, by dedicating more funds to treatment programmes in these countries, PEPFAR privileged a budget line that could, in theory, produce the right kinds of health outcomes. Meanwhile, the organisation has left other programmes and countries sorely underfunded.

14.4   An Exit Strategy

Amid the reprioritisation of programme areas and countries to 'control' the epidemic, PEPFAR has also begun to devise a 'sustainability plan' for recipient countries and an 'exit strategy' for US bilateral support for HIV. The basic idea of the exit strategy was to allow individual countries to transition from dependence on US bilateral aid to greater utilisation of domestic resources. This was considered a 'sustainable' solution for the ongoing management of the HIV epidemic in any given country. The strategy has been strengthened by the United Nation's action plan to attain universal health coverage (UHC), which catalysed the formation of new mechanisms of accountability for greater domestic resource mobilisation. However, the exit strategy has raised significant questions about the transition to country ownership and how success could be ensured (Collins and Beyrer 2013; Esser 2014).

The clinical logics of TasP helped PEPFAR map its exit strategy and define the terms of success. If the epidemic control countries could achieve the goal of lowering new infections below HIV-related deaths, PEPFAR would begin to transfer responsibility for managing the epidemic to the countries. Thus, the estimates of infections and deaths that were inspired by epidemiological models about the population-level effects of TasP, and which PEPFAR sourced from UNAIDS, are key to articulating success. Meeting the metrics would also be the key trigger for handing over responsibility for managing the epidemic to national governments.

However since the clinical logics of TasP had influenced the organisation to devote a disproportionate amount of resources to a select group of countries, and to treatment programmes, over and above all other programme areas, the exit strategy was troubled by a central irony: namely, the programmes and countries that have been systematically under-funded would need to be funded at significant higher levels before the organisation could exit. That is, before transferring responsibility to countries, PEPFAR would need to ensure local partners had sufficient health infra-structures in place, and to do that, the organisation would need to increase the budget for governance and systems as well as management and operations. Indeed, the exit plan hinged on revitalising programme areas that have been in decline for nearly a decade.

The exit strategy also raised concerns about who would be left behind, which epidemiological models based on TasP could not adequately address. Along with the vision to 'end AIDS', PEPFAR had adopted the UNAIDS ethic to 'leave no one behind' which was applied universally across all populations for whom HIV care services could be beneficial. However, as advocates and scholars have contended, in the transition to 'country ownership' some would clearly be left behind, including sex workers, transgender people, and gay and other men who have sex with men in countries that criminalise these populations or otherwise allow lawful discrimination against them (Davis et al. 2017). In the transition toward country ownership, who would care for these key populations? This question challenged any claims to a 'sustainable' solution (Committee on the Outcome and Impact Evaluation of Global HIV/AIDS Programs 2013). This was not an issue that could be resolved by increasing funding for treatment, or other programme areas, but was exacerbated by plans for PEPFAR to pull aid.

Extending trends in planned spending associated with the strategy of epidemic control, the exit plan also stitched together the science of biomedical HIV prevention with the geopolitical interests of the USA in ways that obscured the nation's declining investments in HIV abroad. However, in this case, the over-reliance on a biomedical approach to the epidemic also presented obstacles for a successful exit.

14.5   Conclusion

The clinical logics of TasP structured PEPFAR's latest strategic initiative to achieve 'epidemic control' including the organisation's use of metrics for evaluating perfor-mance, and decisions for allocating funds to specific programs and countries. While TasP was initially conceptualised as an 'evidence-based' solution for effectively treating *and* preventing HIV, which could be consistently measured and reported on, its ability to produce the right kinds of evidence remained abstract and hypothetical. Nevertheless, PEPFAR relied on these metrics to make big claims about its own impact on the epidemic.

The effects of TasP have also been evident in the budget since PEPFAR launched the strategy to achieve 'epidemic control'. Whereas under previous initiatives to 'lead to the global response' to the epidemic, PEPFAR supported a wider variety of program areas, including by strengthening health systems, under the strategy of epidemic control PEPFAR has prioritised treatment programs over and above all others. TasP also justified disproportionate spending on a subset of countries. While this subset of 13 countries has received significantly more support since the initiative began, long-term trends in the budget also reveal that PEPFAR has prioritised these countries since its establishment as an organisation.

By adopting the clinical logics of TasP, PEPFAR justified spending on a limited number of programmes in a small set of countries that could produce what it defined as the right kinds of outcomes, and laid the groundwork for the retreat of US foreign aid. However, PEPFAR must now reckon with the blind spot of an overly biomedical approach, and answer difficult questions about who, and what, has and will be left behind.

Funding Statement Research for this chapter was supported by the European Research Council under the European Union's Seventh Framework Programme (FP7/2007–2013), ERC grant agreement 617,930, and the Swiss National Science Foundation, project grant 189,186.

References

Adams, V. (2016). *Metrics: What counts in Global Health.* (Reprint ed.). Durham, NC: Duke University Press Books.

amfAR, The Foundation for AIDS Research. (2020). *Program areas.* PEPFAR Country/Regional Operational Plans (COPs/ROPs) Database. Retrieved February 20, 2020, from https://copsdata.amfar.org/about/stratareas.

Basu, S., Carney, M. A., & Kenworthy, N. J. (2017). Ten years after the financial crisis: The long reach of austerity and its global impacts on health. *Social Science & Medicine, 187,* 203–207. https://doi.org/10.1016/j.socscimed.2017.06.026.

Biden, J. (2008). *S.2731 – 110th Congress (2007–2008): Tom Lantos and Henry J. Hyde United states global leadership against HIV/AIDS, tuberculosis, and malaria reauthorization act of 2008.* Legislation, July 16, 2008. https://www.congress.gov/bill/110th-congress/senate-bill/2731.

Cambiano, V., Lampe, F. C., Rodger, A. J., Smith, C. J., Geretti, A. M., Lodwick, R. K., et al. (2010). Use of a prescription-based measure of antiretroviral therapy adherence to predict viral rebound in HIV-infected individuals with viral suppression. *HIV Medicine, 11*(3), 216–224. https://doi.org/10.1111/j.1468-1293.2009.00771.x.

Cohen, M. S. (2000). Preventing sexual transmission of HIV – New ideas from sub-Saharan Africa. *New England Journal of Medicine, 342*(13), 970–972. https://doi.org/10.1056/NEJM200003303421311.

Cohen, J. (2010). Treatment as prevention. *Science, 327*(5970), 1196–1197. https://doi.org/10.1126/science.327.5970.1196-b.

Collins, C., & Beyrer, C. (2013). Country ownership and the turning point for HIV/AIDS. *The Lancet Global Health, 1*(6), e319–e320. https://doi.org/10.1016/S2214-109X(13)70092-5.

Committee on the Outcome and Impact Evaluation of Global HIV/AIDS Programs Implemented Under the Lantos-Hyde Act Of 2008, Board on Global Health, youth board on children, and Institute of Medicine. (2013). *Progress toward transitioning to a sustainable response in partner countries.* National Academies Press (USA). Retrieved December 11, 2020, from https://www.ncbi.nlm.nih.gov/books/NBK207016/.

Davis, S. L. M., Goedel, W. C., Emerson, J., & Guven, B. S. (2017). Punitive Laws, key population size estimates, and global AIDS response Progress reports: An ecological study of 154 countries. *Journal of the International AIDS Society, 20*(1), 21386. https://doi.org/10.7448/IAS.20.1. 21386.

Erikson, S. (2016). Metrics and market logics of Global Health. In V. Adams (Ed.), *Metrics: What counts in Global Health* (pp. 147–162). Durham, NC: Duke University Press.

Esser, D. E. (2014). Elusive accountabilities in the HIV scale-up: 'Ownership' as a functional tautology. *Global Public Health, 9*(1–2), 43–56. https://doi.org/10.1080/17441692.2013. 879669.

Granich, R. M., Gilks, C. F., Dye, C., De Cock, K. M., & Williams, B. G. (2009). Universal voluntary HIV testing with immediate antiretroviral therapy as a strategy for elimination of HIV transmission: A mathematical model. *The Lancet, 373*(9657), 48–57. https://doi.org/10.1016/S0140-6736(08)61697-9.

Hyde, H. J. (2003). H.R.1298 – 108th Congress (2003–2004): United States leadership against HIV/AIDS, tuberculosis, and malaria act of 2003. May 27, 2003. https://www.congress.gov/bill/108th-congress/house-bill/1298.

Kenworthy, N., Thomann, M., & Parker, R. (2018). From a global crisis to the 'end of AIDS': New epidemics of signification. *Global Public Health, 13*(8), 960–971. https://doi.org/10.1080/17441692.2017.1365373.

Lock, M., & Nguyen, V.-K. (2018). *An anthropology of biomedicine* (2nd ed.). Oxford: John Wiley & Sons.

Nguyen, V.-K., Bajos, N., Dubois-Arber, F., O'Malley, J., & Pirkle, C. (2011). Remedicalizing an epidemic: From HIV treatment as prevention to HIV treatment is prevention. *AIDS, 25*(3), 291–293. https://doi.org/10.1097/QAD.0b013e3283402c3e.

Oni-Orisan, A. (2016). The obligation to count: The politics of monitoring maternal mortality in Nigeria. In V. Adams (Ed.), *Metrics: What counts in Global Health* (pp. 82–103). Durham, NC: Duke University Press.

PEPFAR. (2005). *First annual report to congress*. Washington, DC: PEPFAR.

PEPFAR. (2006). *Second annual report to congress*. Washington, DC: PEPFAR.

PEPFAR. (2007a). *Third annual report to congress*. Washington, DC: PEPFAR.

PEPFAR. (2007b). *Indicators reference guide. FY2007 reporting/FY2008 planning. Indicators, reporting requirements, and guidelines*. Washington, DC: PEPFAR.

PEPFAR. (2008). *Fourth annual report to congress*. Washington, DC: PEPFAR.

PEPFAR. (2009a). *Fifth annual report to congress*. Washington, DC: PEPFAR.

PEPFAR. (2009b). *Indicators reference guide. FY2009 reporting/FY2010 planning. Indicators, reporting requirements, and guidelines*. Washington, DC: PEPFAR.

PEPFAR. (2010). *Sixth annual report to congress*. Washington, DC: PEPFAR.

PEPFAR. (2011a). *Seventh annual report to congress*. Washington, DC: PEPFAR.

PEPFAR. (2011b). *Indicators reference guide. FY2011 reporting/FY2012 planning. Indicators, reporting requirements, and guidelines*. Washington, DC: PEPFAR.

PEPFAR. (2012). *Eighth annual report to congress*. Washington, DC: PEPFAR.

PEPFAR. (2013a). *Ninth annual report to congress*. Washington, DC: PEPFAR.

PEPFAR. (2013b). *Indicators reference guide. FY2013 reporting/FY2014 planning. Indicators, reporting requirements, and guidelines*. Washington, DC: PEPFAR.

PEPFAR. (2014a). *Tenth annual report to congress*. Washington, DC: PEPFAR.

PEPFAR. (2014b). *Indicators reference guide. FY2014 reporting/FY2015 planning. Indicators, 452 reporting requirements, and guidelines*. Washington, DC: PEPFAR.

PEPFAR. (2015a). *Eleventh annual report to congress*. Washington, DC: PEPFAR.

PEPFAR. (2015b). *Indicators reference guide. FY2015 reporting/FY2016 planning. Indicators, reporting requirements, and guidelines*. Washington, DC: PEPFAR.

PEPFAR. (2016). *Twelfth annual report to congress*. Washington, DC: PEPFAR.

PEPFAR. (2017a). *Thirteenth annual report to congress*. Washington, DC: PEPFAR.

PEPFAR. (2017b). *Strategy for accelerating HIV/AIDS epidemic control, 2017–2020*. Washington, DC: PEPFAR.

PEPFAR. (2018). *Fourteenth annual report to congress*. Washington, DC: PEPFAR.

PEPFAR. (2019). *Fifteenth annual report to congress*. Washington, DC: PEPFAR.

PEPFAR. (2020). *PEPFAR reports to congress 2005–2018*. United States Department of State (blog). Retrieved January 29, 2020, from https://www.state.gov/pepfar-reports-to-congress-2005-2017/.

PEPFAR. (2020b). *Additional data*. PEPFAR Panorama Spotlight. Retrieved February 20, 2020, from https://data.pepfar.gov/additionalData.

Pfeiffer, J. (2013). The struggle for a public sector: PEPFAR in Mozambique. In J. Biehl & A. Petryna (Eds.), *When people come first* (pp. 166–181). Princeton, NJ: Princeton University Press.

Quinn, T. C., Wawer, M. J., Sewankambo, N., Serwadda, D., Li, C., Wabwire-Mangen, F., et al. (2000). Viral load and heterosexual transmission of human immunodeficiency virus type 1. *New England Journal of Medicine, 342*(13), 921–929. https://doi.org/10.1056/NEJM200003303421303.

U.S. Department of State. (2020). *Reports and guidance – PEPFAR*. Retrieved January 29, 2020, from https://www.state.gov/reports-pepfar/.

UNAIDS. (2010). *Getting to zero: 2011–2015 strategy*. Retrieved February 20, 2020, from https://www.unaids.org/sites/default/files/sub_landing/files/JC2034_UNAIDS_Strategy_en.pdf.

UNAIDS. (2014). *90-90-90: An ambitious treatment target to help end the AIDS epidemic*. Retrieved February 19, 2020, from https://www.unaids.org/sites/default/files/media_asset/90-90-90_en.pdf.

UNAIDS. (2018). *Resources and funding*. Retrieved January 15, 2020, from https://www.unaids.org/en/keywords/resources-and-funding.

UNAIDS. (2019). *UNAIDS HIV data and estimates*. Retrieved January 15, 2020, from https://www.unaids.org/en/dataanalysis/knowyourresponse/HIVdata_estimates.

Wendland, C. (2016). Estimating death: A close Reading of maternal mortality metrics in Malawi. In V. Adams (Ed.), *Metrics: What counts in Global Health* (pp. 57–81). Durham, NC: Duke University Press Books.

Whitacre, R. (2020). From advocacy to austerity: The new role of the U.S. public sector in HIV drug development and access. *Global Public Health, 15*(5), 627–637. https://doi.org/10.1080/17441692.2019.1704820.

Open Access This chapter is licensed under the terms of the Creative Commons Attribution 4.0 International License (http://creativecommons.org/licenses/by/4.0/), which permits use, sharing, adaptation, distribution and reproduction in any medium or format, as long as you give appropriate credit to the original author(s) and the source, provide a link to the Creative Commons license and indicate if changes were made.

The images or other third party material in this chapter are included in the chapter's Creative Commons license, unless indicated otherwise in a credit line to the material. If material is not included in the chapter's Creative Commons license and your intended use is not permitted by statutory regulation or exceeds the permitted use, you will need to obtain permission directly from the copyright holder.

Chapter 15
Getting Real on U=U: Human Rights and Gender as Critical Frameworks for Action

Laura Ferguson, William Jardell, and Sofia Gruskin

15.1 Background

HIV treatment has been shown to lead to improved clinical outcomes while yielding the additional benefit of preventing onward transmission once viral suppression is achieved. This process is widely known in the scientific community as 'Treatment as Prevention' (TasP). In 2006, the 'Swiss Statement'—an authoritative statement that people living with HIV who are in receipt of effective antiretroviral therapy (ART), and who do not have any sexually transmitted infections (STIs), cannot transmit HIV through sexual contact—explicitly called on courts to consider this information in criminal HIV transmission cases, noting that unprotected sex between a person living with HIV and an HIV-negative partner 'does not comply with the criteria for an attempt to spread a dangerous disease under section 231 of the Swiss Penal Code, nor for an attempt to cause serious bodily harm under section 122, 123 or 125 of the Swiss Penal Code' (Vernazza et al. 2008).

Since then, several large studies have confirmed the accuracy of the science (Rodger et al. 2016; Eisinger et al. 2019), setting the foundation for global acceptance of the message that undetectable viral load leads to negligible risk of HIV transmission. Importantly, however, distinct from the Swiss Statement, there is no reference to legal implications, human rights principles or gender considerations in the write-up of any of these later studies. Yet, decades of experience have shown the need to pay attention not just to new technologies in relation to HIV but also to the people who are their intended beneficiaries, and, consequently, to human rights and gender in the rollout of any new HIV-related intervention.

L. Ferguson (✉) · W. Jardell · S. Gruskin
USC Institute on Inequalities in Global Health, University of Southern California, Los Angeles, California, USA
e-mail: laura.ferguson@med.usc.edu; jardell@usc.edu; gruskin@med.usc.edu

© Springer Nature Switzerland AG 2021   201
S. Bernays et al. (eds.), *Remaking HIV Prevention in the 21st Century*, Social Aspects of HIV 5, https://doi.org/10.1007/978-3-030-69819-5_15

In 2019, the Prevention Access Campaign launched the 'Undetectable equals Untransmittable' or 'U=U' initiative, now supported by more than 990 organisations from over a hundred countries. More recently, the Campaign has added a third 'U' for 'Universal', urging advocates to use U=U as a platform for demanding universal access to HIV diagnosis, treatment and healthcare for all people living with HIV (Prevention Access Campaign 2019). To reduce the potential for discrimination against people whose viral load is not undetectable (whether through choice or factors beyond their control), another slogan has been introduced: namely 'Viral load does not equal value' (V $\neq$ V) (Stephens 2019). These initiatives have been explicit in recognising barriers such as stigma, discrimination, criminalisation and inadequate health care infrastructure and call for increased access to needed treatment by removing these barriers. U=U in particular has been key in strengthening advocacy efforts for universal access to treatment, care and diagnostics, even as neither human rights nor gender dynamics are explicitly addressed in its original messaging or approach (Prevention Access Campaign 2019).

For U=U to be inclusive, to benefit everyone, and to avoid the potential of creating divisions between those who are virally suppressed and those who are not, addressing the structural factors that shape people's ability to access and adhere to ART is critical. Although the campaign has successfully united community and medical experts, additional attention is still needed to ensure gender and rights are adequately considered in discourse, programming and activities relating to both TasP and U=U.

For TasP and U=U to fulfil their potential, attention to gender and human rights, not only in rhetoric but, critically, in implementation is key. The long history of HIV and human rights has repeatedly made this clear. And yet it seems that in efforts to make U=U and TasP a reality, the focus of research, programming and activities has been predominantly biomedical, with insufficient attention to these issues. In this chapter, we seek to assess the ways in which relevant organisations explicitly consider rights and gender in their U=U and TasP programming and statements. We hope the analysis can help to inform how rights and gender will support future TasP and U=U work both at global and national levels, deliver improved HIV-related outcomes, and ensure support for the most vulnerable populations.

15.2 Why Gender and Human Rights?

15.2.1 Gender

In the context of HIV, gender has long been understood to affect access to resources and decision-making power, vulnerability to HIV infection and people's willingness and ability to access HIV-related services. With respect to both TasP and U=U, if gender relations and dynamics are ignored, many of the structural barriers that impede equitable access and use of HIV-related services are likely to remain unchallenged and unaddressed even if ART is available. On the flip side, systematic efforts to address gender-related barriers can help to ensure these strategies work for everyone: women, men and transgender populations alike.

15.2.2 Human Rights

The application of human rights principles to HIV research and programming is a way to reach those most vulnerable, and to increase positive health outcomes for all. The legal and policy environment shapes the availability of HIV-related services and programmes and the degree to which they are responsive to individual needs and aspirations (Gruskin et al. 2007a). With respect to U=U and TasP, consideration of human rights principles alongside attention to the legal and policy environment can help identify and overcome challenges to increasing and sustaining access to treatment and services, as well as promote accountability and transparency for what is done and how (Gruskin et al. 2007b).

Table 15.1 identifies the range of human rights principles commonly considered relevant to HIV responses and provides an overview of their relevance to HIV within the specific context of U=U/TasP.

15.3 Non-Governmental Organisations' Attention to Gender and Rights in U=U and TasP

Since U=U began to get traction, the need for attention to gender and human rights in U=U interventions has been advocated by a wide range of non-governmental organisations (NGOs). NGOs, often activist and community-led, play a unique role in advancing HIV programming and policy development, and civil society concerns usefully frame the issues that need to be addressed for these interventions to have their intended benefits.

We looked at three large-scale HIV-related NGOs to explore their current messages with regards to gender and rights in the context of U=U and TasP. All three NGOs voice support for U=U but express concern about the barriers that still exist for people living with HIV, especially women and other marginalised populations, to benefit from this development. In addition, they call for increased understanding of structural barriers that prevent access to health services and accurate and rights-based information.

Citing concerns that treatment as prevention might be prioritised over treatment as treatment, that responsibility for HIV prevention might be placed solely on people living with HIV, and that continuing inequities impede access to HIV treatment and services, in 2017, the Global Network of People Living with HIV (GNP+) initially refused to endorse the U=U campaign (GNP+ 2017). Following discussion and at times heated debate, GNP+ ultimately did endorse the statement, but pointed to the

Table 15.1 Human Rights Principles Relevant to TasP and U=U

Human Right/s	Relevance to HIV	Relevance to TasP/U=U
Human rights/rights	Human rights are legally guaranteed under international human rights law. Relevant to HIV, they protect against actions that interfere with fundamental freedoms and human dignity and support the agency of individuals and populations.	Human rights norms and standards provide mechanisms to guarantee equal access to health care services, and treatment information to understand TasP/U=U.
Participation	The inclusion and full participation of all key stakeholders and affected communities, with particular attention to the greater involvement of people living with HIV, is key to HIV responses.	Meaningful participation of communities and people living with HIV in policies and programmes can help ensure their acceptability and effectiveness. This should also include the participation of the HIV negative partners of people living with HIV in decision-making regarding care and treatment options.
Equality and non-discrimination	HIV programmes should respect, protect, promote and fulfil the rights to equality and to non-discrimination for all people living with and affected by HIV.	Attention is needed to ensure no discrimination against people living with HIV who continue to have a detectable viral load. Equitable distribution of services to the most marginalised on a non-discriminatory basis is essential.
The right to health in relation to goods and services	The right to health includes the availability, accessibility, acceptability and quality of the goods and services provided (UN Committee on Economic, Social and Cultural Rights 2000).	
	Availability: Facilities, goods and services should address the underlying determinants of health.	*Availability*: ART (and accompanying diagnostics etc.), which U=U/TasP rely on, must be available to all people living with HIV.
	Accessibility: Accessibility of health facilities, goods and services to all, especially the most vulnerable and affected, encompasses: (i) Non-discrimination (ii) Physical accessibility (iii) Affordability (iv) Access to information	*Accessibility*: Information and services should be available without fear of stigma, discrimination or abuse from government, communities, health care providers or individuals and should be promoted in laws and policies to increase physical accessibility and, importantly, affordability.
	Acceptability: Health facilities, goods and services must be respectful of the culture of individuals, minorities, peoples and communities, sensitive to sex and life-course requirements, as well as designed to respect confidentiality.	*Acceptability*: Success rests on the acceptability of the services on offer to people living with HIV, to support adherence to treatment and regular visits to the health facility.

(continued)

Table 15.1 (continued)

Human Right/s	Relevance to HIV	Relevance to TasP/U=U
	Quality: Goods and services must be scientifically and medically appropriate and of good quality.	*Quality*: Poor quality services, drugs or diagnostics, for example, might hamper individuals' ability to maintain or even monitor viral suppression.
Accountability	If states fail to uphold human rights, individuals and communities should be able to take action to seek accountability for violations.	Governments should be held accountable for laws and policies criminalising people living with HIV that conflict with the scientific basis, the steps they take towards ensuring better treatment and prevention outcomes for all, including the most marginalised, the ability to access ART, regular viral load testing and information.

barriers that exist in many parts of the world to universal optimal treatment options, viral load detection and diagnostic access for all people living with HIV. It advocates for increased dialogue about ways in which the U=U message can address current political and economic barriers using human rights principles including accessibility, decreased stigma, informed decision-making, affordability, respect and quality of care, and participation by people living with HIV at global, regional and national levels. U=U is therefore framed as useful but with many important caveats to be addressed (GNP+ 2012).

The International Community of Women Living with HIV North America (ICW-NA) has recognised that U=U is powerfully changing the lives of millions of people living with HIV. However, ICW-NA holds that most U=U messaging falls short of acknowledging the structural barriers that women face in being able to benefit from U=U. ICW-NA put into place their own 'U=U: Don't Forget Women' campaign, which calls for action to better understand the impact of being undetectable for women with HIV, and in relation to sexual and reproductive health and rights, bodily autonomy, pregnancy and breastfeeding. ICW-NA advocates for women-led research and advocacy to ensure that women's stories and experiences are included in U=U approaches and relevant dialogues (ICW-NA 2020).

The International Council of AIDS Service Organizations (ICASO) has endorsed the U=U campaign since January 2017. Consistent with the approach taken by the Swiss Statement, ICASO recommends the use of up-to-date scientific evidence to reform or repeal laws that criminalise people living with HIV for non-disclosure of their HIV status, including in cases where there is no transmission or risk of transmission. ICASO sees rights as a necessary tool to advocate for stigma reduction, increased affordability, informed decision making and widespread accessibility, and calls for the U=U movement to rally behind women's rights and gender equality to tackle these concerns (ICASO 2017). It notes that power and gender inequalities create additional barriers for women living with HIV to access health services, impacting their ability to benefit from U=U. ICASO views the current application of U=U with respect to women, which it understands to include transgender men, gender queer people and others identified female at birth, as too narrow, suggesting that it has the potential to catalyse much needed conversations about gender inequalities and violence, women's self-determination, access to treatment, women's involvement in research, bodily autonomy and informed choice, irrespective of viral load (ICASO 2018).

There is striking and consistent clarity in the stance taken by these NGOs: namely, that attention to gender and rights in U=U is critical for success. Entirely consistent with the history of the HIV response, this in turn raises the question as to whether this same sensibility exists in the public statements of the international institutions responsible for relevant research and programming. We sought to explore this by analysing the websites of selected global-level institutions working on HIV.

15.4 Global Institutional Approaches to Human Rights and Gender in the Context of U=U and TasP

Global institutions play a range of different roles in the HIV response from setting norms, standards and guidelines to establishing funding priorities and structures that affect the implementation of services and programmes as well as research. The Joint United Nations Programme on HIV and AIDS (UNAIDS), the World Health Organization (WHO), The Global Fund to Fight AIDS, Tuberculosis and Malaria (Global Fund), and the US President's Emergency Plan For AIDS Relief (PEPFAR) are four key organisations. Table 15.2 presents an overview of each organisation's current language around U=U and TasP.

Each of these institutions uses the science behind U=U/TasP to promote the use of ART to help people living with HIV achieve and maintain a suppressed viral load and prevent further transmission. UNAIDS is the only organisation that has both explicitly endorsed and developed guidelines around the U=U message (UNAIDS 2018). Among all four institutions, only WHO explicitly uses the language of TasP. In a programmatic update titled 'Antiretroviral Treatment as Prevention (TasP) of HIV and TB', WHO, in detailing guidance for achieving a suppressed viral load, recognises gaps in accessibility of ART treatment services in low- and middle-income countries as well as in rural areas (WHO 2012).

While these global organisations recognise the importance of gender in terms of HIV as well as the need to address gender dynamics in HIV programming, they have not yet included these dimensions in their materials specific to U=U or TasP. The Global Fund is the most explicit in regards to gender and gender dynamics in the context of U=U, and recognises that a biomedical approach to HIV is insufficient and that responses must address the root causes of vulnerability for women and key populations as well as the barriers to accessing health services faced by heterosexual men (Global Fund 2019a; Global Fund 2020).

Table 15.2 International institutions' published materials on U=U, TasP, gender and human rights

Institution	U=U	TasP	Gender	Human Rights
UNAIDS	U=U is an explicitly named and recognised key message as a way to address HIV transmission, stigma and discrimination, and end the AIDS epidemic. A U=U 'explainer' document outlines U=U messaging and key actions.	TasP is not recognised by name. Treatment for people living with HIV has been showcased in the 90-90-90 by 2020 targets.	Gender as specific to U=U or TasP is not discussed in UNAIDS documents however a U=U 'explainer' discusses the need for a range of treatment and preventive services inclusive of services based on gender (male and female condoms, PrEP, voluntary medical male circumcision).	Human rights as specific to U=U are discussed in the U=U 'explainer' calling for the scale up of comprehensive responses, awareness and knowledge of U=U, access to quality testing and treatment, stigma- and discrimination-free testing and treatment, affordable testing and treatment and the need to address unjust criminalisation that violates human rights and deters people living with HIV from accessing services
WHO	U=U is not recognised by name within WHO guidelines, toolkits, or documents, however WHO does explicate the science behind it.	TasP is explicitly recognised within WHO guidelines, toolkits, and documents. WHO has specific guidelines on TasP.	Gender as specific to U=U or TasP is not discussed, however general HIV guidelines and documents promote gender equality and a woman-centered approach to health care and ART. TasP is discussed in terms of populations (pregnant women, men who have sex with men (MSM), transgender people, sex workers, people who inject drugs (PWID)) but with no	Human rights as specific to U=U are not discussed however general HIV-related guidance promotes human rights-based approaches to ART and pushes for greater efforts in providing primary prevention and addressing structural barriers. Human rights as specific to TasP are discussed in TasP guidelines outlining the importance of a rights framework to control and

(continued)

Table 15.2 (continued)

Institution	U=U	TasP	Gender	Human Rights
			consideration of gender dynamics.	eliminate HIV, with special attention to stigma and discrimination, equity, accessibility, data and monitoring systems.
Global Fund	U=U is named explicitly by the Global Fund and with respect to efforts to prevent new infections. The website information directly links to the UNAIDS 'explainer' document noted above.	TasP is not recognised by name within Global Fund documents, however it recognises treatment paired with other innovative prevention efforts as important to end the HIV epidemic.	Gender as specific to U=U is discussed explicitly. In this context, the Global Fund strongly supports efforts to address gender inequalities, gender-based violence, educational disadvantages, economic disempowerment and structural barriers preventing access to treatment and prevention services by women and girls and key populations (MSM, transgender people, PWID, sex workers).	Attention to human rights as specific to U=U focuses on stigma and discrimination and addressing human-rights barriers. Accountability is also discussed in terms of appropriate data collection and investing in treatment monitoring systems.
PEPFAR	U=U is recognised by name and PEPFAR purports to adopt it enthusiastically. PEPFAR promotes U=U through the MenStar initiative[a] and in guidance documents. PEPFAR-supported programmes for HIV testing amplify the U=U message. PEPFAR directly links to the	TasP is not recognised by name but PEPFAR utilises the TasP science. Its general HIV response includes addressing the unmet need for comprehensive prevention, care, and treatment.	Gender as specific to U=U or TasP is not discussed even as more general HIV-related guidance prioritises preventing new HIV infections in women, adolescent girls and children. PEPFAR states its dedication to continued implementation of the 2013 gender strategy that calls for providing gender-equitable HIV	Human rights are not mentioned in the specific context of U=U or TasP, but more general HIV-related guidance notes the underlying social and cultural issues that prevent people from accessing HIV prevention and treatment services, especially human rights

(continued)

Table 15.2 (continued)

Institution	U=U	TasP	Gender	Human Rights
	UNAIDS 'explainer' document.		prevention, care, treatment, and support.	barriers, stigma and discrimination.

ªMenStar is a public-private partnership launched in 2018 that aims to reach men in sub-Saharan Africa with HIV diagnosis and treatment services

Each of the global institutions reviewed, to varying degrees, include human rights principles in their more general HIV-related documentation and, to some extent, there is also mention of rights among discussion of U=U or TasP. The UNAIDS U=U 'Explainer' document, for example, explicitly addresses the need to dismantle the human rights barriers faced by key populations. Within their TasP guidance, WHO discusses the importance of a rights framework to treat and eliminate HIV, highlighting rights-related barriers including stigma and discrimination, inequity, lack of accessibility, and weak data and monitoring systems (WHO 2012). The Global Fund discusses rights, specifically stigma and discrimination, accountability for data and the need to address human-rights related barriers in the design and delivery of products and programmes (Global Fund 2019b). Each of these organisations recognises the need to address human rights barriers especially as they relate to stigma/discrimination, access to health services, and affordability when it comes to U=U/TasP. However, none of them present clear action steps as to what this should look like in practice. PEPFAR does not specifically discuss human rights in relation to U=U or TasP.

15.5   Discussion

The analyses above lay the groundwork for exploring what needs to be done to make a difference on the ground. Through the prism of gender and rights, three broad areas of concern emerge: (1) the extent to which overarching structural factors impede the effectiveness of U=U/TasP; (2) the extent to which gender and rights concerns are addressed within existing health system approaches to U=U/TasP; and (3) the extent to which gender and rights concerns at both individual and community levels impact access to and use of relevant health services, goods and commodities.

15.5.1   Structural Factors Impacting U=U/TasP

15.5.1.1   Laws and Policies Affecting the Potential of U=U/TasP

In the context of U=U/TasP, increased attention has been paid to the legal and policy barriers that inhibit the sustained access to treatment necessary for people living with

HIV to achieve and maintain a suppressed viral load. The overly broad criminalisation of HIV transmission has not only been shown to be detrimental to the overall HIV response, but also to contribute to fear and anxiety among people living with HIV in ways that have a direct impact on U=U. The adoption of U=U as a strategy highlights the need for legal reform in the many contexts where HIV remains criminalised, and the promotion of U=U/TasP could be used to lead to legal and policy changes, including the removal of HIV non-disclosure criminalisation laws.

Other types of laws create barriers to U=U/TasP, including laws that criminalise sex between men, or harm reduction programmes for people who use drugs (Bereczky 2019). Removing laws that criminalise people living with HIV and members of key populations can shift public attitudes and reduce stigma, in turn helping to support sustained access to treatment (Rendina and Parsons 2018). In addition to the larger legal environment, a range of policies can impact the effectiveness of U=U/TasP. For example, national policies limiting comprehensive sexuality education restrict access to basic information about sex, sexuality, HIV and HIV programmes, resulting in limited awareness of U=U even when services are available. Policies intended to address U=U/TasP in and of themselves can be both facilitators and barriers.

A range of HIV-specific government policies can make it impossible for people living with HIV to achieve an undetectable viral load. For example, in 2019, while 182 countries reported that ART is initiated irrespective of CD4 count, seven countries reported not initiating ART until a client's CD4 count dropped below 500 cells/mm^3 (WHO 2019). Thus, for some people living with HIV, U=U is unattainable simply because of how government shapes relevant policy. Additional policies that can either facilitate or hinder the accessibility of treatment include the frequency of required clinic visits, particularly when people live far from where services are available.

Conversely, official government policies can improve accessibility to treatment and remove barriers to access. For example, the removal of upfront copayments for treatment or providing access to free ART to all people living with HIV can radically enhance access to the means of achieving an undetectable viral load (Callander et al. 2016).

15.5.1.2   Gender Dynamics and Relations

A review of current literature suggests that there is minimal U=U/TasP research being done with women living with HIV or transgender populations even though it is widely understood that the barriers may be greatest for these populations. Gay and other men who have sex with men appear to be the main populations studied in current U=U/TasP research (Jungwirth and Helfand 2020). The intersection of race and gender is evident and adds one more layer of complexity to be addressed.

Widespread power inequalities can delay women's access to viral load testing which is necessary for U=U to be effective (ICASO 2018). Fear of intimate partner violence and economic dependency may also deter women from seeking treatment and care (Chikovore et al. 2016; Kalichman et al. 2018). In line with one of ICASO's stated concerns, a study, focusing on women in Kenya, Zimbabwe, and South Africa, found that providing HIV treatment to women was perceived as approving increased sexual freedom for women, a notion that is highly stigmatised, consequently leading to lower access to and adherence to treatment (Minnis et al. 2019).

From a gender perspective, the exclusive focus of U=U messaging on sexual transmission of HIV, as noted by ICASO, constitutes a real limitation. In the absence of relevant information, women of reproductive age around the world have struggled to understand the implications of U=U for the prevention of vertical transmission of HIV if their viral load is undetectable (ICW 2020) suggesting clearer messaging is required.

Transgender and gender diverse people are at high risk for HIV infection due to lack of knowledge and sensitivity among healthcare providers as well as stigma and discrimination associated with poor mental health, substance use, violence, lack of family support, homelessness and unemployment all of which can compromise access to HIV care and treatment and ultimately a suppressed viral load (Teti et al. 2019). Tackling the gender stereotypes and dynamics that disadvantage specific groups is critical to the success of U=U/TasP, and frames the health system, community and individual level factors that influence the effectiveness of these interventions.

15.5.2   Health System Factors Affecting the Potential of U=U/ TasP

Within the health system, many different issues impact the success of U=U/TasP strategies. A human rights lens draws attention to the availability, accessibility, acceptability and quality of the services delivered, as well as the access people have to the information needed for informed decision-making. All of these issues are, of course, also gendered with gender dynamics playing out and intersecting in relation to each one of them.

15.5.2.1   The Right to Health: Availability, Accessibility, Acceptability and Quality

Concerns have been raised about a potential disconnect between the spreading of U=U/TasP messaging and the limited availability or accessibility of ART in some contexts. Caution is needed: generalising the effectiveness of U=U/TasP models and assuming their results will play out similarly in all countries, and contexts, is not particularly helpful. There is a need to evaluate U=U/TasP interventions on a country by country basis, and also at sub-national levels, taking into account the health system, and in particular the availability of free or affordable treatment and viral load monitoring (Barrow and Barrow 2015). Where ART is available and accessible, the acceptability of TasP has been found to increase with people's exposure to its success such as with regular testing and exposure to positive testimonials disseminated in person or through mass media (Mooney et al. 2017; Kalichman et al. 2018).

Taking this one step further, there is a need to ensure the availability, accessibility, acceptability and quality of a wide range of health services to ensure the success of U=U/TasP. This could include not only pre-exposure prophylaxis (PrEP) but family planning, STI and sexual health information and services in the context of condomless sex, as well as mental health services. The right to health reminds us that U=U/TasP cannot be implemented in isolation. While U=U/TasP offers opportunities for individuals to manage HIV and prevent onward transmission, these same individuals also need access to quality health services that can support their overall health and ability to reach and maintain viral suppression.

15.5.2.2   Access to Health Information

Barriers exist to up to date, comprehensive, and culturally-tailored information about U=U/TasP. The language used by researchers, NGOs, global institutions, public health officials and healthcare providers matters and impacts both attitudes and access to care (Brett 2020). An analysis across 25 countries found that people living with HIV with adequate knowledge about U=U had more favourable health outcomes, including in relation to mental health, sexual health, treatment satisfaction and viral suppression, than those who did not (Okoli 2020).

The science behind U=U tells us that negligible risk is zero risk in the context of sexual transmission. Yet this messaging seems to acquire greater credibility, at least in the USA, after endorsement by the national Centers for Disease Control, illustrating the important role that key agencies play not only in prioritising interventions but how they are understood (Rendina and Parsons 2018). However, in some settings the medical community has been accused of withholding U=U/TasP messaging from patients due to fears that negligible is not zero (Ford 2019). Scientists now promote the use of phrasing such as 'effectively zero', 'no risk' or 'cannot transmit' to resolve earlier incorrect or biased communications around U=U (i-Base 2017). Even with these semantic shifts, however, messages still need to be tailored to individual clients and their partner(s).

As noted above, withholding of information about U=U/TasP has occured among health care providers, particularly with patients from marginalised populations. Documented factors include not only lack of provider knowledge, but disbelief in U=U/TasP, and negative and discriminatory attitudes (Ford 2019; Calabrese and Mayer 2020). Providers have also acknowledged concern around providing information about U=U/TasP to patients for fear of being blamed if transmission were to occur (Calabrese and Mayer 2020). Research has found that while Black men who have sex with men expect their providers to initiate conversations around HIV transmission and U=U, racial discrimination makes health providers less likely to share information and decision-making power with their Black clients in this context (Calabrese and Mayer 2020).

15.5.2.3   Prioritisation within the Health System

Resource constraints impacting HIV responses are real, whether driven by decreases in international donor funding, reluctance to fund services related to sexual and reproductive health, or the inability to ensure the sustainability of free treatment. Some settings have seen 'AIDS fatigue' and a decrease in political will. Even if a U=U/TasP strategy is in place, funding shortfalls can negatively impact service availability and accessibility resulting in drug stock outs, high costs, and a lack of consistent and reliable (or indeed any) viral load testing (Bereczky 2019).

15.5.3   Community Factors Affecting the Potential of U=U/ TasP

15.5.3.1   Stigma and Discrimination

In the context of U=U, studies have documented that the stigma faced by people from vulnerable communities as well as internalised stigma can lead to greater barriers to accessing relevant HIV information, treatment and care (Prado Generoso 2020; Prevention Access Campaign 2020).

In line with its original intention, however, U=U can serve as a means to begin to dismantle both external and internalised stigma and discrimination. Knowledge of U=U has been found to be associated with lower presence of anxiety and depression and also impacts internalised stigma (Reyes-Diaz et al. 2020). In Vietnam, adopting U=U was found to reduce stigma and discrimination because it increased collaboration and information sharing between people living HIV and key population communities, healthcare providers, international organisations, and leaders and influencers in society (Nguyen 2020).

15.5.3.2   Access to Information within the Community

The provision of accurate information regarding U=U/TasP in health services is critical but so too is community education and messaging. Widespread understanding can help reduce HIV-related stigma and discrimination within communities but promoting such understanding often requires nuanced approaches. Millions of people living with HIV, as well as those at risk of infection, remain unaware of the facts and potential implications of U=U for their lives as well as for their sexual partners. Differences have been found in the perceived accuracy of U=U messaging across various subgroups, based on such factors as socioeconomic status, race/ethnicity, geographic location, drug use, engagement in sex work, being on PrEP and/or HIV status (Rendina and Parsons 2018).

These variations call for nuanced, subgroup-specific health promotion (Rendina and Parsons 2018). The involvement of NGOs in government community health programmes, so that activism and targeted messaging can shape prevention responses and allow for public participation is critical (Monteiro et al. 2019). Even within identified population groups, no group is monolithic nor has uniform and predictable behaviours (Chikovore et al. 2016), highlighting the need for any community-level U=U/TasP messaging to be designed as an entry point for individual level discussion.

15.6   Moving Forward

Even as NGOs have been vocal about many of these issues, there remains a lack of explicit attention to gender dynamics and human rights among global institutions and in research and programming concerned with U=U/TasP. While the epidemiological risks of HIV transmission during different types of sexual intercourse have been explored, far less attention has been given to the rights- and gender-related factors that play key roles in influencing people's ability to reach and maintain an undetectable viral load.

The success of U=U/TasP is contingent on an array of factors beyond individuals' control including a protective legal environment, access to acceptable and quality health services that deliver an uninterrupted supply of antiretroviral drugs and regular access to viral load testing, and supportive community environments. Increased focus on ensuring the availability and accessibility of functional mechanisms of accountability can help promote attention to all of these issues, drawing attention to who is responsible for each element, where they are succeeding, and, importantly, where they are falling short.

U=U has had a great impact where it has been boldly embraced, clearly articulated and tailored to reach those who need it most. Using gender and rights as frameworks to understand and address the structural, health system and community factors that create barriers to the full achievement of U=U/TasP can help inform interventions at all levels. There is sufficient evidence to press for changes in laws, policies and practices to ensure that as these interventions roll out on a large scale, they do not cause harm but create benefits, and that these benefits accrue to all populations, not just those who are easiest to reach.

References

Barrow, G., & Barrow, C. (2015). HIV treatment as prevention in Jamaica and Barbados: Magic bullet or sustainable response? *Journal of the International Association of Providers of AIDS Care, 14*(1), 82–87. https://doi.org/10.1177/2325957413511113.

Bereczky, T. (2019). U=U is a blessing: But only for patients with access to HIV treatment: An essay by Tamás Bereczky. *British Medical Journal (Clinical Research Ed.), 366*, l5554. https://doi.org/10.1136/bmj.l5554.

Brett, A. (2020). *Messaging transmission: A qualitative analysis of factors in the uptake of U=U in Canadian public health messaging (abstract).* International AIDS conference 2020.

Calabrese, S. K., & Mayer, K. H. (2020). Stigma impedes HIV prevention by stifling patient-provider communication about U = U. *Journal of the International AIDS Society, 23*(7), e25559. https://doi.org/10.1002/jia2.25559.

Callander, D., Stoové, M., Carr, A., Hoy, J. F., Petoumenos, K., Hellard, M., et al. (2016). A longitudinal cohort study of HIV 'treatment as prevention' in gay, bisexual and other men who have sex with men: The treatment with Antiretrovirals and their impact on positive and negative men (TAIPAN) study protocol. *BMC Infectious Diseases, 16*(1), 752. https://doi.org/10.1186/s12879-016-2073-2.

Chikovore, J., Gillespie, N., McGrath, N., Orne-Gliemann, J., Zuma, T., & ANRS 12249 TasP Study Group. (2016). Men, masculinity, and engagement with treatment as prevention in KwaZulu-Natal, South Africa. *AIDS Care, 28*(Suppl 3), 74–82. https://doi.org/10.1080/09540121.2016.1178953.

Eisinger, R. W., Dieffenbach, C. W., & Fauci, A. S. (2019). HIV viral load and transmissibility of HIV infection: Undetectable equals Untransmittable. *JAMA, 321*(5), 451–452. https://doi.org/10.1001/jama.2018.21167.

Ford, O. G. (2019). *Understanding undetectable equals Untransmittable – a growing global community builds a movement.* POZ. Retrieved August 27, 2020, from https://www.poz.com/article/understanding-undetectable-untransmittable.

Global Fund. (2019a). *HIV, human rights and gender equality. The Global Fund to Fight AIDS, Tuberculosis and Malaria.* Retrieved August 27, 2020, from https://www.theglobalfund.org/media/6348/core_hivhumanrightsgenderequality_technicalbrief_en.pdf.

Global Fund. (2019b). *Step up the fight: Focus on human rights. The Global Fund to Fight AIDS, Tuberculosis and Malaria.* Retrieved August 27, 2020, from https://www.theglobalfund.org/media/8119/publication_humanrights_focuson_en.pdf?u=637321467292270000.

Global Fund. (2020). *HIV & AIDS. The Global Fund to Fight AIDS, Tuberculosis and Malaria.* Retrieved August 27, 2020, from https://www.theglobalfund.org/en/hivaids/..

GNP+. (2012). *GNP+ position paper: ART for prevention.* Global Networks of People Living with HIV. GNP+. Retrieved August 27, 2020, from https://www.gnpplus.net/assets/wbb_file_updown/4513/ART%20for%20Prevention.pdf.

GNP+. (2017). *Follow up on previous article: On fear, infectiousness, Undetectability.* Global Network of People Living with HIV. GNP+. Retrieved August 19, 2020, from https://www.gnpplus.net/follow-up-on-previous-article-on-fear-infectiousness-undetectability/.

Gruskin, S., Ferguson, L., & O'Malley, J. (2007a). Ensuring sexual and reproductive health for people living with HIV: An overview of key human rights, policy and health systems issues. *Reproductive Health Matters, 15*(29 Suppl), 4–26. https://doi.org/10.1016/S0968-8080(07)29028-7.

Gruskin, S., Mills, E. J., & Tarantola, D. (2007b). History, principles, and practice of health and human rights. *The Lancet, 370*(9585), 449–455. https://doi.org/10.1016/S0140-6736(07)61200-8.

i-Base. (2017). *The evidence for U=U (Undetectable = Untransmittable): Why negligible risk is zero risk.* i-Base. Retrieved August 27, 2020, from https://i-base.info/htb/32308.

ICASO. (2017). *Undetectable = Untransmittable: A community brief.* International Council of AIDS Service Organizations. Retrieved August 19, 2020, from http://icaso.org/wp-content/uploads/2017/11/UU-brief-EN-2.pdf.

ICASO. (2018). *Understanding U=U for women living with HIV: ICASO community brief.* International Council of AIDS Service Organizations. Retrieved August 19, 2020, from http://icaso.org/wp-content/uploads/2018/09/Understanding-UU-for-Women.pdf.

ICW. (2020). *Webinar: Topic U=U + women: Minding the gaps – June 18, 2020.* International Community of Women Living with HIV. Retrieved August 27, 2020, from https://www.thewellproject.org/groups/hiv-eventsconferences/webinar-topic-uu-women-minding-gaps-june-18-2020.

ICW-NA. (2020). *U=U: Not without women.* International Community of Women Living with HIV. Retrieved August 27, 2020, from https://icwnorthamerica.org/portfolio-items/uu-not-without-women/?portfolioCats=43.

Jungwirth, B., & Helfand, M. (2020). *This week in HIV research: Do you believe in U=U? TheBodyPro.* Retrieved August 27, 2020, from https://www.thebodypro.com/slideshow/week-hiv-research-undetectable-equals-untransmittable-belief.

Kalichman, S. C., Cherry, C., Kalichman, M. O., Eaton, L. A., Kohler, J. J., Montero, C., & Schinazi, R. F. (2018). Mobile health intervention to reduce HIV transmission: A randomized trial of behaviorally enhanced HIV treatment as prevention (B-TasP). *Journal of Acquired Immune Deficiency Syndromes, 78*(1), 34–42. https://doi.org/10.1097/QAI.0000000000001637.

Minnis, A. M., Montgomery, E. T., Napierala, S., Browne, E. N., & van der Straten, A. (2019). Insights for implementation science from 2 multiphased studies with end-users of potential multipurpose prevention technology and HIV prevention products. *Journal of Acquired Immune Deficiency Syndromes, 82*(Suppl 3), S222–S229. https://doi.org/10.1097/QAI.0000000000002215.

Monteiro, S. S., Brigeiro, M., Vilella, W. V., Mora, C., & Parker, R. (2019). Challenges facing HIV treatment as prevention in Brazil: An analysis drawing on literature on testing. Desafios do tratamento Como prevenção do HIV no Brasil: Uma análise a partir da literatura sobre testagem. *Ciencia & Saude Coletiva, 24*(5), 1793–1807. https://doi.org/10.1590/1413-81232018245.16512017.

Mooney, A. C., Gottert, A., Khoza, N., Rebombo, D., Hove, J., Suárez, A. J., et al. (2017). Men's perceptions of treatment as prevention in South Africa: Implications for engagement in HIV care and treatment. *AIDS Education and Prevention, 29*(3), 274–287. https://doi.org/10.1521/aeap.2017.29.3.274.

Nguyen, A. (2020). *Undetectable = Untransmittable (U=U) to drive stigma reduction and epidemic control in Vietnam: A global model for political and program innovation (abstract).* International AIDS conference 2020.

Okoli, C., Richman, B., Allan, B., Brough, G., Castallanos, E., Young, B., et al. (2020). *A tale of two "U" s and their use by healthcare providers: A cross-country analysis of information-sharing about 'Undetectable = Untransmittable' (U=U) (abstract).* International AIDS conference 2020.

Prado Generoso, I. (2020). *The relation of internalized homonegativity with HIV prevention strategies: Results from Latin-America MSM internet survey (LAMIS) in Brazil (abstract).* International AIDS conference 2020.

Prevention Access Campaign. (2019). *Consensus statement: Risk of sexual transmission of HIV from a person living with HIV who has an undetectable viral load.* Prevention Access Campaign. Retrieved August 17, 2020, from https://www.preventionaccess.org/consensus.

Prevention Access Campaign. (2020). *The third U=unequal.* Prevention Access Campaign. Retrieved August 19, 2020, from https://www.preventionaccess.org/3rdu.

Rendina, H. J., & Parsons, J. T. (2018). Factors associated with perceived accuracy of the undetectable = Untransmittable slogan among men who have sex with men: Implications for messaging scale-up and implementation. *Journal of the International AIDS Society, 21*(1), e25055. https://doi.org/10.1002/jia2.25055.

Reyes-Diaz, M., Schmidt, A. J., Veras, M. A., Stuardo, V., & Caceres, C. F. (2020). *Undetectable=untransmissible (U=U) knowledge and sexual behavior during the most recent sexual encounter with non-steady partners among MSM in the Latin-American MSM internet survey (LAMIS) (abstract). International AIDS conference 2020.*

Rodger, A. J., Cambiano, V., Bruun, T., Vernazza, P., Collins, S., van Lunzen, J., et al., for the PARTNER Study Group. (2016). Sexual activity without condoms and risk of HIV transmission in Serodifferent couples when the HIV-positive partner is using suppressive antiretroviral therapy. JAMA, 316(2), 171–181. https://doi.org/10.1001/jama.2016.5148.

Stephens, C. (2019). *Viral load does not equal value*. POZ. Retrieved August 27, 2020, from https://www.poz.com/article/viral-load-equal-value-charles-stephens.

Teti, M., Bauerband, L. A., & Altman, C. (2019). Adherence to antiretroviral therapy among transgender and gender nonconforming people living with HIV: Findings from the 2015 U.S. trans survey. *Transgender Health, 4*(1), 262–269. https://doi.org/10.1089/trgh.2019.0050.

UN Committee on Economic, Social and Cultural Rights. (2000). *General comment 14 on the right to the highest attainable standard of health*. United Nations. Retrieved August 27, 2020, from https://www.refworld.org/pdfid/4538838d0.pdf.

UNAIDS. (2018). *Undetectable = Untransmittable: Public health and viral load suppression*. Geneva: UNAIDS. Retrieved August 27, 2020, from https://www.unaids.org/sites/default/files/media_asset/undetectable-untransmittable_en.pdf.

Vernazza, P., Hirschel, B., Bernasconi, E., & Flepp, M. (2008). Les personnes séropositives ne souffrant d'aucune autre MST et suivant un traitement antirétroviral efficace ne transmettent pas le VIH par voie sexuelle. *Bulletin des Médecins Suisses, 89*, 165–169.

WHO. (2012). *Programmatic update: Antiretroviral treatment as prevention (TasP) of HIV and TB*. Geneva: World Health Organization. Retrieved August 27, 2020, from https://apps.who.int/iris/bitstream/handle/10665/70904/WHO_HIV_2012.12_eng.pdf;jsessionid=513A43DC8ECB7D0DDB31C51DCA4A23D0?sequence=1.

WHO. (2019). *WHO policy data 2019: Recommended ART CD4 initiation threshold in adults and adolescents. Global, most recent data*. Geneva: World Health Organization. Retrieved August 27, 2020, from http://lawsandpolicies.unaids.org/topicresult?i=38.

Chapter 16
Falling Short of 90-90-90: How Missed Targets Govern Disease Elimination

Kari Lancaster and Tim Rhodes

16.1 Introduction

In 2014 the Joint United Nations Programme on HIV/AIDS (UNAIDS) established a new target for HIV treatment scale-up globally, with the goal of ending the AIDS epidemic as a public health threat by 2030. In what was at the time called 'a new, final, ambitious, but achievable target', it was declared that by 2020 90% of all people living with HIV would know their HIV status, 90% of all people diagnosed with HIV infection would receive sustained antiretroviral therapy, and 90% of all people receiving antiretroviral therapy would have viral suppression (UNAIDS 2014: see Fig. 16.1). In 2016, the 90-90-90 target was given further articulation in the World Health Organization's (WHO) *Global Health Sector Strategy on HIV 2016–2021*. Designed to contribute to the attainment of the Sustainable Development Goal on health (Goal 3), the WHO strategy outlined a set of 'Global Targets for 2020' aimed at taking 'a decisive leap' towards ending the AIDS epidemic (WHO 2016b, p. 23). The 2016 HIV strategy specified areas for 'fast track action' essential for meeting the targets, including via bolstering combination prevention, new testing approaches, filling the treatment gap, holistic care, reaching vulnerable and at risk populations, reducing costs and improving efficiencies (WHO 2016b, p. 14). It was said that an 'immediate, fast-tracked global response that achieves the targets set out in this strategy will effectively end the epidemic as a global public health threat' (WHO 2016b, p. 15). Enacting a future in which 'ending AIDS' was not only conceivable but achievable, the experts assured that '90-90-90 can happen'

K. Lancaster (✉)
Centre for Social Research in Health, UNSW Sydney, NSW, Australia
e-mail: k.lancaster@unsw.edu.au

T. Rhodes
University of New South Wales, Sydney, Australia

London School of Hygiene and Tropical Medicine, London, UK

© Springer Nature Switzerland AG 2021   219
S. Bernays et al. (eds.), *Remaking HIV Prevention in the 21st Century*, Social
Aspects of HIV 5, https://doi.org/10.1007/978-3-030-69819-5_16

THE TREATMENT TARGET

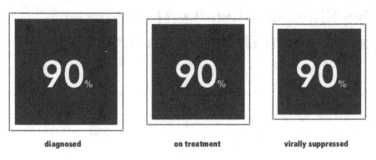

Fig. 16.1 90-90-90 The Treatment Target. Reproduced from UNAIDS (2014, p. 1)

(UNAIDS 2014, p. 16). Through the 90-90-90 target, the 'roadmap for ending the AIDS epidemic is clear' (Sidibé et al. 2016).

Writing in 2020 in the midst of the COVID-19 pandemic, we are faced with an immeasurably more uncertain global public health landscape. The promise of disease elimination futures imagined within global health strategies appears tenuous, not least due to ever-more stretched resources and disruptions to health services and supplies (WHO 2020b). In the case of HIV, as at July 2020, 73 countries had reported being at risk of stock-outs of antiretroviral medicines (WHO 2020c). Of these countries, 24 reported critically low stocks, meaning an estimated 8.3 million people in those regions – or one third of all people receiving HIV treatment globally – were potentially affected by supply shortages. Modelling teams estimated that if these treatment interruptions were not mitigated, disruptions could lead to an additional 500,000 deaths from AIDS-related illness in sub-Saharan Africa in 2020–2021 alone, effectively 'setting the clock back' to 2008 (Hogan et al. 2020; Jewell et al. 2020; WHO 2020a). The WHO noted that 'despite steady advances in scaling up treatment coverage – with more than 25 million people in need of ARVs receiving them in 2019 – key 2020 global targets will be missed' (WHO 2020c).

As the anticipated future of 2020 imagined in the 90-90-90 target becomes the past, and in a moment of major disruption and crisis in global health, we want to pose a question: what do *missed* targets *do*? On the surface, this might seem like an odd question. Surely the power-of-acting of global health targets is in their achievement and success? After all, 90-90-90 had been called a *final* target – we had been told that 'ending the AIDS epidemic is both achievable and an outcome that will serve not only as a fitting coda to the long AIDS struggle but also as an inspiration to the broader global health and international development fields' (UNAIDS 2014, p. 11). The achievability of the treatment target was said to be a realistic expectation, based on 'scientific knowledge and implementation evidence' and 'better understanding of the full potential of available tools' (UNAIDS 2014, p. 11). However, we suggest that the unprecedented global events of 2020 offer an opportunity to reflect differently on *how* these enumerated targets do their governing, in more complex ways. Missed targets are, after all, ubiquitous. More often than not, global health targets are not met. In many ways, we might say that global health is governed through failure (or, more precisely, *failing*). Thus, how might *missed* targets be seen as performative actors with governing potential in the constitution of health? What possibilities can global health targets as enumerated entities afford *even now*? And what might noticing the performativity and governing potential of missed targets tell us about how global health targets do their work, and how it might be done well?

16.2 Numbering Practices and Governance

To notice how global health targets do their work, even as they appear to fall short, we turn to the study of number and numbering practices (Verran 2010, 2012, 2015; Day et al. 2014). Our orientation towards *practices* is in keeping with scholarship in the field of science and technology studies (STS) which has sought to draw renewed attention to matters of ontology, highlighting the performativity of everyday practices and the '*accomplished* ontology of entities' (Mol 2002; Law 2004; Woolgar and Lezaun 2013, p. 333, emphasis original). By focusing on the generative power of the practices involved in the enactment of realities, this mode of analysis helps probe seemingly mundane, finished or ready-made objects which might not appear controversial, interfering with the assumption of a singular, complete, stable and ordered world (Woolgar and Lezaun 2013). Doing away with the assumption of singularity opens up distinctly ontopolitical possibilities in so far as 'different constellations of practice and their hinterlands might make it possible to enact realities in different ways' (Law 2004, p. 66). Things could be made otherwise (Mol 2002; Law and Urry 2004).

   Numbers might be considered amongst the ordinary, mundane, unproblematic entities that seemingly transcend context. However, by attuning our attention to the constitutive effects of practices and the relations involved in the enactments of realities, we can say that numbers 'are not simply representations of an external reality but also *produce* actors, objects and relationships' (Hansen and Porter 2012, p. 410, emphasis added). Far from being referents of an exogenous world, we find that numbers are 'made in the materials of science and other practices, and furthermore, they make effects, including beyond calculus, in the "real worlds" of action, intervention and policy' (Rhodes and Lancaster 2020, p. 1). Thus, thinking about *numbering practices* shifts our focus towards 'what numbers *do*, what they *become*, and the effects they *make*, through their implementations', thus appreciating numbers as situated *evidence-making interventions* (Rhodes and Lancaster 2019, 2020 p. 1, emphasis original).

   A growing body of critical scholarship has destabilised positivist conceptions of numbers as 'representations of the world' by illuminating the ontopolitical effects of numbering practices and how numbers constitute the objects of governance (Rose 1991; Rose and Miller 1992; Porter 1996; Miller 2001; Rowse 2009; Merry 2011, 2016; Hansen and Porter 2012; Day et al. 2014; Rottenburg et al. 2015; Shore and Wright 2015; Verran 2015; Holtrop 2018; Kovacic 2018). Philosopher of science,

Helen Verran, suggests that we can think about numbers '*as materialised relations*' (Verran 2010, p. 171, emphasis original). Just as people are and have kin, in both a material and semiotic sense, so too numbers both *are* and *have* relations (Verran 2010). Mobilising a performativist approach, Verran (2015, pp. 367–368) distinguishes between a number and what she calls an *enumerated entity*:

> Enumerated entities as objects known in a performative analytic, are particular relational beings; they are events or happenings in some actual present here and now. Importantly there are quite strict conditions under which enumerated entities come into existence as relational entities in our worlds. Part of the wonder of enumeration is that sets of very specific practices can indeed happen just as exactly as they need to, again and again, as repetitions. Sets of routine practices must be collectively, and more or less precisely, enacted in order for an enumerated entity to come to life. So, in looking 'inside,' what most people would simply call numbers (and probably not imagine as having an inside), I elaborate the every day techniques by which they come to life.

Verran's emphasis here is on noticing the materialising routines and collective actions by which enumerated entities are 'done' and constituted, including the metaphysical commitments embedded in those actions. In doing so, it becomes possible to interrogate the means by which governing is made possible. Enumerated entities have effects and as they circulate: 'they begin to change our worlds, at a minimum this occurs by directing our attentions to some things and not others' (Verran 2015, p. 371). There is a *politics* at work.

16.3   Targets and the Making of Disease Elimination

Building on this thinking, we can begin to notice how enumerated global health targets do their governing in practice, and how targets participate relationally as actors in global health assemblages. By 'assemblages' we refer to the coming together of multiple elements, both human and nonhuman, which through their entanglements materialise realities (Deleuze and Guattari 1988; Duff 2014), in this case realities of disease elimination. Assemblages are arrangements 'connoting active and evolving practices rather than a passive or static structure' (Watson-Verran and Turnbull 1995, p. 117). This means assemblages are 'tentative and hesitant and unfolding', a 'recursive process', in which 'the elements put together are not fixed in shape, do not long belong to a larger pre-given list, but are constructed at least in part as they are entangled together' (Law 2004, p. 42). Numbering practices – including metrics, models and targets – are one of many elements in the assembling of disease elimination, for instance, bundling together with policies, governments, discourses, laws, science, expertise, communities, cultures, viruses and so on (Erikson 2012; Taylor-Alexander 2017; Tichenor 2017; Lancaster et al. 2020; Rhodes and Lancaster 2020; Rhodes et al. 2020). But numbering affords a particular power of acting in the governing of population health and infectious disease (Porter 1996; Bauer 2013; Rhodes and Lancaster 2020). As Adams (2016, p. 9) argues, numbers can 'move policy, confer political allegiance, guarantee funding, even bring about health. But they do so not simply by claiming truth about the empirical world. They do so because of the ways they are "produced" and the ways they are circulated'. Numbers are afforded their agency through their entanglements in evolving assemblages.

Epidemics, infection and viral pandemics are 'typical of the kinds of events that attract numbers and number practices' (Mackenzie 2014, p. 191; Rhodes et al. 2020). In epidemics, and especially pandemics, there is a heightened sense of knowing the future as uncertain and needing to know with greater certainty in order to bring about infection control. Within the imaginaries of global public health, it might be suggested that one cannot eliminate that which is not measured. Enumerated global health targets (and the modelling informing them) therefore do particularly significant performative work. As an effect of their enumeration, targets constitute 'disease elimination' and 'health' as objects of governance (Lancaster et al. 2020; Rhodes and Lancaster 2020). As technologies of governance, global targets work to make the problem of disease elimination recognisable and manageable as a 'global problem', amenable to structuring, action, and multilateral global management (Shore and Wright 2015; Merry 2016; Lancaster and Rhodes 2020; Lancaster et al. 2020; Rhodes and Lancaster 2020). Numerical targets bring the object of disease elimination 'into the real'. The intrinsic future orientation of targets, in particular, has ontopolitical effects, orienting action in-the-now and working to govern the present to shape possible futures (Lancaster and Rhodes 2020).

16.4   Missing the Mark, Falling Short

Despite the growing interest in the performativity of numbers, metrics and targets in global health, there has been comparatively little critical attention paid to *missed* or *failed* targets. In some ways this is surprising, given that the story of disease elimination is so often told with reference to a 'threshold' of success or failure. When it comes to public health targets, we are either 'on' or 'off track' (WHO 2015; Boseley 2018; Polaris Observatory 2020). Storied accounts of successful interventions into smallpox and polio are alive in the imaginaries of global health, travelling alongside accounts of failures to adequately respond to the Ebola outbreak in West Africa or premature declarations of leprosy elimination, for instance (Caplan 2009; Pai 2019; Center for Global Development 2020). The failure to acknowledge – and learn from – the ubiquity of 'failure' in global health has been seen as a cultural problem in the field, perpetuated in part by global health systems of governance (Rajkotia 2018). Invariably the response to failure in global health is to explain it away, and locate it, as a problem of systems, complexity, implementation or coordination (Mackenbach and McKee 2013; Charan and Paramita 2016). It has been suggested that high stakes, expectation and collective ambition to improve global health has precipitated 'enormous pressure' to achieve targets and that there is a need to 'break open the "success cartel"' (Rajkotia 2018, p. 2). Although there is an imperative to advance and progress swiftly towards imagined futures of disease elimination, the complexity of global health challenges means that, more often than not, 'failure is guaranteed' (Pai 2019).

However, categorising these stories according to a binary 'threshold' of 'success' and failure' obscures a more complex picture. Read another way, we can notice how global health targets govern not through arrival or achievement but rather through *progression*; an almost-there-ness holding ontologically open the possibility of *success even in failure*. Here, it is the open process of assembling, and the anticipation that this affords, that makes-up and keeps vital realities of disease control. The earlier '3 by 5' initiative launched by the WHO is one example. '3 by 5' aimed to connect three million people living with HIV/AIDS in low- and middle-income countries with antiretroviral treatment (ART) by the end of 2005. We could say that this initiative missed its mark. In June 2005 the WHO reported that 'overall progress is unlikely to be fast enough to reach the target set by WHO and UNAIDS of treating 3 million people by the end of 2005' (WHO 2005). But in these accounts of failing and falling short, we can begin to notice how it is that targets do their work. Even in 2005, as the future imagined in the global initiative became a failure of the present, it was *progression* towards the possibility of an alternative future that was made to matter, over and above any sense of arrival or completion: 'the number of people receiving ART is *increasing* in every region of the world, and the rate of scale-up is also *accelerating*' (WHO 2005, emphasis added). More recently, of the 3 by 5 initiative it was said that 'despite considerable scepticism regarding the advisability and feasibility of expanding access to ART in low and middle income settings, as of mid-2014 over 12 million PLHIV were on ART' (Fast Track Cities n.d.). The story of 'falling short' was simultaneously told as a story of achievement and success, for example here in the *New England Journal of Medicine*: 'This "3 by 5" initiative *fell short of its target but resulted in* antiretroviral-drug treatment for 1.3 million patients, preventing an estimated 250,000 to 350,000 deaths. In 2005 alone, \$8.3 billion was spent on AIDS — about 30 times as much as at the creation of UNAIDS' (Merson 2006, emphasis added). Through stories of global health failure, targets are nonetheless being *made present*, continuing to solidify. Not only are targets being made present, but we can begin to see one of the reasons why they never really fail. Targets perform a governance and generate action even as they fall short because *progression* (and not completeness), an *aim* (not necessarily an outcome), is fundamental to how targets do their work. Success or failure has a *latitude* which makes ongoing governance possible. This hits home our earlier point that assemblages of disease elimination, in which numbers circulate to do their performative work, are unfolding and becoming, with targets, progress, success and failure always situated and never fixed; and thus open rather than closed.

16.5 Vague Predicates

But how is this openness achieved? How do numbers afford latitude? After all, are numbers not precise? Is it not the case that numerical targets hone precision in relation to a single point of measurable accomplishment? By noticing how missed targets do their work through progression, in a process of assembling towards a something which remains open, we can see how it is that as enumerations targets are afforded an ongoing power-of-acting by enacting, managing and stabilising their object of governance (disease elimination) as a 'vague whole' (Rhodes and Lancaster 2020). Helen Verran (2015, p. 370) argues that enumerated entities, in different ways, offer a means for 'managing the sorites paradox in rendering the vague whole of what is governed into the specific units in and through which governance proceeds'. The sorites (or heap) paradox invoked here is a classic logic paradox which arises when a term or predicate has vague, fuzzy or unclear boundaries, for example a 'heap' or a 'pile'. One grain of rice is not a heap; and one grain of rice is too small to make a difference to whether something is or is not a heap: 'if one starts with a pile of rice and begins taking grains away, when does it stop being a pile?' (Verran 2015, p. 369). While this is on the surface a logic problem, we can also see that vague predicates like 'heap' are vague in a *useful* way. Verran argues that the workings of enumerated entities offer *enough certainty* to otherwise fuzzy boundaries to *enact a governance*.

The object of 'disease elimination' made up within global health targets is a vague predicate. In many ways this is quite obvious in that enumerating HIV and other disease elimination targets is a methodological challenge characterised by empirical uncertainty. The 90-90-90 targets signalling the 'end of AIDS', for instance, are not necessarily measurable measures (for discussion of some of these complexities, see Marsh et al. 2019). How is 90% of all people living with HIV knowing their HIV status, 90% of all people diagnosed with HIV infection receiving sustained antiretroviral therapy, and 90% of all people receiving antiretroviral therapy having viral suppression to be evidenced? How is this to be done across settings in which surveillance and other data vary dramatically in terms of quality and availability? Even assuming these data indicators were measurable in uniform and standardised ways, how are they to be performed into a meaningful global analysis which transforms their combined enumeration into evidence of disease elimination? Here then, we articulate the vague predicates of disease elimination targets as an epistemological problem for implementation science in terms of how target measures might relate, with any certainty or precision, to imagined realities of the end of AIDS.

Our concern here though, is not so much whether targets can be measured precisely against a particular imagined reality, but how targets *do their work* as vague predicates that also afford a sense of evidence-based precision. Just how much latitude do targets have when doing their work to enumerate progress towards a particular imagined future? This is why the case of *missed targets* is illuminating. The generative capacity of fluid boundaries becomes all the more obvious when we notice what missed targets do. How far short of the target (whether or not this can be precisely measured) can we fall before the possibility of a disease elimination future becomes undone? It is notable that the 'end of AIDS' as a public health threat is not defined as *zero* cases, or stopping transmission entirely. Rather, the end of AIDS is made up through a *combination* of *proportional* targets, each set at 90%. There are two elements at work here – *combinations* and *proportions*. Through their potential for combination, numbers 'can generate uniformity among different objects counted (three apples and two oranges makes five fruits)' (Hansen and Porter 2012, p. 413). The 90-90-90 target recombines different interventions and establishes new relations between them (the ubiquitous figure of the 'cascade of care' in global health does similar work: see WHO 2016b, p. 20). But further to this, the possibility of disease elimination imagined in the target is constituted not in relation to absolute numbers or cases, but as a percentage (90%). The percentage implies a 'completion, or wholeness of some kind, to the category-name – the denominator – that equals the "100"' (Guyer 2014, p. 156). However, the denominator – for example all people receiving HIV treatment globally – remains an empirical unknown, and is especially difficult to measure with certainty in the context of a global health emergency when health services and surveillance systems are challenged. The complexities of enumerating population-level HIV treatment access (as with the other 90s) are masked through proportionality, affording a 'virtual precision' in the face of uncertainty (Verran 2015; Rhodes and Lancaster 2020).

The combination of proportional targets which make-up '90-90-90' thus enact 'elimination' or 'the end of AIDS' as a vague predicate – a vague whole; akin to a heap or a pile. Returning, then, to the sorites paradox we can ask the question again: in the global health assemblage of 2020, as health services and treatment access are profoundly disrupted by the COVID-19 pandemic, how much HIV treatment can be taken away before the ontological possibility of disease elimination ceases to exist? That is, when does the disease elimination target fall short? The logic paradox fails as it always does – a definitive cut-off or threshold is not possible (one more person receiving antiretroviral therapy, or one more person with viral suppression, does not tip the balance between declaring whether we are 'on track' in the race to 'the end of AIDS' or not). But the *proportion* manages the problem of the quantification, managing uncertainty and the impossibilities of measureable cut-offs. The latitude afforded by the vague predicate allows for progression towards the possibility of an imagined disease elimination future to be retained, and claimed, even within the bounds of evidence-based science.

In the context of the possibility of *missed targets,* the impossibility or illogic of a cut-off not only usefully makes governance at a distance possible but enacts a *continued hope* in the possibility of elimination as a future to be attained. The vague predicate allows for an imagined disease elimination future to continue to govern and have effects in the uncertain present. The possibility of a breakthrough which might change the situation for better or worse remains open; action is still possible and progress imperative. We can see this even in recent estimates of progress towards the 90-90-90 target, generated before the COVID-19 pandemic. Although it was estimated that many countries were 'unlikely' to reach the target, the very possibility of progress nonetheless generated a call for 'urgency' (Marsh et al. 2019, pp. S213, S224). This demonstrates the power-of-acting afforded through targets; the enumerated target makes up elimination as an object of governance, even as it seems to slip from future to past, and entangles with fresh matters of concern.

16.6   Timescapes and Disease Elimination Futures

We have argued that targets continue to govern even as they fall short because, as enumerated entities, targets do their work through progression and not completion, and enact disease elimination as a vague predicate. Disease elimination targets, including those constituting the ending of AIDS, are often also predicated in relation to a measure of time, usually a calendar year. The year 2030 is a point in calendar time that looms large, for it is set as a uniform horizon across global development and health sector strategies relating to HIV, viral hepatitis, and sexually transmitted infections (STI), and accordingly incorporated into related disease elimination targets (WHO 2016a). More than disease elimination, 2030 is the target in time by which the world is to be 'transformed' through the implementation of 17 sustainable development goals and 169 linked targets which together seek to 'end poverty and hunger everywhere', 'combat inequalities', 'build peaceful, just and inclusive societies', 'protect human rights and promote gender equality', and 'ensure lasting protection of the planet' (United Nations (UN) 2015). What is it about 2030 that serves as *the* time by which progress across all sorts of health and social developments complete? How is this precise point in calendar time evidence-based as the measure of time from now by which the speed and nature of target developments – from disease to poverty eliminations – come to be? Again, we find enacted a vague predicate which performs an apparent precision. The calendar year 2030 is not vague in the sense of being beyond absolute or actual measure once this threshold passes, as in the case of the virtual precision of immeasurable disease eliminations known instead by proportionate targets (see above, and Rhodes and Lancaster 2020). Rather, it is vague because it is *arbitrary*. It may even be random, aside from the sense that its selection is rooted in the performance of a matter of concern in relation to urgency, and the need to act in time, according to measures of global development which appear to be indexed in tens of years and even numbered decades. We emphasise then, that while there are ever more sophisticated approaches to measurement, evaluation, auditing, and estimating incidence and prevalence in relation to the precision of disease elimination targets, the thresholds in time which delineate success or failure, being 'on track' or 'falling short', are remarkably detached and without precision. Time matters for governing potential. And yet time goes largely unquestioned in the work that targets do and the time-based futures that they imagine. We take our cue here from Marsha Rosengarten who asks us to attend to time as an entangled element in assemblages of disease elimination. As she says: 'What is proposed in the name of time has remained unquestioned in public health and the sciences concerned with infection' (Rosengarten 2019, p. 3).

How then, do missed targets do time? All targets, as we have noted above, invoke a progressive futurity (Michael 2000; Adam and Groves 2007; Puig de la Bellacasa 2017; Lancaster and Rhodes 2020). In this sense, they perform, in the present, a particular future that is different from that of the now or times past. Targets not only anticipate but *make-up* a sense of time-space. When target futures, such as a world without AIDS, are indexed to points in calendar time, such as 2020 or 2030, they become open to enumeration in relation to binary measures of success or failure. There are, then, multiple forms of temporality at play in how time-based targets do time: there is a move across time towards a different future (a timescape of progressive futurity with its own particular features) measured in relation to linear calendar time (a designated date or number of years). These temporalities do not necessarily entangle in ways that make sense to the other, or in ways that matter to the actualised progression of infections and their eliminations. This is to say, that when disease elimination targets are 'missed', and fall short of their dates of completion, futures without disease are nonetheless still imagined and have affective implications. Missed targets do not 'fail' in performing anticipated progress. In fact, missed targets, especially those which 'just miss', are arguably especially good at keeping alive the possibility of a different better future to the time of now. By not quite keeping to time, time is being done, futures are protected, and advances can continue. For instance, while the disruptions of the COVID-19 pandemic to health services and medical supplies threaten to 'stall progress' towards 2020 disease elimination targets (WHO 2020c), this does not mean that these missed targets fail to afford a future without AIDS. Because they are necessarily future oriented, and in the case of treatment targets especially technoscientifically so, targets perform an 'inexhaustible pull' (Puig de la Bellacasa 2017, p. 174) of continued 'advance' in time. Missed targets that nearly succeed, and that fail without extinguishing all imagined potential, will always 'work' for they at once invoke a fear of regression to an earlier time (Puig de la Bellacasa 2017). With targets, we have *hope*, and thus, what matters is less that target dates are missed (like 2020 or 2030), but whether we are generally, more or less, moving ahead or falling behind (Michael 2000; Lancaster and Rhodes 2020). A particular timescape of progressive futurity is what matters. Even while the 90-90-90 targets might be evidenced as now unachievable by their 2020 threshold (WHO 2020c), the future anticipated in the targets nonetheless demands a response (Adams et al. 2009). Clock time, an arbitrary predicate, is detached from, but nonetheless points towards, what matters.

This temporal distinction, that can go unnoticed, brings into question whether disease elimination targets need calendar time at all. Diseases and infections do not live or transform according to calendar time. They are situated in time, of course, and they make-up different and distinct timescapes, as we have witnessed in the periodic evolution of HIV and AIDS through times of pandemic emergency, chronic disease management, and viral elimination. A future without disease does not need a calendar date to be imagined and neither does the calendar date make a material difference to its realisation. Diseases do not behave in this way, and in fact, make their own time situated in nature irrespective of universal clock time (Rosengarten 2019). So why is an arbitrary calendar date performed as if having evidence-based precision in the global science and policy of ending AIDS? Does anyone actually believe that 2020 or 2030 are, in themselves, meaningful benchmarks for bringing about disease eliminations in practice, and that they therefore make empirical sense to build into disease elimination models and enumerations? No. Rather, these arbitrary predicates are *made meaningful* in how they are *put-to-use* as measures to afford action and make progress. We need a calendar date in order that targets can be missed. A fear of regression, which within reason serves to maintain hope, needs a threshold. Without the potential to miss, targets do not work. It is through clock time that missed targets enact their futures.

Calendar time is thus made meaningful in relation to a particular timescape. When progress towards the realisation of '2020' targets is said to be falling behind to the treatment rates of '2008' as a consequence of COVID-19 (see above), what is being invoked by the missed target is not a matter of calendar concern (the date is insignificant in itself) but a concern in relation to temporal location according to sociotechnical and everyday arrangements (Puig de la Bellacasa 2017). Calendar dates here perform a 'time in practice', that is, an alternative timescape of global health assemblage (Adam 1998). Falling behind reconnects to an alternative generational assemblage of global health materiality and practices – not '2008' per se, but a time, for example, before ready ART access in low and middle income countries. This is a different 'lived, embodied, historically and socially experienced' temporality (Puig de la Bellacasa 2017, p. 175). This (and our earlier example of 3 by 5) tells us that while targets are deployed in relation to numbered calendar years – 2005, 2020, 2030 – they do not necessarily perform this way. Missed targets help us to notice how the timescape of futurity enacted through targets is in tension with alternative timescapes of viral and global health assemblage. It tells us that calendar time, or the inexhaustible and linear pull of a progressive and technoscientific futurity, need not be the only timescape through which the governance of targets work. We can already see that the enumerated calendar time of 2020 and 2030 is coexisting with other viral and global health assemblages, enacting time in practice in other ways which might be disruptive. This disruption, we suggest, might be seen as a resource for resistance through which targets might continue to govern even as the futures imagined within them become past, according to but one measure of time.

This leads us to ask how we might imagine and better situate the next ecological future of disease elimination. Is there a way that targets could be made more sensitive to the co-presence of different temporalities and timescapes? And if we could, would targets do their governing work even more effectively, and perhaps, more carefully? Borrowing from Puig de la Bellacasa (2017), we might speculate as to how the practices of maintenance and repair done within global health strategy (including efforts to 'stay on track' amidst crises) might work to enact a *temporality of care*. This temporality of care might be more fitting as we think about the proposal of a 'fourth 90', which calls for good health-related quality of life (Lazarus et al. 2016; Harris et al. 2018), or the need for other indicators and targets that go beyond the biomedical treatment paradigm. Such targets are not readily measured, but allow for the possibility of missing to allow for progress to be made, and, importantly, index to ethico-political and embodied matterings that might ordinarily be obscured.

The suggestion that alternative timescapes (Adam 1998) could work to perform hope and imagined futures with effects in the present is to better attune targets to their situated contexts and entanglements (that is, in the temporalities of global health assemblages and care, not bureaucratic cycles). These alternative timescapes might alter the relevance and virtual precision of targets, and how they open up or close down possible futures.

16.7   Conclusion

As discussion of viral control takes a new turn in the COVID-19 era, and well-trodden strategic challenges of global health governance become entangled with fresh matters of concern, there are lessons to be learned. In this extraordinary moment of global disruption and dis-ease, we have sought to consider how targets do their work through missing and falling short. We do this not to 'rationalise' failure in global health, as others have suggested (Rajkotia 2018; Pai 2019). Rather, our engagement with the performativity of targets – even in their falling short – has been driven by a critical intent to notice what is already going on, so as to speculate as to how targets and strategies might be enacted in a different, and more careful, mode.

We find that even in the midst of a global health crisis in 2020 when modelling and fractured health systems would seemingly signal otherwise, the 90-90-90 target as an enumerated entity continues to 'govern the present in relation to an imagined future through practices of virtual precision giving rise to *virtual elimination*' (Rhodes and Lancaster 2020, p. 4). Situated as we are in 2020, we find that the possibility of a missed or failing target is no less real, and does no less governing work, than the possibility of an achievable target. As an enumerated entity the 90-90-90 target constitutes disease elimination as a vague predicate and these fuzzy boundaries are *useful* – they make governing possible.

While the enumerated entity of the 90–90-90 target affords the possibility of a virtual elimination – even as it falls short in 2020 – we might also speculate as to what alternative futures it might close down. Is this virtual elimination done well, with care, or could it be made otherwise, in ways that attends to other more divergent worlds? We have tentatively proposed that thinking differently about the timescapes of disease elimination and global health, might be one way of extending the affordances of targets and their governing potential.

Certainly, the events of 2020 prompt consideration of the complex entanglements of global health ecologies and precarity of futures without disease. Most of all, it prompts consideration of how to live better with uncertainty in the race to elimination and remain open to multiple contingencies (Lancaster and Rhodes 2020). Beyond the question of what targets *do* and *how* they govern, we may also consider whether another object of elimination is possible, and how varied numbering practices and enumerations might afford different possibilities for intervention and the governance of health.

References

Adam, B. (1998). *Timescapes of modernity: The environment and invisible hazards*. London: Routledge.

Adam, B., & Groves, C. (2007). *Future matters: Action, knowledge, ethics*. Leiden: Brill.

Adams, V. (2016). *Metrics: What counts in global health*. Durham: Duke University Press.

Adams, V., Murphy, M., & Clarke, A. E. (2009). Anticipation: Technoscience, life, affect, temporality. *Subjectivity, 28*(1), 246–265.

Bauer, S. (2013). Modeling population health. *Medical Anthropology Quarterly, 27*, 510–530.

Boseley, S. (2018). *Food industry in England fails to meet sugar reduction target. The Guardian.* https://www.theguardian.com/society/2018/may/22/food-industry-in-england-fails-to-meet-sugar-reduction-target

Caplan, A. L. (2009). Is disease eradication ethical? *The Lancet, 373*(9682), 2192–2193.

Center for Global Development. (2020). *Millions saved*. Retrieved August 18, 2020, from http://millionssaved.cgdev.org.

Charan, M., & Paramita, S. (2016). Health programs in a developing country—Why do we fail. *Health Systems and Policy Research, 3*(3), 27.

Day, S., Lury, C., & Wakeford, N. (2014). Number ecologies: Numbers and numbering practices. *Distinktion: Journal of Social Theory, 15*(2), 123–154.

Deleuze, G., & Guattari, F. (1988). *A thousand plateaus*. London: Athlone.

Duff, C. (2014). *Assemblages of health*. London: Springer.

Erikson, S. L. (2012). Global Health business: The production and performativity of statistics in Sierra Leone and Germany. *Medical Anthropology, 31*(4), 367–384.

Fast Track Cities. (n.d.). *Frequently asked questions about 90-90-90 targets, the HIV care continuum, the updated national HIV AIDS strategy (NHAS), and the fast-track cities initiative.* Retrieved August 18, 2020, from http://www.fast-trackcities.org/sites/default/files/FAQ%20FTCI%20and%20updated%20NHAS.pdf.

Guyer, J. I. (2014). Percentages and perchance: Archaic forms in the twenty-first century. *Distinktion: Scandinavian Journal of Social Theory, 15*(2), 155–173.

Hansen, H. K., & Porter, T. (2012). What do numbers do in transnational governance? *International Political Sociology, 6*(4), 409–426.

Harris, T. G., Rabkin, M., & El-Sadr, W. M. (2018). Achieving the fourth 90: Healthy aging for people living with HIV. *AIDS (London, England), 32*(12), 1563–1569.

Hogan, A. B., Jewell, B., Sherrard-Smith, E., Vesga, J., Watson, O. J., Whittaker, C., et al. (2020). *Report 19: The potential impact of the COVID-19 epidemic on HIV, TB and malaria in low- and middle-income countries*. Retrieved August 18, 2020, from https://www.imperial.ac.uk/mrc-global-infectious-disease-analysis/covid-19/report-19-hiv-tb-malaria/.

Holtrop, T. (2018). 6.15%: Taking numbers at Interface value. *Science & Technology Studies, 31*(4), 75–88.

Jewell, B. L., Mudimu, E., Stover, J., Kelly, S. L., Phillips, A. (2020). *Potential effects of disruption to HIV programmes in sub-Saharan Africa caused by COVID-19: Results from multiple mathematical models.* https://figshare.com/articles/preprint/Potential_effects_of_disruption_to_HIV_programmes_in_sub-Saharan_Africa_caused_by_COVID-19_results_from_multiple_mathematical_models/12279914

Kovacic, Z. (2018). Conceptualizing numbers at the science–policy Interface. *Science, Technology, & Human Values, 43*(6), 1039–1065.

Lancaster, K., & Rhodes, T. (2020). Futuring a world without disease: Visualising the elimination of hepatitis C. *Critical Public Health*, 1–15. https://doi.org/10.1080/09581596.2020.1787347.

Lancaster, K., Rhodes, T., & Rance, J. (2020). "Towards eliminating viral hepatitis": Examining the productive capacity and constitutive effects of global policy on hepatitis C elimination. *International Journal of Drug Policy, 80*, 102419.

Law, J. (2004). *After method: Mess in social science research*. Oxon: Routledge.

Law, J., & Urry, J. (2004). Enacting the social. *Economy and Society, 33*(3), 390–410.

Lazarus, J. V., Safreed-Harmon, K., Barton, S. E., Costagliola, D., Dedes, N., del Amo Valero, J., et al. (2016). Beyond viral suppression of HIV – The new quality of life frontier. *BMC Medicine, 14*(1), 94.

Mackenbach, J., & McKee, M. (2013). *Successes and failures of health policy in Europe: Four decades of divergent trends and converging challenges.* Open University Press. Retrieved August 18, 2020, from https://www.euro.who.int/__data/assets/pdf_file/0007/215989/Suc cesses-and-Failures-of-Health-Policy-in-Europe.pdf.

Mackenzie, A. (2014). Multiplying numbers differently: An epidemiology of contagious convolu- tion. *Distinktion: Journal of Social Theory, 15*(2), 189–207.

Marsh, K., Eaton, J. W., Mahy, M., Sabin, K., Autenrieth, C. S., Wanyeki, I., et al. (2019). Global, regional and country-level 90-90-90 estimates for 2018: Assessing progress towards the 2020 target. *AIDS (London, England), 33 Suppl, 3*(Suppl 3), S213–S226.

Merry, S. E. (2011). Measuring the world: Indicators, human rights, and global governance: With CA comment by John M. Conley. *Current Anthropology, 52*(S3), S83–S95.

Merry, S. E. (2016). *The seductions of quantification: Measuring human rights, gender violence, and sex trafficking.* Chicago: University of Chicago Press.

Merson, M. H. (2006). The HIV–AIDS pandemic at 25 — The global response. *New England Journal of Medicine, 354*(23), 2414–2417.

Michael, M. (2000). Futures of the present: From performativity to Prehension. In N. Brown, B. Rappert, & A. Webster (Eds.), *Contested futures: A sociology of prospective techno-science* (pp. 21–42). Aldershot: Ashgate Publishing.

Miller, P. (2001). Governing by numbers: Why calculative practices matter. *Social Research, 68*(2), 379–396.

Mol, A. (2002). *The body multiple: Ontology in medical practice.* Durham: Duke University Press.

Pai, M. (2019). *Archives of failures in global health.* Retrieved August 18, 2020, from https:// naturemicrobiologycommunity.nature.com/posts/51659-archive-of-failures-in-global-health.

Polaris Observatory. (2020). *Countries on track to achieve WHO elimination targets.* Retrieved August 18, 2020, from https://cdafound.org/dashboard/polaris/maps.html.

Porter, T. M. (1996). *Trust in numbers: The pursuit of objectivity in science and public life.* Princeton: Princeton University Press.

Puig de la Bellacasa, M. (2017). *Matters of care: Speculative ethics in more than human worlds.* Minneapolis: University of Minnesota Press.

Rajkotia, Y. (2018). Beware of the success cartel: A plea for rational progress in global health. *BMJ Global Health, 3*(6), e001197.

Rhodes, T., & Lancaster, K. (2019). Evidence-making interventions in health: A conceptual framing. *Social Science and Medicine, 238*(October), 112488.

Rhodes, T., & Lancaster, K. (2020). How to think with models and targets: Hepatitis C elimination as a numbering performance. *International Journal of Drug Policy, 1–11.* https://doi.org/10. 1016/j.drugpo.2020.102694.

Rhodes, T., Lancaster, K., & Rosengarten, M. (2020). A model society: Maths, models and expertise in viral outbreaks. *Critical Public Health, 30*(3), 253–256.

Rose, N. (1991). Governing by numbers: Figuring out democracy. *Accounting, Organizations and Society, 16*(7), 673–692.

Rose, N., & Miller, P. (1992). Political power beyond the state: Problematics of government. *British Journal of Sociology, 43*(2), 173–205.

Rosengarten, M. (2019) *In the name of time: Ebola, securitization and the insistence of novel occurrences, paper presented at the workshop 'infection and time'.* Faculty of Arts and Social Science Distinguished Visitors Program, Centre for Social Research in Health, University of New South Wales, Sydney, 10 December, 2019.

Rottenburg, R., Merry, S. E., Park, S.-J., & Mugler, J. (2015). *The world of indicators: The making of governmental knowledge through quantification.* Cambridge: Cambridge University Press.

Rowse, T. (2009). The ontological politics of 'closing the gaps'. *Journal of Cultural Economy, 2* (1–2), 33–48.

Shore, C., & Wright, S. (2015). Governing by numbers: Audit culture, rankings and the new world order. *Social Anthropology, 23*(1), 22–28.

Sidibé, M., Loures, L., & Samb, B. (2016). The UNAIDS 90-90-90 target: A clear choice for ending AIDS and for sustainable health and development. *Journal of the International AIDS Society, 19* (1), 21133–21133.

Taylor-Alexander, S. (2017). Ethics in numbers: Auditing cleft treatment in Mexico and beyond. *Medical Anthropology Quarterly, 31*(3), 385–402.

Tichenor, M. (2017). Data performativity, performing health work: Malaria and labor in Senegal. *Medical Anthropology, 36*(5), 436–448.

UN. (2015). *Transforming our world: the 2030 Agenda for Sustainable Development.* Retrieved October 22, 2020, from https://sdgs.un.org/2030agenda.

UNAIDS. (2014). *90-90-90 An ambitious treatment target to help end the AIDS epidemic.* Retrieved August 18, 2020, from https://www.unaids.org/sites/default/files/media_asset/90-90-90_en_0.pdf.

Verran, H. (2010). Number as an inventive frontier in knowing and working Australia's water resources. *Anthropological Theory, 10*(1–2), 171–178.

Verran, H. (2012). Number. In C. Lury & N. Wakefield (Eds.), *Inventive methods: The happening of the social* (pp. 110–124). London: Routledge.

Verran, H. (2015). Enumerated entities in public policy and governance. In E. Davis & P. J. Davis (Eds.), *Mathematics, substance and surmise: Views on the meaning and ontology of mathematics* (pp. 365–379). Cham: Springer International Publishing.

Watson-Verran, H., & Turnbull, D. (1995). Science and other indigenous knowledge systems. In S. Jasanoff, G. Markle, J. Peterson, & T. Pinch (Eds.), *Handbook of science and technology studies* (pp. 115–139). Thousand Oaks, CA: Sage.

WHO. (2005). *Access to HIV treatment continues to accelerate in developing countries, but bottlenecks persist, says WHO/UNAIDS report [Press release].* Retrieved August 18, 2020, from https://www.who.int/3by5/progressreportJune2005/en/.

WHO. (2015). *Global vaccination targets 'off-track' warns WHO [Press release].* Retrieved August 18, 2020, from https://www.who.int/mediacentre/news/releases/2015/global-vaccination-targets/en/.

WHO. (2016a). *Global Health Sector Strategies for HIV, viral hepatitis, STIs, 2016–2021 [Development of the strategy].* Retrieved August 18, 2020, from http://www.who.int/hepatitis/strategy2016-2021/en/.

WHO. (2016b). *Global health sector strategy on HIV, 2016–2021.* Geneva: WHO.

WHO. (2020a). *The cost of inaction: COVID-19-related service disruptions could cause hundreds of thousands of extra deaths from HIV [Press release].* Geneva: WHO. Retrieved August 18, 2020, from https://www.who.int/news-room/detail/11-05-2020-the-cost-of-inaction-covid-19-related-service-disruptions-could-cause-hundreds-of-thousands-of-extra-deaths-from-hiv.

WHO. (2020b). *Pulse survey on continuity of essential health services during the COVID-19 pandemic. Interim report.* Geneva: WHO. Retrieved August 18, 2020, from https://www.who.int/publications/i/item/WHO-2019-nCoV-EHS_continuity-survey-2020.1

WHO. (2020c). *WHO: Access to HIV medicines severely impacted by COVID-19 as AIDS response stalls [Press release].* Retrieved August 18, 2020, from https://www.who.int/news-room/detail/06-07-2020-who-access-to-hiv-medicines-severely-impacted-by-covid-19-as-aids-response-stalls.

Woolgar, S., & Lezaun, J. (2013). The wrong bin bag: A turn to ontology in science and technology studies? *Social Studies of Science, 43*(3), 321–340.

Part IV
Anticipating and Understanding the Consequences of Biomedicine

Chapter 17
Stigma and Confidentiality Indiscretions: Intersecting Obstacles to the Delivery of Pre-Exposure Prophylaxis to Adolescent Girls and Young Women in East Zimbabwe

Morten Skovdal, Phyllis Magoge-Mandizvidza, Rufurwokuda Maswera, Melinda Moyo, Constance Nyamukapa, Ranjeeta Thomas, and Simon Gregson

17.1 Introduction

At the start of 2019, Zivai's story, a fictitious girl in a relationship with an older man, was discussed by adolescent girls and young women (AGYW) in a series of interviews and focus group discussions. One participant, Jackeline, summarised a core theme running through many of the reflections emerging from this vignette: 'Community norms will make Zivai fail to access Pre-Exposure Prophylaxis (PrEP) because Zivai will be judged if people know that she is using PrEP. In the community there will be several teachings telling them how to behave and not to have sex before marriage. If people find out that Zivai is actually having sex and using prevention methods like PrEP, this is something she will be scolded for. Zivai would have made her life very difficult because health professionals will make sure that they tell Zivai's mother that her daughter is being mischievous and is having sex when the time isn't yet ripe for her to do so.' In this chapter we unpack the fear of AGYW to be associated with, or 'outed' as, someone seeking out or accessing PrEP for HIV prevention, and the implications of this for their utilisation of PrEP.

M. Skovdal (✉)
Department of Public Health, University of Copenhagen, Copenhagen, Denmark

P. Magoge-Mandizvidza · R. Maswera · M. Moyo
Manicaland Centre for Public Health Research, Biomedical Research and Training Institute, Harare, Zimbabwe

C. Nyamukapa · S. Gregson
Manicaland Centre for Public Health Research, Biomedical Research and Training Institute, Harare, Zimbabwe

Department of Infectious Disease Epidemiology, Imperial College London, London, UK

R. Thomas
Department of Health Policy, London School of Economics and Political Science, London, UK

© The Author(s) 2021
S. Bernays et al. (eds.), *Remaking HIV Prevention in the 21st Century*, Social Aspects of HIV 5, https://doi.org/10.1007/978-3-030-69819-5_17

PrEP is a pill, which, when taken daily, significantly reduces the risk of HIV taking hold and spreading in the body, should it enter the bloodstream. PrEP is efficacious and trials show that PrEP can reduce risk of HIV by over 90% when taken consistently (McCormack et al. 2016). While PrEP is associated with reductions in HIV acquisition amongst men who have sex with men (MSM) in both high and low-income countries, PrEP trials with African women in the general population have found adherence levels so low, particularly amongst young women, that efficacy could not be ascertained (Marrazzo et al. 2015). Studies suggest that uptake and adherence to PrEP amongst women may be low due to low risk perception and ambivalence around using antiretrovirals for prevention. The FEM-PrEP study, for example, observed that women often underestimated their risk of infection and that perceived risk was associated with greater adherence to PrEP (Corneli et al. 2015).

PrEP is still a relatively new HIV prevention method in many country contexts and settings, including sub-Saharan Africa. Although more than 300,000 people took up PrEP at least once in 2018, this is far short of a global target of 3 million people by 2020 (Joint United Nations Programme on HIV/AIDS (UNAIDS) 2019), and reflects challenges, both to make make PrEP available and accessible, as well as to motivate people 'at risk' to engage with PrEP. While 'correcting' risk perception and addressing ambiguity around availability, usability and effectiveness of PrEP is central to the uptake of PrEP, little has been done to unpack the socio-cultural norms at stake in sub-Saharan Africa, which may prevent AGYW from accessing PrEP.

17.2 PrEP-Related Stigmas

The fear of 'being outed' as a PrEP user suggests there are stigmas related to PrEP use. According to Goffman (1963, p. 9), stigma refers to 'the situation of the individual who is disqualified from full social acceptance.' Individuals who are 'disqualified' often inhabit an attribute, which a social context has defined to be devaluing. Individuals who inhabit one or more devalued attributes, may be subject to labelling, stereotyping, status loss and discrimination, depending on the context (Link and Phelan 2001). While stigma in large parts takes place within broader social and structural contexts and inequalities (Parker and Aggleton 2003), how stigma manifests in the lives of discredited people also depends on how they are able to manage stigma. According to Goffman (1963), people adopt strategies to avoid revealing their association with devalued attributes, as has been observed in relation to people's concealing strategies when engaging with and managing ART. We draw on these ideas both to unpack the socio-cultural norms and attitudes that give rise to PrEP-related stigmas, and to demonstrate how declining PrEP is a rational strategy to manage such stigmas.

PrEP-related stigma is however not a new phenomenon. It is present in a small, but expanding number of studies reporting on the experience of men who have sex with men (MSM) in the global North (Eaton et al. 2017; Dubov et al. 2018; Schwartz and Grimm 2019). Only a small number of studies from sub-Saharan Africa allude to the potential social risks of taking PrEP. A study in Kenya, for example, explored PrEP use amongst two 'key' population groups: sex workers and MSM. The study found that some participants feared disclosing their PrEP use to family and friends, often out of a concern that daily pill-taking could lead others to think they are HIV positive (Van der Elst et al. 2013). PrEP is an antiretroviral pill, taken daily, and often accessed through HIV services, making it easy to mistake PrEP for antiretroviral therapy, affecting people's engagement with PrEP. Whilst this association did not deter these 'high-risk' individuals from taking PrEP, it did encourage them to carefully manage whom they disclosed their PrEP use to.

PrEP, because of its convenient protection against HIV, is also regularly linked to 'socially unacceptable' behaviour, and is, by some, believed to promote 'risky' sexual behaviour (Knight et al. 2016). A study from the USA has found such stigmatising rhetoric to prevent socially more isolated MSM or transgender women from engaging with PrEP (Mehrotra et al. 2018). In Zimbabwe, a recent study has found that similar perceptions of PrEP meant that young women either declined to engage with PrEP, or opted to discontinue PrEP, fearing their partners would find out and accuse them of extramarital affairs (Gombe et al. 2020). It appears that the decision of some at-risk individuals to reject PrEP is a strategy to manage related stigmas, warranting further attention.

17.3 The Qualitative Study

It is our aim to explore (1) the socio-cultural norms that give rise to PrEP-related stigmas; and (2) the implications of these norms and stigmas on AGYWs engagement with PrEP. The study obtained ethical approvals from the Medical Research Council of Zimbabwe (REF: MRCZ/A/2243), the institutional review board of the Biomedical Research and Training Institute in Zimbabwe (REF: AP140/2017), and the Imperial College London Research Ethics Committee (REF: 17IC4160).

17.3.1 Study Setting and Participants

The qualitative explorations were conducted in two communities of Manicaland province in east Zimbabwe. The communities were selected for the qualitative study because of their rural/urban location, and for being randomly chosen as intervention sites in the larger study trial. This allowed us to recruit participants with different levels of exposure to PrEP. Half had participated in an intervention introducing them to PrEP (see Thomas et al. 2019), the other half had only heard of PrEP peripherally from other sources. Both communities are characterised by high levels of poverty and HIV. The average HIV prevalence of Manicaland was 11% in 2015–2016, down from over 25% at the end of the 1990s (Gregson et al. 2017).

Thirty AGYW from the two settings were invited to participate in either individual interviews (n = 12) or focus group discussions (FGD) (n = 18) with the aim of revealing how they encounter, respond to, and negotiate PrEP uptake and engagement. The AGYW were chosen from a baseline survey by purposeful sampling following the criteria that they had to be between the age of 18 and 24, HIV-negative, sexually active, and considered 'at risk' (according to a risk screening tool under development by the World Health Organization (WHO)). Individual interviews with HIV prevention service providers (n = 12)—recruited from health facilities in the two communities—were also conducted.

17.3.2 Producing and Making Sense of the Data

The different methods were applied by a team of experienced qualitative researchers in Shona, the local language of the study area. Interviews and focus group discussions were semi-structured and steered by topic guides. The topic guides for AGYW sought to elicit their experiences and perspectives on HIV risk, relationships, sexuality, HIV prevention practices, services and technologies. The topic guide directed at HIV prevention service providers opened up for a discussion on young people's HIV prevention practices, as well as the opportunities and challenges for young people to access available HIV prevention services and technologies. Interviews and focus groups were digitally recorded, and scheduled to last 60 and 90 min respectively, a time that was kept and ultimately reflects the length of the interviews.

All interview and focus group recordings were transcribed and translated into English, before being imported into NVivo 12 for thematic coding and interrogation. A cluster of codes, which were deemed relevant for this analysis, were subjected to a thematic network analysis (Attride-Stirling 2001). This involved clustering the codes, or basic themes, into organising themes (or parent nodes in NVivo). We generated three organising themes, providing detail on sexuality stigmas, PrEP stigmas and confidentiality indiscretions. We present each of the organising themes in turn.

17.4 Findings

17.4.1 Sexuality Stigmas: 'A "Child" Shouldn't Be Having Sex'

Our interviews expose a generational rift when it comes to girls' sexuality. Both AGYW and the healthcare providers spoke about a socio-cultural perception that unmarried AGYW should not be having sex. A number of AGYW said that it was shameful to access HIV prevention methods, 'as they should not be having sex' or because 'parents won't accept it because this promotes promiscuity.' Much of the shame was linked to what older people—and their parents in particular—thought about their 'children' being sexually active. However, there was recognition that some parents, whilst struggling to accept their children's sexuality, may also find comfort in knowing that their 'children' are protecting themselves against HIV.

> She will be disappointed that I am having sexual relationships before marriage [. . .] Okay, on one side she might be disappointed and on the other side she will be comforted knowing that I am preserving my life and reducing chances of getting HIV. (Jocelyn, AGYW in interview)

As AGYW consider PrEP they need to weigh up their perceived risk of acquiring HIV with the social risk of their parents passing judgement or being disappointed by their child's decision to engage in pre-marital sex. AGYW are not only the 'children' of their biological parents. They are also 'children' of their community, which means some healthcare providers may pass similar judgement to 'the kids'. One healthcare provider, who, upon reflection, recognises their role in preventing AGYW from accessing PrEP services, illustrates this:

> The other thing that demotivates the children to access PrEP services is that when they get to the hospital gate and asks for PrEP, they will be met by someone older, like me, who will judge them for being sexually active at that age, when in fact they should be getting assisted. So yes, health staff can be demotivating. When children come looking for PrEP there is no need to start asking why they are sexually active, just focus on talking them through PrEP. (Healthcare provider (3))

There is a clear tension between how the health system classifies AGYW as adults who do not require guardian permission to access PrEP, and the operational practices, which, shaped by social norms and moralising discourses circulating within the health system, approach AGYW as 'children'. Relatedly, and given the fact that PrEP in this context is being delivered within one place to everyone (at the opportunistic infection clinic), a healthcare provider calls for youth-friendly corners, staffed with personnel not much older than the AGYW themselves.

> Middle-aged healthcare providers still have that connotation of fatherhood and motherhood. This should be addressed [. . .] I think we should have adolescent clinics. I think this will help because the young will go to a place where they can see people of their own age. If they are too old people working there, with the mentality that this client is a child, they will not assist a person as a client. A person who comes for services, should be provided with the services. (Healthcare provider (2))

It is evident from our interviews that there is a fear of AGYW to be seen as sexually active by parents or healthcare providers of a similar age to their parents, which inhibit their engagement with health clinics offering PrEP. PrEP use, however, does not only signal a sexuality, but is associated with a range of other stigmatising attitudes, some of which we will now elucidate.

17.4.2 PrEP Stigmas: 'PrEP is for Women with a "Loose Moral"'

Due to research showing that PrEP might be cost-effective in high-risk populations and less so in the wider population, WHO (2015) developed guidance that PrEP should be offered to population groups with HIV incidence above 3%. This meant that when PrEP was first rolled out in Zimbabwe, as in many other sub-Saharan African countries, it targeted female sex workers. Such messaging and targeting meant that for many of our young female participants, PrEP was considered a prevention method primarily for 'high risk' individuals, including female sex workers, or women with a so-called 'loose moral'. One AGYW stated that if on PrEP, 'they will think I am being mischievous.' Another AGYW drew a direct parallel between being on PrEP and assumed to be a sex worker.

> They will be saying things like. . . let's say it's a woman. . . her husband occasionally travels or maybe goes to South Africa. Imagine being seen going to get PrEP. The assumption will be that you are a prostitute and you are sleeping around in your husband's absence. (Jocelyn, AGYW in interview)

Another common perception, resonating with observations made elsewhere in Zimbabwe (Gombe et al. 2020), was that PrEP can easily be misunderstood as HIV treatment, demonstrating that residual fears of acquiring HIV still persist. Because PrEP is an antiretroviral drug, accessed through sexual health clinics, just like antiretroviral drugs for HIV treatment, a number of AGYW spoke about their fear of being seen as HIV positive and on treatment.

> People are scared of taking PrEP because the tablets look like the ones that are taken by HIV positive people so one may be scared of what people will say about the person taking tablets that are similar to that. (Alice, AGYW in interview)

Healthcare workers noted similar concerns, and offered insights to alternative ways of delivering PrEP.

> PrEP, should be dispensed in another container. They don't want it to be dispensed in its original containers which are easily identified. (Healthcare providers (W1))

The stigmatising attitudes highlighted above underline the importance of PrEP delivery discretion.

17.4.3 Confidentiality Indiscretions: 'The Issue of Confidentiality is Their Greatest Worry'

AGYW worry about walking into clinic spaces where PrEP is on offer. Many of our young female participants said that they would be 'shy to go to health facilities to look for these methods'—worrying about being seen or heard seeking out PrEP services, or, as noted above, mistaken as someone on HIV treatment. These concerns indicate that many AGYW do not feel that community-embedded clinics, although accessible because of their proximity, can ensure confidentiality. Both healthcare workers and the young women themselves noted a fear amongst AGYW to run into neighbours or community members at the clinic, believing they may inform their parents or partners about their clinic visit.

They [AGYW] do not want to go to the clinic, particularly when it is busy. They always feel that there will be someone who can recognize them and report them to their parents [...] I don't know what we can do because some say when they get to the hospital they will be seen by neighbours. (Healthcare provider (3))

A girl will feel shy or embarrassed to be seen by community members or other close people accessing these methods from the local clinic. She will also fear for her partner knowing that she is using PrEP or condoms, which leads to her being dumped by her partner because of that. (Mercy, AGYW in FGD)

The participants not only noted that confidentiality is hard to maintain in public clinic spaces, but also alluded to AGYW's lack of trust in the ability of healthcare providers to maintain confidentiality. Like Jackeline, a number of participants believed there was a chance that some healthcare providers may disclose details of AGYW's use of, or interest in, PrEP to relatives or acquaintances in the community. Mary stressed the importance of healthcare providers maintaining confidentiality.

Upholding privacy is important, especially to the nurses who would have served someone who has visited the clinic to access HIV prevention methods. They should be told that it is not allowed for them to go and spread the word that so and so has come to the clinic to access PrEP or condoms or getting tested. (Mary, AGYW in FGD)

Healthcare providers recognised this concern and went to great lengths in the interviews to explain their efforts to ensure that the young women felt safe and comfortable to open up about their sexual risk practices and need for PrEP.

We are trying by all means to offer services in a cheerful manner so that the patient feels free to open up. We give them a platform, a confidential space, for whatever discussion we are going to have; it will be between the two of us and no-one else will hear about what we have discussed. So maybe that will give the patient confidence in us that anyone in the street will not know what we are talking about. (Healthcare provider (2))

Our findings suggest that AGYW and healthcare providers are acutely aware of the community-embeddedness of local clinics delivering PrEP. This embeddedness, coupled with the stigmas associated with PrEP, heightens the social risk of confidentiality indiscretions. The decision of AGYW not to go to the clinic during busy times, or all together, or not to disclose details about at-risk behaviours to healthcare providers is a strategic one. A conscious choice of 'information management' (Goffman 1963) to minimise their association with PrEP and related stigmas.

17.5 Discussion

Our study reveals two prevailing socio-cultural norms around girls' sexuality and use of HIV prevention methods. One, a norm that girls should not be having sex before marriage; two, a norm that uptake of PrEP signals promiscuity. According to our participants, girls who have sex before marriage, or make use of PrEP may be subject to stigmatising attitudes and rhetoric. Out of fear of being associated with these stigmas, heightened by concerns of clinic-level confidentiality indiscretions, AGYW, as a way of managing stigma, may actively avoid seeking out local PrEP services. Stigma and the worry of AGYW that privacy and confidentiality cannot be maintained in local health clinics and by local healthcare providers, presents a major barrier to the uptake of PrEP.

These findings are constrained by some methodological limitations. First, the study relies on self-reported data. Future research may consider adopting a more in-depth and longitudinal ethnographic approach. Second, our study was cross-sectional and only provides a brief snapshot of perspectives at a particular moment in time. Third, whilst our rural and urban findings were broadly similar, the generalisability of our findings is limited and may not apply to other country settings, as the socio-cultural norms and PrEP service delivery structures characteristic of our setting may vary from others. This study only reports on the perspectives of AGYW and healthcare providers. In future studies we will broaden the scope and include the perspectives and experiences of parents, community members and young men.

Nonetheless, our findings resonate with observations made elsewhere. Public discourses of PrEP as a 'promiscuity pill' have also been noted amongst gay men in north America (Eaton et al. 2017) and in Malaysia (Bourne et al. 2017), with implications for their interest in adopting PrEP. Our observation that potential PrEP users express a fear of stigma by healthcare providers, because of their socio-cultural values and norms, has been noted elsewhere. In San Francisco, USA, many men on PrEP have reported feeling stigmatised by healthcare providers (Liu et al. 2014), and accounts from female sex workers in South Africa stress the importance of health clinics being safe spaces, free of judgement from healthcare providers (Eakle et al. 2018). Resonating with an argument made by Müller et al. (2016) in relation to sexual and reproductive health policies and services for adolescents in South Africa, our observations suggest that front-line healthcare providers, by virtue of how their own moral compasses and values influence their delivery of PrEP, act as gate-keepers for the implementation of PrEP policies and services. Müller et al. (2016) go on to argue that nurse morals and judgments can result in uneven policy trans-lations and service provisions, jeopardising sexual and reproductive health services for adolescents.

Our findings are not wholly unexpected. 'Not unexpected' because our observa-tions resonate with earlier and broader discussions of adolescents' uptake of sexual and reproductive health services (Bearinger et al. 2007), and reflect long-standing challenges pertaining to family planning (Tavrow et al. 2012), condom use (MacPhail and Campbell 2001) and treatment of sexually transmitted infections

(Sales et al. 2007). It is disappointing that we do not seem to have managed to learn very much from the plethora of evidence concerning social and structural approaches to HIV prevention (Campbell et al. 2005; Gupta et al. 2008). The enthusiasm to harness recent biomedical and health service successes in HIV treatment and expand PrEP to AGYW is understandable. Not least because PrEP is considered cost-effective in averting HIV infection (Schackman and Eggman 2012) and because it offers women the opportunity to take control over sexual risks. However, efforts to scale up PrEP must build on decades of social science research that have scrutinised the intersections between socio-cultural norms of youth sexuality, stigma and engagement with a variety of sexual and reproductive health services.

For instance, there have been numerous calls for 'youth-friendly' sexual and reproductive health services (Kennedy et al. 2013). It is evident from our findings that PrEP also needs to be delivered in youth friendly corners, where (young) health care providers are trained to welcome and engage young people in ways that foster trustful relations and make young people feel they are in a safe space. Mmari and Magnani (2003) have found youth-friendly corners to increase sexual and reproductive health services uptake in Zambia, but also noted that health services do not operate in a vacuum, and addressing socio-cultural norms and barriers at a community-level, may have an even greater impact. In an action research project in Kenya, Chubb (2018) innovatively explores the role of traditional meeting and dialogue structures (like the Kenyan *mabaraza*) for intergenerational dialogues on sex-related issues. She concludes that 'community conversations' about young people's sexuality, introduced in, and supported by, traditional structure, are key for breaking down community-level barriers to young people's sexual health.

While most of our observations reflect long-standing challenges to young people's engagement with sexual and reproductive health services, PrEP-specific factors hindering uptake did emerge. More broadly, it appears that PrEP, and how the technology was historically introduced to MSM and female sex workers, is shaping the public imagination about PrEP in a way that might be quite distinctive. Our findings suggest that PrEP for AGYW in the general population, it is saddled with an additional layer of social resistance. This resistance requires health service providers to carefully consider how best to deliver PrEP, for instance through youth-friendly corners, and re-thinking how PrEP pills are packed and handed over to AGYW. The 'V' initiative in southern Africa is looking to address this challenge by repackaging PrEP tablets in containers that look like lip-gloss (www.conrad.org/launchingv). More broadly however, it also calls for critical reflection on how PrEP has become an intervention for AGYW in sub-Saharan Africa and the implications of this for AGYW.

17.6   Conclusions

The biomedical nature of PrEP heightens the impact of socio-cultural norms as they relate to adult attitudes to HIV prevention methods and sex. PrEP may provide AGYW with control over their sexual risks, but the journey to access PrEP involves a series of social risks, which appear to outweigh the perceived benefits of engaging with PrEP amongst AGYW in eastern Zimbabwe. To shift this balance there is an urgent need to tackle the range of socio-cultural norms and social practices that interact to form the context that prevents AGYW from taking advantage of PrEP. We have previously noted that approaching engagement with PrEP as a social practice is key to identifying and responding to the combination of social and structural interventions needed to make engagement with PrEP a possible and desirable thing to do for AGYW (Skovdal 2019).

Acknowledgments   We would like to thank all the participants for their time and valuable insight. We would also like to thank Rangarirayi Primrose Nyamwanza, Douglas Muchemwa, Rumbidzai Bangidza and Moreblessing Mangwiro for research support. The study was supported by the National Institute of Mental Health (NIMH) (Grant R01MH114562–01) and the Bill and Melinda Gates Foundation (BMGF) (OPP1161471). The content is solely the responsibility of the authors and does not necessarily represent the official views of the NIMH or the BMGF. CN and SG acknowledge joint MRC Centre for Global Infectious Disease Analysis funding from the UK Medical Research Council and Department for International Development (MR/R015600/1).

References

Attride-Stirling, J. (2001). Thematic networks: An analytic tool for qualitative research. *Qualitative Research, 1*(3), 385–405. https://doi.org/10.1177/146879410100100307.

Bearinger, L. H., Sieving, R. E., Ferguson, J., & Sharma, V. (2007). Global perspectives on the sexual and reproductive health of adolescents: Patterns, prevention, and potential. *The Lancet, 369*(9568), 1220–1231. https://doi.org/10.1016/S0140-6736(07)60367-5.

Bourne, A., Cassolato, M., Thuan Wei, C. K., Wang, B., Pang, J., Lim, S. H., et al. (2017). Willingness to use pre-exposure prophylaxis (PrEP) for HIV prevention among men who have sex with men (MSM) in Malaysia: Findings from a qualitative study. *Journal of the International AIDS Society, 20*(1), 21899.

Campbell, C., Foulis, C., Maimane, S., & Sibiya, Z. (2005). The impact of social environments on the effectiveness of youth HIV-prevention: A south African case study. *AIDS Care, 17*(4), 471–478.

Chubb, L. (2018). *Struggle for a sustainable solution: Building safe sex-talk spaces with a rural kenyan community*. PhD thesis, Auckland: The University of Auckland. Available from: https://researchspace.auckland.ac.nz/handle/2292/44012

Corneli, A., Perry, B., Agot, K., Ahmed, K., Malamatsho, F., & Van Damme, L. (2015). Facilitators of adherence to the study pill in the FEM-PrEP clinical trial. *PLoS One, 10*(4), e0125458–e0125458. https://doi.org/10.1371/journal.pone.0125458.

Dubov, A., Galbo, P., Jr., Altice, F. L., & Fraenkel, L. (2018). Stigma and shame experiences by MSM who take PrEP for HIV prevention: A qualitative study. *American Journal of Men's Health, 12*(6), 1843–1854.

Eakle, R., Bourne, A., Mbogua, J., Mutanha, N., & Rees, H. (2018). Exploring acceptability of oral PrEP prior to implementation among female sex workers in South Africa. *Journal of the International AIDS Society, 21*(2), e25081.

Eaton, L. A., Kalichman, S. C., Price, D., Finneran, S., Allen, A., & Maksut, J. (2017). Stigma and conspiracy beliefs related to pre-exposure prophylaxis (PrEP) and interest in using PrEP among black and white men and transgender women who have sex with men. *AIDS and Behavior, 21* (5), 1236–1246.

Goffman, E. (1963). *Stigma: Notes on the management of spoiled identity.* Englewood Cliffs, NJ: Prentice-Hall.

Gombe, M. M., Cakouros, B. E., Ncube, G., Zwangobani, N., Mareke, P., Mkwamba, A., et al. (2020). Key barriers and enablers associated with uptake and continuation of oral pre-exposure prophylaxis (PrEP) in the public sector in Zimbabwe: Qualitative perspectives of general population clients at high risk for HIV. *PLoS One, 15*(1), e0227632. https://doi.org/10.1371/journal.pone.0227632.

Gregson, S., Mugurungi, O., Eaton, J., Takaruza, A., Rhead, R., Maswera, R., et al. (2017). Documenting and explaining the HIV decline in East Zimbabwe: The Manicaland general population cohort. *BMJ Open, 7*(10), e015898.

Gupta, G. R., Parkhurst, J. O., Ogden, J. A., Aggleton, P., & Mahal, A. (2008). Structural approaches to HIV prevention. *The Lancet, 372*(9640), 764–775.

Kennedy, E. C., Bulu, S., Harris, J., Humphreys, D., Malverus, J., & Gray, N. J. (2013). "Be kind to young people so they feel at home": A qualitative study of adolescents' and service providers' perceptions of youth-friendly sexual and reproductive health services in Vanuatu. *BMC Health Services Research, 13*(1), 455.

Knight, R., Small, W., Carson, A., & Shoveller, J. (2016). Complex and conflicting social norms: Implications for implementation of future HIV pre-exposure prophylaxis (PrEP) interventions in Vancouver, Canada. *PLoS One, 11*(1), e0146513.

Link, B. G., & Phelan, J. C. (2001). Conceptualizing stigma. *Annual Review of Sociology, 27,* 363–385. https://doi.org/10.1146/annurev.soc.27.1.363.

Liu, A., Cohen, S., Follansbee, S., Cohan, D., Weber, S., Sachdev, D., et al. (2014). Early experiences implementing pre-exposure prophylaxis (PrEP) for HIV prevention in San Francisco. *PLoS Medicine, 11*(3), e1001613.

MacPhail, C., & Campbell, C. (2001). 'I think condoms are good but, aai, I hate those things': Condom use among adolescents and young people in a southern African township. *Social Science & Medicine, 52*(11), 1613–1627. https://doi.org/10.1016/s0277-9536(00)00272-0.

McCormack, S., Dunn, D. T., Desai, M., Dolling, D. I., Gafos, M., Gilson, R., et al. (2016). Pre-exposure prophylaxis to prevent the acquisition of HIV-1 infection (PROUD): Effectiveness results from the pilot phase of a pragmatic open-label randomised trial. *Lancet, 387*(10013), 53–60. https://doi.org/10.1016/S0140-6736(15)00056-2.

Marrazzo, J. M., Ramjee, G., Richardson, B. A., Gomez, K., Mgodi, N., Nair, G., et al. (2015). Tenofovir-based preexposure prophylaxis for HIV infection among African women. *New England Journal of Medicine, 372*(6), 509–518.

Mehrotra, M. L., Amico, K. R., McMahan, V., Glidden, D. V., Defechereux, P., Guanira, J. V., et al. (2018). The role of social relationships in PrEP uptake and use among transgender women and men who have sex with men. *AIDS and Behavior, 22*(11), 3673–3680.

Mmari, K. N., & Magnani, R. J. (2003). Does making clinic-based reproductive health services more youth-friendly increase service use by adolescents? Evidence from Lusaka, Zambia. *Journal of Adolescent Health, 33*(4), 259–270. https://doi.org/10.1016/S1054-139X(03) 00062-4.

Müller, A., Röhrs, S., Hoffman-Wanderer, Y., & Moult, K. (2016). "You have to make a judgment call" – Morals, judgments and the provision of quality sexual and reproductive health services for adolescents in South Africa. *Social Science & Medicine, 148,* 71–78. https://doi.org/10.1016/j.socscimed.2015.11.048.

Parker, R., & Aggleton, P. (2003). HIV and AIDS-related stigma and discrimination: A conceptual framework and implications for action. *Social Science & Medicine, 57*(1), 13–24.

Sales, J. M., DiClemente, R. J., Rose, E. S., Wingood, G. M., Klein, J. D., & Woods, E. R. (2007). Relationship of STD-related shame and stigma to female adolescents' condom-protected inter-course. *Journal of Adolescent Health, 40*(6), 573.e571–573.e576. https://doi.org/10.1016/j.jadohealth.2007.01.007.

Schackman, B. R., & Eggman, A. A. (2012). Cost–effectiveness of pre-exposure prophylaxis for HIV: A review. *Current Opinion in HIV/AIDS, 7*(6), 587–592.

Schwartz, J., & Grimm, J. (2019). Stigma communication surrounding PrEP: The experiences of a sample of men who have sex with men. *Health Communication, 34*(1), 84–90. https://doi.org/10.1080/10410236.2017.1384430.

Skovdal, M. (2019). Facilitating engagement with PrEP and other HIV prevention technologies through practice-based combination prevention. *Journal of the International AIDS Society, 22* (S4), e25294. https://doi.org/10.1002/jia2.25294.

Tavrow, P., Withers, M., & McMullen, K. (2012). Age matters: Differential impact of service quality on contraceptive uptake among post-abortion clients in Kenya. *Culture, Health and Sexuality, 14*(8), 849–862.

Thomas, R., Skovdal, M., Galizzi, M., Schaefer, R., Moorhouse, L., Nyamukapa, C., et al. (2019). Improving risk perception and uptake of pre-exposure prophylaxis (PrEP) through interactive feedback-based counselling with and without community engagement in young women in Manicaland, East Zimbabwe: Study protocol for a pilot randomised trial. *Trials, 20*, 668. https://doi.org/10.1186/s13063-019-3791-8.

UNAIDS. (2019). *Global AIDS update 2019 — Communities at the Centre*. Geneva: Joint United Nations Programme on HIV/AIDS.

Van der Elst, E. M., Mbogua, J., Operario, D., Mutua, G., Kuo, C., Mugo, P., et al. (2013). High acceptability of HIV pre-exposure prophylaxis but challenges in adherence and use: Qualitative insights from a phase I trial of intermittent and daily PrEP in at-risk populations in Kenya. *AIDS and Behavior, 17*(6), 2162–2172. https://doi.org/10.1007/s10461-012-0317-8.

WHO. (2015). *Guideline on when to start antiretroviral therapy and on pre-exposure prophylaxis for HIV*. https://www.who.int/hiv/pub/guidelines/earlyrelease-arv/en/. Accessed 7 January 2019.

Open Access This chapter is licensed under the terms of the Creative Commons Attribution 4.0 International License (http://creativecommons.org/licenses/by/4.0/), which permits use, sharing, adaptation, distribution and reproduction in any medium or format, as long as you give appropriate credit to the original author(s) and the source, provide a link to the Creative Commons license and indicate if changes were made.

The images or other third party material in this chapter are included in the chapter's Creative Commons license, unless indicated otherwise in a credit line to the material. If material is not included in the chapter's Creative Commons license and your intended use is not permitted by statutory regulation or exceeds the permitted use, you will need to obtain permission directly from the copyright holder.

Chapter 18
Imagined Futures and Unintended Consequences in the Making of PrEP: An Evidence-Making Intervention Perspective

Martin Holt

18.1 Introduction

Pre-exposure prophylaxis (PrEP), the regular use of antiretroviral medications to prevent HIV acquisition, has been endorsed by global agencies as a highly effective prevention strategy (World Health Organization (WHO) 2016). Ten years after the first positive trial results in PrEP's favour (Grant et al. 2010), there is a growing body of 'evidence' about PrEP's effects on individuals, communities, health services and epidemics. In this chapter, I consider the way in which PrEP was imagined before it was widely used, the evidence that has been generated as it has been trialled and implemented, and how these knowledge-making practices have been incorporated into the ongoing making of PrEP as an HIV prevention strategy (Rhodes and Lancaster 2019). The aim is to show that varied effects and unintended consequences should be considered an *expected* and vital part of developing an HIV prevention strategy, and the way in which these are incorporated and adjusted to affect what the strategy becomes as it is implemented. The manner in which we respond to unintended consequences and incorporate them (or not) into an intervention's making is a political as well as a technical process. This approach rejects the idea of PrEP as a singular, stable object (as would be suggested in evidence-based medicine or implementation science), and instead proposes that it is multiple and relational (Mol 2002). In fact, in order for PrEP to be effective and useful for affected populations in different parts of the world, I suggest it must change, adapt and multiply, including to unintended consequences.

M. Holt (✉)
Centre for Social Research in Health, UNSW, Sydney, Australia
e-mail: m.holt@unsw.edu.au

© Springer Nature Switzerland AG 2021   249
S. Bernays et al. (eds.), *Remaking HIV Prevention in the 21st Century*, Social
Aspects of HIV 5, https://doi.org/10.1007/978-3-030-69819-5_18

18.2   PrEP's Beginnings (or the Beginning of PrEP)

The first successful trial results demonstrating PrEP's efficacy in preventing HIV acquisition were published in 2010 (Grant et al. 2010). This announcement followed at least a decade of preparatory, lobbying and advocacy work to create the conditions in which PrEP trials were seen as legitimate and necessary, and for funding to be secured. This earlier period also saw a number of halted trials in low- and middle-income countries where participants and communities had protested against inadequate access to existing prevention methods and treatment (Haire 2011). Therefore, before any trials had been (successfully) completed, PrEP's future was highly speculative and politicised (Rosengarten and Michael 2009).

Many involved in PrEP trials were keenly aware of the uncertainty about what PrEP might become and were active in considering potential issues with its implementation (Youle and Wainberg 2003; Rosengarten and Michael 2009; Holt 2015). A variety of issues and doubts were raised by researchers, such as how efficacious PrEP might be, how much it would cost, how easy it would be to adhere to a regular pill regime, whether users would experience side effects or toxicity, how PrEP might be targeted, and how its use would be supported and monitored (Paxton et al. 2007). PrEP was seen as a potential means of prevention for people at risk of HIV who found it difficult to use existing strategies like condoms, although it was unclear how people who struggled with strategies like condoms would find it easier to use a pill-based strategy like PrEP (Youle and Wainberg 2003; Holt 2015). There were also concerns that a strategy like PrEP might encourage people to use condoms less often (often referred to as 'risk compensation'), which would be particularly problematic if PrEP was only partially effective in preventing HIV (Holt and Murphy 2017). However, the promise of a strategy that could be temporally separated from the event when sex occurred (i.e. taking pills in private), was seen as a potentially valuable addition to prevention options, particularly for women.

18.3   PrEP as Stable Object or Emergent Process

During the trial period, the anticipation of PrEP's potential and the possibilities of what it could become demonstrated that it was considered as both a stable object and an emergent process, including by those tasked with testing its efficacy in trials (Rosengarten and Michael 2009). This is worth considering in more detail, as it highlights a key difference or tension between traditional public health and implementation science approaches to HIV prevention, and relational or process approaches from science and technology studies (STS; Mol 2002; Law and Singleton 2005; Rhodes and Lancaster 2019).

In a traditional public health approach, an intervention like PrEP is a known and stable entity, from the trial period through to its implementation, and on into the future as it becomes more widely used. PrEP was initially characterised as the regular (daily) use of antiretroviral drugs in pill form (specifically tenofovir and emtricitabine) by a person who saw themselves (or was judged to be) at risk of HIV (Youle and Wainberg 2003). In this traditional framing, PrEP was seen as a minimum as a pharmaceutical agent in pill form, ingested by a willing patient (what Auerbach and Hoppe (2015) pithily referred to as 'getting drugs into bodies'). The trials of PrEP were set up to test whether the chemical agent of PrEP was sufficiently potent to prevent HIV acquisition, with the assumption that the pharmaceutical drug is the core or primary agent in PrEP (its essence, if you will). If proven to be sufficiently efficacious at preventing HIV, then PrEP as a stable entity could be extracted from the trial setting and administered to patients in health systems across the world, with the assumption that PrEP would produce the same effect (HIV prevention) in multiple populations and settings.

However, this characterisation of PrEP as a stable object is difficult to sustain considering the multiple elements that are required in order to make PrEP 'work'. Even in the narrow conception of PrEP outlined above, there are multiple elements posited as necessary for PrEP's success. These elements are arguably inseparable from what PrEP is. There are the drugs, combined in a pill. There is the person who is supposed to take pills as directed but may not do so, whose (sexual) behaviour is expected to remain relatively unchanged, and who is expected to stay engaged in the trial and its monitoring. There are the clinics which engage and support patients, dispense the drug, and conduct monitoring and testing. These elements alone suggest that PrEP is far more than a drug in a body and is, at the very least, a combination of drug, trial participant and clinic: a drug-participant-clinic assemblage, actor-network or network of associations (Law and Singleton 2005; Rhodes and Lancaster 2019).

If we cast our gaze wider, the assemblage that comprises PrEP (and makes it work or fail) is much more complex and variable, depending on where PrEP is trialled or implemented. There are the manufacturers that sell to government or private buyers, international and local supply chains, and state policies that encourage or restrict PrEP use. The health system may be intensively or poorly resourced, easily accessible or out of reach. Where PrEP is introduced will have a particular HIV epidemic and history, in which some affected communities will have galvanised an effective response while others will be frustrated by neglect, ignorance, gender-based violence and stigma (Kippax and Stephenson 2016). HIV literacy and knowledge may be actively generated by open discussion and education, or stymied by paternalism and moralism.

In a traditional public health or implementation science framing, all the elements outlined above are seen as *external* to the intervention, a background that is controlled for in a trial, or simply the context to which PrEP is 'added' when it is implemented. But if we recognise these elements as an integral part of the PrEP assemblage, then our expectation of what PrEP implementation should look like and the effects it should have will change. Rather than seeing PrEP as a discrete object that travels unchanged across contexts and countries, unaffected by the systems through which it is made and delivered, or by the people who use it, we could instead see it as an intervention that unfolds and is constituted in practice (Rhodes and Lancaster 2019). Arguably, we could think of the focus on intervention 'fidelity' in implementation science as an attempt to make PrEP an 'immutable mobile' (following Latour), a discrete object that is reproduced as a stable set of relations despite its travels (Law and Singleton 2005; Carroll et al. 2007). However, PrEP may be better thought of as a fluid object that needs to shift and adapt to local relations while retaining a certain 'coreness' or recognisability (Rod et al. 2014), or a fire object that is enacted differently in different networks and contexts, creating multiple and possibly incommensurable PrEPs (Mol 2002; Law and Singleton 2005). All of these versions of PrEP (immutable, fluid, fire) are possible, and all rely on networks of socio-material relations.

18.4   Trial Results and PrEP in Transition

The release of the first main PrEP trial results in 2010 illustrates the tension between the idea of PrEP as a stable object and a process that could result in multiple PrEPs. The iPrEx study involved nearly 2500 cisgender men who have sex with men and transgender women in five middle income countries and the USA (Grant et al. 2010). The main study analysis found that HIV infections were 44% lower in the arm receiving the active study drug (tenofovir and emtricitabine or TDF-FTC) versus those given a placebo. However, the research team (and many commentators) noted the high degree of variability in adherence to the daily pill regimen and how this had affected efficacy. Efficacy in preventing HIV was calculated to be over 90% in participants who had taken the daily pill sufficiently often to maintain detectable drug levels (at least four pills a week). Detectable drug levels were much more likely to be found in trial participants in the USA than in Peru or Ecuador, among older men, and those who reported condomless receptive sex (Liu et al. 2014).

In a traditional public health understanding of PrEP, the variability in adherence and efficacy observed for different types of people and places is seen as external to the intervention. However, a relational understanding of PrEP encourages close attention to this variability, suggesting there may be critical elements other than the drug itself (or even the narrow drug-user-clinic assemblage) that are necessary to make PrEP effective in practice. The iPrEx investigators speculated that older, US gay men who took part in the study appeared to have greater research literacy and engagement with HIV prevention trials, which encouraged them to take the study drug as directed (Liu et al. 2014). This suggests that taking a drug in a high income country like the USA, with a sophisticated, well-resourced health system, a culture that embraces pharmaceuticals (Dumit 2002), and in a location with highly visible gay and HIV-positive populations (San Francisco), could be a great deal easier than in other locations. Meeting a basic income and survival needs, easy access to and resourcing of health care, a supportive culture of medicine-taking, and a relative lack of stigma towards HIV-affected populations may also be necessary to make adherence possible and sustainable over time. In a STS characterisation, all PrEPs are fashioned in and reliant on elaborate networks of relations. To be successful, PrEP may need to be made with a number of these so-called 'external' elements.

The variability of PrEP's efficacy in different locations and populations was later underscored by trials that were completed in sub-Saharan Africa and with heterosexual men and women. The Partners PrEP study, conducted in Kenya and Uganda, assessed the efficacy of TDF-FTC (or tenofovir on its own) versus placebo in preventing HIV acquisition for HIV-negative partners in serodiscordant relationships when the HIV-positive partner was not receiving treatment (Baeten et al. 2012). The trial found that PrEP was 67–75% efficacious, with high levels of adherence observed. The TDF2 trial enrolled heterosexual men and women in Botswana but suffered from poor levels of retention. Among those who remained in the study and could be followed up, it found that PrEP was 62% efficacious in preventing HIV (Thigpen et al. 2012). In contrast, the FEM-PrEP trial, of over 2000 women in Kenya, South Africa and Tanzania was stopped early because of a lack of efficacy of TDF-FTC versus placebo, with low detectable drug levels observed in the TDF-FTC group (Van Damme et al. 2012). Similarly, the VOICE study of over 5000 women in South Africa, Uganda and Zimbabwe, comparing TDF-FTC, tenofovir on its own and placebo found that none of the drugs reduced HIV acquisition risk, and adherence to all of the PrEP options was poor (Marrazzo et al. 2015). Qualitative research conducted alongside the study suggested a number of barriers to taking PrEP, such as forgetting doses, fearing or experiencing side effects, the association of antiretroviral drugs with HIV stigma and illness, and unsupportive partners and families (van der Straten et al. 2014).

Other PrEP studies that had successful outcomes in this period appeared to replicate the well-resourced conditions experienced in the US arm of the iPrEx study. They included the IPERGAY study of on-demand dosing among French and Canadian gay and bisexual men (Molina et al. 2015), and the PROUD open-label study of daily TDF-FTC among British gay and bisexual men (McCormack et al. 2016). These studies were concluded early because of the high level of efficacy found in the active drug arms (86% in both studies) and to avoid further HIV infections in the placebo and control groups.

What do these mixed trial results tell us about PrEP's efficacy and the networked elements required to make PrEP efficacious? The US Centers for Disease Control decided relatively swiftly after the iPrEx study results that PrEP could be offered to gay and bisexual men at high risk of HIV (Centers for Disease Control and Prevention 2011). The following year the US Federal Drug Administration approved PrEP for all adults at risk of HIV (US Food and Drug Administration 2012). The FDA announcement both acknowledged and downplayed the mixed results from the trials. The FDA approval and media coverage focused on the two successful trials (iPrEx and Partners PrEP) as evidence that daily PrEP worked, if taken as directed (US Food and Drug Administration 2012). The announcements then stressed the importance of adherence in order to achieve a protective effect, tacitly acknowledging the failed trials. This is, of course, consistent with a narrow public health understanding of PrEP as a stable object and pharmaceutical agent. But a broader understanding of PrEP as a process suggests a number of other necessary conditions to make PrEP work in practice. There is, for example, one's perceived risk of getting HIV (such as in the Partners PrEP study, in which HIV-negative participants were aware that they might acquire HIV from their untreated serodiscordant partners). The FEM-PrEP and VOICE studies suggest it is more difficult to make PrEP work in settings in which HIV remains highly stigmatised, and antiretroviral drugs can signify that one already has HIV. Supportive partners and family members may also be helpful (suggesting that PrEP is not necessarily an individual intervention, as is commonly understood, but may need to be collectively owned and supported to work). These results suggested that in resource-poor, stigmatised or high prevalence settings, additional effort is needed to enmesh users in social networks and routines that support regular pill-taking; something that was not guaranteed to work in the post-trial period.

18.5   Implementation Fidelity and Adaptation

It is well recognised in implementation science that the transition from the trial stage of an intervention to its implementation in practice can be challenging. Some in the field emphasise the need for 'fidelity' to be maintained between the way an intervention is tested or administered in a trial and its implementation in the 'real world':

> Evidence-based practice assumes that an intervention is being implemented in full accordance with its published details. This is particularly important given the greater potential for inconsistencies in implementation of an intervention in real world rather than experimental conditions (Carroll et al. 2007, p. 2).

This approach assumes that if an intervention is sufficiently discrete that it can be extracted from the trial setting (and that it can reproduced in multiple locations with sufficient resemblance to the trialled intervention that its positive effects will be replicated). As noted above, this assumes that the core of the intervention can travel unchanged across contexts and achieve similar effects, and that the surrounding conditions in which the trial was conducted are less important in achieving an intervention's efficacy. With PrEP, it is relatively easy to imagine it as a discrete, immutable object if one focuses on the pharmaceutical drug or pill and ignores the other conditions and relations that make taking PrEP possible.

In implementation science, the emphasis on intervention fidelity is not without its detractors. Some have noted a tension between maintaining an intervention's fidelity (or closeness to the original trial conditions) and the need for local adaptation: 'Without fidelity, valid claims cannot be made about the effects of a programme and yet, without adaptation a programme cannot be put into practice' (Rod et al. 2014, p. 297). Reflecting on local contingencies and the process of implementation, they conclude that 'an intervention may assume numerous forms in the course of social interaction and that the relationship between these forms may not be adequately captured by the fidelity/adaptation distinction' (Rod et al. 2014, p. 304).

Bearing this fidelity/adaptation dynamic in mind, and the tension between the idea of PrEP as a stable object or a relational process, can assist us in understanding the success (or failure) of PrEP in the post-trial period, and the different PrEPs that may be locally generated. As Rosengarten and Michael (2009) observed, it was common for those involved in PrEP's development to sometimes view PrEP as a stable, discrete object, and at other times conceptualise it as a process that would evolve and change. This tension has continued as PrEP has been introduced in multiple settings, and has shaped how experts have responded to the consequences of PrEP's introduction, including whether effects regarded as unintended or undesirable are incorporated into our understanding of what PrEP is, or quarantined from it.

18.6   Post-Trial PrEPs, (Unintended) Consequences and Quarantining/Adaptation

As noted earlier, many of those involved in the development of PrEP had speculated about its potential consequences, particularly unwanted or undesirable effects. The primary hope for PrEP was that it would be effective in preventing HIV, and therefore reduce individual risk and population levels of transmission. However, there were concerns about efficacy, adherence, side effects and PrEP's effects on condom use and sexually transmitted infections, among others (Youle and Wainberg 2003; Paxton et al. 2007; Holt 2015).

'Unintended consequences' are commonly understood in implementation research as unwanted or undesirable effects that may or may not have been anticipated, but there can also be unexpected but beneficial consequences of interventions. In all of these situations, anticipated or not, beneficial or not, the ways in which consequences and effects are incorporated or not into our understanding of what an intervention is can affect what it becomes (Rhodes and Lancaster 2019). In debates about PrEP's consequences and effects, we can see an ongoing tension between the idea of PrEP as a stable object or an unfolding process. The acceptance or rejection of consequences as part of the intervention by researchers and other interlocutors demonstrates a tacit understanding of 'ontological politics' (Mol 2002); that there are multiple options for what PrEP could become, and some of these may be better for its users and HIV prevention than others (Holt et al. 2019).

One of the major changes in the post-trial period was that potential PrEP users could be told the intervention would work, if they took it as recommended. In high income countries like Canada, France and the USA, participants in the iPrEX and IPERGAY studies were offered PrEP in open label extensions of the original randomised trials. In these extension studies, the efficacy of PrEP in preventing HIV increased to 97–100% if participants took the pills as directed (Grant et al. 2014; Molina et al. 2017). These findings, along with those pooled from other studies, have generally led experts and international agencies to conclude that PrEP is highly effective when correctly used (Fonner et al. 2016; WHO 2016). However, even in these open label studies there have been issues with adherence, with some participants taking very few pills or stopping PrEP altogether, despite knowing that it could protect them from HIV (Grant et al. 2014). Lower levels of PrEP use were found among younger, less educated participants with fewer sexual partners. This suggests that the conditions necessary to facilitate drug adherence (or to make a successful PrEP-user assemblage, as noted before) remain critical to implementing PrEP.

Broader than the issue of adherence are the issues of PrEP uptake and ongoing use. Despite its protective capacity, it appears that it is not straightforward to facilitate and sustain widespread PrEP use without concerted effort and supportive conditions. In the USA, where PrEP has been publicly available for longest, uptake has been characterised as 'slow' with widely varying levels of use throughout the country, with approximately 20% of gay and bisexual men reporting PrEP use by 2017 (Finlayson et al. 2019; Sullivan et al. 2020). Men who appear at higher risk of HIV are more likely to use PrEP, while Black, Hispanic and younger men, those without health insurance and those living in non-urban areas are less likely to use it. Rates of use are also noticeably higher in cities with large gay communities that took part in earlier PrEP studies (Nwokolo et al. 2017; Grulich et al. 2018; Chen et al. 2019; Psomas and Kinloch 2020).

However, achieving high levels of PrEP use and sustaining them appears to be difficult in many other locations. Researchers have started discussing PrEP 'persistence' and 'discontinuation' and recommending various interventions to promote adherence and ongoing use (Coy et al. 2019). This has been prompted by reports of high levels of users trying but then stopping PrEP, with the majority of users discontinuing use after a year in South Africa, the USA and Zimbabwe (Celum et al. 2019; Coy et al. 2019; Scott et al. 2019). In the USA, transgender women, Black people, those who reported injecting drug use and those who lacked comprehensive health insurance were the most likely to stop (Coy et al. 2019; Scott et al. 2019). Sex workers and gay and bisexual men in South Africa have identified side effects and feeling stigmatised for using PrEP as common reasons for stopping use (Pillay et al. 2020). Collectively, these studies suggest sustaining PrEP use is difficult, particularly for marginalised populations or people without health insurance, and in settings which lack community support for PrEP. This does not appear to be particularly different from the situations experienced in the early PrEP trials. This is an unwanted situation, given how effective PrEP can be in a favourable context, but maybe it should not be considered unexpected, if we take seriously the idea that constructing an effective PrEP assemblage requires more than simply providing pills to patients.

Concerns about reduced condom use as a result of people using PrEP were raised early in its development, along with the related idea that sexually transmitted infections could become more common (Youle and Wainberg 2003; Paxton et al. 2007). The idea that users might reduce one form of protective behaviour (condoms) after taking up another intervention (PrEP) is often referred to as 'risk compensation' (Holt and Murphy 2017). Debate about PrEP and condom use has been most visible and febrile in the USA. After PrEP had been approved for general prescribing in the USA, some gay men, HIV experts and public commentators questioned its efficacy and appropriateness as an alternative to condoms. One now infamous commentary, titled 'Truvada whores?', suggested that gay men who wanted to use PrEP were 'irresponsible', wanted to 'engage in unsafe practices' and would be exposing themselves to sexually transmitted infections (Duran 2012). Interviewed for a newspaper article about PrEP, the head of the AIDS Healthcare Foundation labelled PrEP a 'party drug' (Associated Press 2014). Both types of commentary recycled a longstanding moralism in some strands of HIV prevention and (gay) community politics, in which condoms are seen as the only acceptable or responsible HIV prevention method. This is often asserted despite (or perhaps because of) evidence that condom use has never been universally practised and has declined in many countries since the availability of effective HIV treatments (Hess et al. 2017). The criticisms of PrEP were called out as 'slut shaming' and stigmatising (Spieldenner 2016), potentially impeding access to an effective prevention method. The debate prompted HIV organisations and community networks in the USA to more aggressively promote and support PrEP use (Calabrese and Underhill 2015). The argument also created a charged atmosphere in which early implementation occurred. Considering PrEP as an evolving assemblage, we could view these public arguments as attempts to attach various affective and biopolitical qualities to PrEP such as promiscuity, recklessness, responsibility or pride, and therefore discourage or encourage its use. In effect, these interlocutors were trying to enfold these qualities with potential PrEP users (or quarantine PrEP from negative associations) and influence its implementation (Holt 2015).

Research evidence about PrEP and condom use has gradually emerged since it became more widely used. Reviews indicate that participants in the early randomised trials, who did not know whether they were receiving PrEP or not, largely did not reduce condom use (Fonner et al. 2016). However, multiple observational studies in the post-trial period have found that PrEP users tend to reduce condom use as they come to rely upon the intervention (Traeger et al. 2018). This is understandable, given that users are now told how well PrEP can work if they establish a regular pattern of use. A few observational studies have also shown that the introduction of PrEP can disrupt condom use at a community level, i.e. that non-PrEP users may use condoms less often as PrEP use becomes more common. This unintended and initially unwanted effect has been observed in Melbourne, Sydney and San Francisco (Holt et al. 2018b; Chen et al. 2019). However, it has generally not created enduring concern in these locations because HIV infections have fallen as PrEP use has increased. Reducing HIV infections at a local level has largely confounded criticisms of PrEP as an inferior strategy to condoms, and encouraged other jurisdictions to consider its introduction (Grulich et al. 2018). The findings do, however, underscore that PrEP and condoms are not discrete interventions, but influence and change each other.

The issue of increased sexually transmitted infections (STIs) as a result of PrEP has also received considerable attention. As PrEP was never intended to prevent STIs other than HIV, sexually transmitted infections are the definition of unintended and unwanted consequences as a result of introducing an intervention. Reviews of multiple studies indicate that PrEP users tend to be diagnosed with bacterial STIs at higher rates than non-users (Traeger et al. 2018). This appears to be because PrEP users tend to use condoms inconsistently or less often after they start using PrEP, and because they undergo more frequent testing for STIs. The issue of STIs appears to have been particularly vexed in the USA, where PrEP researchers and proponents are concerned that eligible patients are not coming forward and doctors are reticent to recommend PrEP, because of stigma and fears about risk compensation and STIs (Calabrese and Underhill 2015; Golub 2018). This has prompted a concerted effort to defend PrEP and reposition it as a way to encourage people to manage their sexual health, and get STIs diagnosed and treated more quickly (Koester and Grant 2015; Golub 2018). In effect, there is an ongoing effort to attach and enfold positive qualities in the making of PrEP and its users (e.g. better sexual health, responsibility, increased pleasure) while at the same time quarantining potentially negative consequences (higher rates of STIs) to one side (Holt 2015). This simultaneously treats PrEP as both a relational process that can be expanded (to include sexual health) and a discrete object that can separated from unwanted relations (STIs).

Finally, it is important to consider the broader effects of PrEP's introduction, and how these are shaping what PrEP becomes as it adapts to and is adapted within different settings and populations. In HIV social research it is well known that the introduction of new technologies throughout the epidemic (e.g. testing, treatment and prevention methods) can foster new forms of identity, affinity, belonging and risk perception, and can generate novel sexual practices and relationships. These biosocial effects are often far broader than the original (and narrow) intended use of a technology (Lock and Nguyen 2018). The classic example is HIV antibody testing, which was developed to identify and diagnose HIV infection but has led to social identities, affiliations and divisions based on HIV status (HIV-negative, HIV-positive). The availability of effective HIV treatments has allowed HIV-positive people to maintain their health, but can create a sense of therapeutic or pharmaceutical citizenship, and a responsibility to adhere to treatment (Nguyen et al. 2007). What biosocial effects is the introduction of PrEP prompting, and how are they incorporated or not into PrEP's unfolding as an intervention?

Qualitative research conducted with PrEP users indicates a range of positive experiences associated with PrEP, such as relief from anxiety about HIV, an enhanced sense of control, greater pleasure from sex and confidence in relationships, including those with HIV-positive partners (Koester et al. 2017; Franks et al. 2018; Grace et al. 2018; Hughes et al. 2018; Camlin et al. 2020). For heterosexual couples in particular, these benefits may be undermined by a lack of trust, or suspicion about sex outside of primary relationships (Camlin et al. 2020). Heterosexual women may also find it harder than men to negotiate and agree on PrEP use with partners, troubling the idea of PrEP as a discreet, empowering intervention under individual control.

Various forms of stigma and stigmatising practices have been raised in relation to PrEP, demonstrating both liberating and constraining effects of PrEP in practice. As noted in South Africa, the use of antiretroviral drugs is heavily associated with being HIV-positive in high prevalence settings, and can be viewed as a sign that one is ill, making it harder to engage in and disclose PrEP use (van der Straten et al. 2014). Gay and bisexual men in North America have faced similar types of HIV stigma and connotations of promiscuity when disclosing PrEP use to partners or family members (Franks et al. 2018; Grace et al. 2018). Some may counter this by asserting pride in PrEP use and sexual pleasure and reclaiming labels such as 'Truvada whore' (Spieldenner 2016). However, it appears more common for PrEP users to assert a sense of responsibility and pharmaceutical citizenship; that in taking PrEP they are transforming HIV prevention, tackling stigma and helping to end the epidemic (Hughes et al. 2018; Philpot et al. 2020). This sense of collective enterprise has perhaps been most evident in countries where advocates have campaigned against limited access and helped each other to import PrEP drugs from overseas (Paparini et al. 2018; Martinez-Lacabe 2019).

Some have seen PrEP as an opportunity to reduce HIV stigma and the 'sero-divide' between HIV-negative and HIV-positive people (Persson et al. 2016; Philpot et al. 2020). There are signs that PrEP users are more comfortable having sex with HIV-positive people, although perhaps not to the extent initially imagined (Holt et al. 2018a). Some PrEP users may perceive an affinity between PrEP and having an undetectable viral load as superior HIV prevention strategies, creating the conditions for new forms of marginalisation and exclusion, such as the rejection of non-PrEP-users or condom users as potential partners (Martinez-Lacabe 2019). In a few high-income settings, there has been a profound and rapid reordering of prevention practices, with PrEP becoming the dominant mode of HIV prevention for gay and bisexual men in cities like San Francisco, London and Sydney (Nwokolo et al. 2017; Grulich et al. 2018; Chen et al. 2019). In these locations PrEP may be considered normative for HIV-negative men, and those who cannot or will not use PrEP may be judged in a similar way to those who did not use condoms in an earlier era. While PrEP's biosocial effects continue to unfold, it is clear that trying to locally fashion PrEP as an effective and sustainable form of prevention inevitably implicates users, communities and researchers in longstanding debates about responsibility, stigma and acceptable forms of sex and relationships.

18.7   Conclusion

In analysing PrEP's development, implementation and various effects, I have argued that considering PrEP as a relational and contingent process can attune us to the socio-material conditions necessary for effective implementation, and the circumstances in which successful HIV prevention may be impeded. PrEP's development indicates a range of local conditions that facilitate PrEP use and acceptance of the intervention, such as engaged and supportive affected communities, reliable and cheap health care, and a culture that views pharmaceutical use as normal and responsible. In contrast, high levels of HIV-related stigma, a lack of affordable health care and judgemental attitudes about alternatives to condoms appear to impede PrEP use. While a traditional public health approach views these conditions as external to an intervention like PrEP, I have suggested that PrEP's local unfolding is dependent on and inseparable from this elaborate network of relations.

As PrEP implementation has proceeded, we have seen a variety of effects associated with its use, and fierce debates about unwanted and unintended consequences such as reduced condom use, STIs, or the potential for new forms of affiliation and exclusion. In responding to these effects, it is possible to see the ontological politics of making interventions like PrEP in certain ways and not others, with proponents keen to acknowledge and celebrate positive consequences of PrEP (like relief from fear, increased pleasure and responsibility) and enfold them into the PrEP assemblage, while critics have tried to contaminate PrEP by associating it with recklessness, the loss of condoms and STIs. The analysis offered here suggests that it is not possible to separate PrEP from existing practices like condoms, or longstanding arguments about appropriate forms of sexual conduct and responsibility. To make PrEP work effectively, we should recognise and embrace the dense networks of relations on which it relies, and the positive and disruptive effects it can simultaneously provoke. These are all part of PrEP's making, and may help us practise a more relational, informed and effective form of implementation science, one that rejects the idea that interventions travel freely without consequence.

References

Associated Press. (2014, April 6). Divide over HIV prevention drug Truvada persists. *USA Today*. Retrieved May 8, 2020, from https://www.usatoday.com/story/news/nation/2014/04/06/gay-men-divided-over-use-of-hiv-prevention-drug/7390879/.

Auerbach, J. D., & Hoppe, T. A. (2015). Beyond "getting drugs into bodies": Social science perspectives on pre-exposure prophylaxis for HIV. *Journal of the International AIDS Society, 18*(4S3), 19983. https://doi.org/10.7448/IAS.18.4.19983.

Baeten, J. M., Donnell, D., Ndase, P., Mugo, N. R., Campbell, J. D., Wangisi, J., et al. (2012). Antiretroviral prophylaxis for HIV prevention in heterosexual men and women. *New England Journal of Medicine, 367*(5), 399–410. https://doi.org/10.1056/Nejmoa1108524.

Calabrese, S. K., & Underhill, K. (2015). How stigma surrounding the use of HIV preexposure prophylaxis undermines prevention and pleasure: A call to destigmatize "Truvada whores". *American Journal of Public Health, 105*(10), 1960–1964. https://doi.org/10.2105/AJPH.2015.302816.

Camlin, C. S., Koss, C. A., Getahun, M., Owino, L., Itiakorit, H., Akatukwasa, C., et al. (2020). Understanding demand for PrEP and early experiences of PrEP use among young adults in rural Kenya and Uganda: A qualitative study. *AIDS and Behavior., 24*(7), 2149–2162. https://doi.org/10.1007/s10461-020-02780-x.

Carroll, C., Patterson, M., Wood, S., Booth, A., Rick, J., & Balain, S. (2007). A conceptual framework for implementation fidelity. *Implementation Science, 2*(1), 40. https://doi.org/10.1186/1748-5908-2-40.

Celum, C., Mgodi, N., Bekker, L. G., Hosek, S., Donnell, D., Anderson, P. L., et al. (2019). *PrEP adherence and effect of drug level feedback among young African women in HPTN 082*. Paper presented at the IAS Conference on HIV Science, Mexico City.

Centers for Disease Control and Prevention. (2011). Interim guidance: Preexposure prophylaxis for the prevention of HIV infection in men who have sex with men. *Morbidity & Mortality Weekly Report, 60*(3), 65–68.

Chen, Y.-H., Guigayoma, J., McFarland, W., Snowden, J. M., & Raymond, H. F. (2019). Increases in pre-exposure prophylaxis use and decreases in condom use: Behavioral patterns among

HIV-negative San Francisco men who have sex with men, 2004–2017. *AIDS and Behavior, 23*(7), 1841–1845. https://doi.org/10.1007/s10461-018-2299-7.

Coy, K. C., Hazen, R. J., Kirkham, H. S., Delpino, A., & Siegler, A. J. (2019). Persistence on HIV preexposure prophylaxis medication over a 2-year period among a national sample of 7148 PrEP users, United States, 2015 to 2017. *Journal of the International AIDS Society, 22*(2), e25252. https://doi.org/10.1002/jia2.25252.

Dumit, J. (2002). Drugs for life. *Molecular Interventions, 2*(3), 124–127.

Duran, D. (2012, November 12). Truvada whores? *The Huffington Post.* Retrieved May 8, 2020, from http://www.huffingtonpost.com/david-duran/truvada-whores_b_2113588.html.

Finlayson, T., Cha, S., Xia, M., Trujillo, L., Denson, D., Prejean, J., et al. (2019). Changes in HIV preexposure prophylaxis awareness and use among men who have sex with men - 20 urban areas, 2014 and 2017. *Morbidity & Mortality Weekly Report, 68*(27), 597–603. https://doi.org/10.15585/mmwr.mm6827a1.

Fonner, V. A., Dalglish, S. L., Kennedy, C. E., Baggaley, R., O'Reilly, K. R., Koechlin, F. M., et al. (2016). Effectiveness and safety of oral HIV pre-exposure prophylaxis (PrEP) for all populations: A systematic review and meta-analysis. *AIDS, 30*(12), 1973–1983. https://doi.org/10.1097/QAD.0000000000001145.

Franks, J., Hirsch-Moverman, Y., Loquere, A. S., Amico, K. R., Grant, R. M., Dye, B. J., et al. (2018). Sex, PrEP, and stigma: Experiences with HIV pre-exposure prophylaxis among new York City MSM participating in the HPTN 067/ADAPT study. *AIDS and Behavior, 22*(4), 1139–1149. https://doi.org/10.1007/s10461-017-1964-6.

Golub, S. A. (2018). PrEP stigma: Implicit and explicit drivers of disparity. *Current HIV/AIDS Reports, 15*(2), 190–197. https://doi.org/10.1007/s11904-018-0385-0.

Grace, D., Jollimore, J., MacPherson, P., Strang, M. J., & Tan, D. H. (2018). The pre-exposure prophylaxis-stigma paradox: Learning from Canada's first wave of PrEP users. *AIDS Patient Care and STDs, 32*(1), 24–30. https://doi.org/10.1089/apc.2017.0153.

Grant, R. M., Lama, J. R., Anderson, P. L., McMahan, V., Liu, A. Y., Vargas, L., et al. (2010). Preexposure chemoprophylaxis for HIV prevention in men who have sex with men. *New England Journal of Medicine, 363*(27), 2587–2599. https://doi.org/10.1056/Nejmoa1011205.

Grant, R. M., Anderson, P. L., McMahan, V., Liu, A., Amico, K. R., Mehrotra, M., et al. (2014). Uptake of pre-exposure prophylaxis, sexual practices, and HIV incidence in men and transgender women who have sex with men: A cohort study. *The Lancet Infectious Diseases, 14*(9), 820–829. https://doi.org/10.1016/S1473-3099(14)70847-3.

Grulich, A. E., Guy, R., Amin, J., Jin, F., Selvey, C., Holden, J., et al. (2018). Population-level effectiveness of rapid, targeted, high-coverage roll-out of HIV pre-exposure prophylaxis in men who have sex with men: The EPIC-NSW prospective cohort study. *The Lancet HIV, 5*(11), E629–E637. https://doi.org/10.1016/S2352-3018(18)30215-7.

Haire, B. G. (2011). Because we can: Clashes of perspective over researcher obligation in the failed PrEP trials. *Developing World Bioethics, 11*(2), 63–74. https://doi.org/10.1111/j.1471-8847.2010.00292.x.

Hess, K. L., Crepaz, N., Rose, C., Purcell, D., & Paz-Bailey, G. (2017). Trends in sexual behavior among men who have sex with men (MSM) in high-income countries, 1990–2013: A systematic review. *AIDS and Behavior, 21*(10), 2811–2834. https://doi.org/10.1007/s10461-017-1799-1.

Holt, M. (2015). Configuring the users of new HIV-prevention technologies: The case of HIV pre-exposure prophylaxis. *Culture, Health & Sexuality, 17*(4), 428–439. https://doi.org/10.1080/13691058.2014.960003.

Holt, M., & Murphy, D. A. (2017). Individual versus community-level risk compensation following preexposure prophylaxis of HIV. *American Journal of Public Health, 107*(10), 1568–1571. https://doi.org/10.2105/ajph.2017.303930.

Holt, M., Draper, B. L., Pedrana, A. E., Wilkinson, A. L., & Stoové, M. (2018a). Comfort relying on HIV pre-exposure prophylaxis and treatment as prevention for condomless sex: Results of an online survey of Australian gay and bisexual men. *AIDS and Behavior, 22*(11), 3617–3626. https://doi.org/10.1007/s10461-018-2097-2.

Holt, M., Lea, T., Mao, L., Kolstee, J., Zablotska, I., Duck, T., et al. (2018b). Community-level changes in condom use and uptake of HIV pre-exposure prophylaxis by gay and bisexual men in Melbourne and Sydney, Australia: Results of repeated behavioural surveillance in 2013–17. *The Lancet HIV, 5*(8), E448–E456. https://doi.org/10.1016/S2352-3018(18)30072-9.

Holt, M., Newman, C. E., Lancaster, K., Smith, A. K., Hughes, S., & Truong, H.-H. M. (2019). HIV pre-exposure prophylaxis and the 'problems' of reduced condom use and sexually transmitted infections in Australia: A critical analysis from an evidence-making intervention perspective. *Sociology of Health & Illness, 41*(8), 1535–1548. https://doi.org/10.1111/1467-9566.12967.

Hughes, S. D., Sheon, N., Andrew, E. V. W., Cohen, S. E., Doblecki-Lewis, S., & Liu, A. Y. (2018). Body/selves and beyond: men's narratives of sexual behavior on PrEP. *Medical Anthropology, 37*(5), 387–400. https://doi.org/10.1080/01459740.2017.1416608.

Kippax, S., & Stephenson, N. (2016). *Socialising the biomedical turn in HIV prevention*. London: Anthem Press.

Koester, K., & Grant, R. M. (2015). Keeping our eyes on the prize: No new HIV infections with increased use of HIV pre-exposure prophylaxis. *Clinical Infectious Diseases, 61*(10), 1604–1605. https://doi.org/10.1093/cid/civ783.

Koester, K., Amico, R. K., Gilmore, H., Liu, A., McMahan, V., Mayer, K., et al. (2017). Risk, safety and sex among male PrEP users: Time for a new understanding. *Culture, Health & Sexuality, 19*(12), 1301–1313. https://doi.org/10.1080/13691058.2017.1310927.

Law, J., & Singleton, V. (2005). Object lessons. *Organization, 12*(3), 331–355. https://doi.org/10.1177/1350508405051270.

Liu, A., Glidden, D. V., Anderson, P. L., Amico, K. R., McMahan, V., Mehrotra, M., et al. (2014). Patterns and correlates of PrEP drug detection among MSM and transgender women in the global iPrEx study. *Journal of Acquired Immune Deficiency Syndromes, 67*(5), 528–537. https://doi.org/10.1097/QAI.0000000000000351.

Lock, M., & Nguyen, V.-K. (2018). *An anthropology of biomedicine* (2nd ed.). Hoboken: Wiley.

Marrazzo, J. M., Ramjee, G., Richardson, B. A., Gomez, K., Mgodi, N., Nair, G., et al. (2015). Tenofovir-based preexposure prophylaxis for HIV infection among African women. *New England Journal of Medicine, 372*(6), 509–518. https://doi.org/10.1056/NEJMoa1402269.

Martinez-Lacabe, A. (2019). The non-positive antiretroviral gay body: The biomedicalisation of gay sex in England. *Culture, Health & Sexuality, 21*(10), 1117–1130. https://doi.org/10.1080/13691058.2018.1539772.

McCormack, S., Dunn, D. T., Desai, M., Dolling, D. I., Gafos, M., Gilson, R., et al. (2016). Pre-exposure prophylaxis to prevent the acquisition of HIV-1 infection (PROUD): Effectiveness results from the pilot phase of a pragmatic open-label randomised trial. *The Lancet, 387*(10013), 53–60. https://doi.org/10.1016/S0140-6736(15)00056-2.

Mol, A. (2002). *The body multiple: Ontology in medical practice*. Durham: Duke University Press.

Molina, J.-M., Capitant, C., Spire, B., Pialoux, G., Cotte, L., Charreau, I., et al. (2015). On-demand preexposure prophylaxis in men at high risk for HIV-1 infection. *New England Journal of Medicine, 373*(23), 2237–2246. https://doi.org/10.1056/NEJMoa1506273.

Molina, J.-M., Charreau, I., Spire, B., Cotte, L., Chas, J., Capitant, C., et al. (2017). Efficacy, safety, and effect on sexual behaviour of on-demand pre-exposure prophylaxis for HIV in men who have sex with men: An observational cohort study. *The Lancet HIV, 4*(9), e402–e410. https://doi.org/10.1016/S2352-3018(17)30089-9.

Nguyen, V.-K., Ako, C. Y., Niamba, P., Sylla, A., & Tiendrébéogo, I. (2007). Adherence as therapeutic citizenship: Impact of the history of access to antiretroviral drugs on adherence to treatment. *AIDS, 21*, S31–S35. https://doi.org/10.1097/01.aids.0000298100.48990.58.

Nwokolo, N., Hill, A., McOwan, A., & Pozniak, A. (2017). Rapidly declining HIV infection in MSM in Central London. *The Lancet HIV, 4*(11), e482–e483. https://doi.org/10.1016/S2352-3018(17)30181-9.

Paparini, S., Nutland, W., Rhodes, T., Nguyen, V.-K., & Anderson, J. (2018). DIY HIV prevention: Formative qualitative research with men who have sex with men who source PrEP outside of clinical trials. *PLoS One, 13*(8), e0202830–e0202830. https://doi.org/10.1371/journal.pone. 0202830.

Paxton, L. A., Hope, T., & Jaffe, H. W. (2007). Pre-exposure prophylaxis for HIV infection: What if it works? *The Lancet, 370*(9581), 89–93.

Persson, A., Ellard, J., & Newman, C. E. (2016). Bridging the HIV divide: Stigma, stories and serodiscordant sexuality in the biomedical age. *Sexuality & Culture, 20*(2), 197–213. https://doi. org/10.1007/s12119-015-9316-z.

Philpot, S., Prestage, G., Holt, M., Haire, B., Maher, L., Hammoud, M., & Bourne, A. (2020). Gay and bisexual men's perceptions of pre-exposure prophylaxis (PrEP) in a context of high accessibility: An Australian qualitative study. *AIDS and Behavior, 24*(8), 2369–2380. https:// doi.org/10.1007/s10461-020-02796-3.

Pillay, D., Stankevitz, K., Lanham, M., Ridgeway, K., Murire, M., Briedenhann, E., et al. (2020). Factors influencing uptake, continuation, and discontinuation of oral PrEP among clients at sex worker and MSM facilities in South Africa. *PLoS One, 15*(4), e0228620. https://doi.org/10. 1371/journal.pone.0228620.

Psomas, C. K., & Kinloch, S. (2020). Highlights of the 17th European AIDS Clinical Society (EACS) conference, 6-9 November 2019, Basel, Switzerland. *Journal of Virus Eradication, 6* (1), 38–44.

Rhodes, T., & Lancaster, K. (2019). Evidence-making interventions in health: A conceptual framing. *Social Science & Medicine, 238*, 112488. https://doi.org/10.1016/j.socscimed.2019. 112488.

Rod, M. H., Ingholt, L., Sørensen, B. B., & Tjørnhøj-Thomsen, T. (2014). The spirit of the intervention: Reflections on social effectiveness in public health intervention research. *Critical Public Health, 24*(3), 296–307. https://doi.org/10.1080/09581596.2013.841313.

Rosengarten, M., & Michael, M. (2009). The performative function of expectations in translating treatment to prevention: The case of HIV pre-exposure prophylaxis, or PrEP. *Social Science and Medicine, 69*, 1049–1055.

Scott, H. M., Spinelli, M., Vittinghoff, E., Morehead-Gee, A., Hirozawa, A., James, C., et al. (2019). Racial/ethnic and HIV risk category disparities in preexposure prophylaxis discontinuation among patients in publicly funded primary care clinics. *AIDS, 33*(14), 2189–2195. https://doi.org/10.1097/QAD.0000000000002347.

Spieldenner, A. (2016). PrEP whores and HIV prevention: The queer communication of HIV pre-exposure prophylaxis (PrEP). *Journal of Homosexuality, 63*(12), 1685–1697. https://doi. org/10.1080/00918369.2016.1158012.

Sullivan, P. S., Sanchez, T. H., Zlotorzynska, M., Chandler, C. J., Sineath, R. C., Kahle, E., & Tregear, S. (2020). National trends in HIV pre-exposure prophylaxis awareness, willingness and use among United States men who have sex with men recruited online, 2013 through 2017. *Journal of the International AIDS Society, 23*(3), e25461. https://doi.org/10.1002/jia2.25461.

Thigpen, M. C., Kebaabetswe, P. M., Paxton, L. A., Smith, D. K., Rose, C. E., Segolodi, T. M., et al. (2012). Antiretroviral preexposure prophylaxis for heterosexual HIV transmission in Botswana. *New England Journal of Medicine, 367*(5), 423–434. https://doi.org/10.1056/ Nejmoa1110711.

Traeger, M. W., Schroeder, S. E., Wright, E. J., Hellard, M. E., Cornelisse, V. J., Doyle, J. S., & Stoové, M. A. (2018). Effects of pre-exposure prophylaxis for the prevention of human immunodeficiency virus infection on sexual risk behavior in men who have sex with men: A systematic review and meta-analysis. *Clinical Infectious Diseases, 67*(5), 676–686. https://doi. org/10.1093/cid/ciy182.

US Food and Drug Administration. (2012). *FDA approves first drug for reducing the risk of sexually acquired HIV infection.* Silver Spring, New Hampshire: US Department of Health & Human Services.

Van Damme, L., Corneli, A., Ahmed, K., Agot, K., Lombaard, J., Kapiga, S., et al. (2012). Preexposure prophylaxis for HIV infection among African women. *New England Journal of Medicine, 367*(5), 411–422. https://doi.org/10.1056/NEJMoa1202614.

van der Straten, A., Stadler, J., Luecke, E., Laborde, N., Hartmann, M., Montgomery, E. T., & VOICE-C Study Team. (2014). Perspectives on use of oral and vaginal antiretrovirals for HIV prevention: the VOICE-C qualitative study in Johannesburg, South Africa. *Journal of the International AIDS Society, 17*(3S2), 19146. https://doi.org/10.7448/ias.17.3.19146.

WHO. (2016). *Consolidated guidelines on the use of antiretroviral drugs for treating and preventing HIV infection* (2nd ed.). Geneva: World Health Organization.

Youle, M., & Wainberg, M. A. (2003). Pre-exposure chemoprophylaxis (PrEP) as an HIV prevention strategy. *Journal of the International Association of Physicians in AIDS Care, 2*(3), 102–105. https://doi.org/10.1177/154510970300200302.

Chapter 19
The Drive to Take an HIV Test in Rural Uganda: A Risk to Prevention for Young People?

Sarah Bernays, Allen Asiimwe, Edward Tumwesige, and Janet Seeley

19.1 Introduction

The effectiveness of recent efforts to scale up universal test and treat (UTT) for HIV to ensure those living with HIV are initiated promptly on antiretroviral treatment (ART), relies on the high uptake of HIV testing (World Health Organization (WHO) 2016). Recent trials and studies of UTT in sub-Saharan Africa have shown modest success in reducing HIV incidence (Iwuji et al. 2018; Abdool Karim 2019; Havlir et al. 2019; Hayes et al. 2019; Havlir et al. 2020), with one longitudinal study in Rakai, Uganda, showing a significant drop in HIV incidence over a 16-year period attributed to HIV combination prevention efforts (Grabowski et al. 2017). Much attention is being focused on those not being tested, and for those who do test and are found to be living with HIV who do not link to care. The missing are often young people, particularly young men (Baisley et al. 2019; Seeley et al. 2019).

S. Bernays (✉)
School of Public Health, Faculty of Medicine and Health, University of Sydney, Sydney, Australia

Department of Global Health and Development, London School of Hygiene and Tropical Medicine, London, UK
e-mail: sarah.bernays@sydney.edu.au

A. Asiimwe · E. Tumwesige
Social Science Department, MRC/UVRU & LSHTM Uganda Research Unit, London School of Hygiene and Tropical Medicine, Entebbe, Uganda

J. Seeley
Department of Global Health and Development, London School of Hygiene and Tropical Medicine, London, UK

Social Science Department, MRC/UVRU & LSHTM Uganda Research Unit, London School of Hygiene and Tropical Medicine, Entebbe, Uganda

African Health Research Institute, Durban, South Africa

© The Author(s) 2021
S. Bernays et al. (eds.), *Remaking HIV Prevention in the 21st Century*, Social Aspects of HIV 5, https://doi.org/10.1007/978-3-030-69819-5_19

Yet, testing HIV-negative is also an entry point into HIV prevention (Hargreaves et al. 2016; Nall et al. 2019), and with HIV testing being more widely available, repeat testing is encouraged to ensure that people know their HIV status and can seek appropriate prevention and care support (Perkins et al. 2018; Harichund et al. 2019). In this chapter we look at young people's engagement with HIV prevention options and how, why and with what consequences some prioritise HIV testing not as an entry into HIV prevention or care options but as their preferred (and often singular) prevention method.

Evidence from a systematic review of the uptake and positivity rate of HIV testing services among children and adolescents (ages 5–19) indicates that approaches evaluated to date have not been tailored to the needs of this age group (Govindasamy et al. 2015). Rather, they replicate strategies for adults and do not consider the specific barriers that adolescents face (Fox et al. 2013), or indeed the ways in which young people may view testing (Gottert et al. 2018). HIV testing is encouraged as the responsible thing to do, infusing the push for testing with a moral tone (Bond et al. 2016).

In 2018, 2.8 million children and adolescents (aged 0–19 years) were living with HIV, the majority (nearly nine out of 10) in sub-Saharan Africa (UNICEF 2019); three in four new HIV infections in adolescents (aged 15–19 years) occur in sub-Saharan Africa (UNICEF 2017). Concern about the high levels of HIV-infection among young people, particularly adolescent girls, has prompted bodies, such as the President's Emergency Plan for AIDS Relief, to support targeted interventions such as DREAMS (Determined, Resilient, Empowered, AIDS-Free, Mentored, and Safe), providing a broad combination of health, educational and social interventions targeting young women and girls to prevent HIV in ten countries in sub-Saharan Africa (Abdool Karim et al. 2017; Saul et al. 2018). Recent data from three districts in Uganda where DREAMS has been implemented show that male partners of the young women in the programme tested for HIV frequently, often after having had sex for the first time with a partner, or when wishing to stop using condoms, but also as a result of concerns after separating from a partner (Gottert et al. 2018). Interestingly, the authors observe that 'for many men, testing seemed to serve as validation for continuing their practice of having multiple partners' (p. 11)—few respondents in that study described changing their behaviour after receiving a negative HIV-test result.

19.2   Methods

We draw on findings from a qualitative methods study with young people (aged 16–24 years old) living in rural South-West Uganda to explore how HIV testing is situated within their portfolio of HIV prevention strategies. We sought to understand these young people's lived experiences in relation to sexual health practices and knowledge, particularly in relation to perceptions of HIV-risk and patterns of engagement with prevention services. We adopted a longitudinal design, using repeat waves of data collection over a year, to both capture some of the dynamism of their lives as well as to develop rapport.

Over a month we conducted a rapid participatory assessment of the study site, holding informal discussions with young and older people we encountered in the community, individually and in groups, to inform our approach to recruitment of young people, many of whom had recently moved into the area. We focused primarily on those who had recently arrived into the fieldwork area because it is very common for youth to move to pursue economic opportunities (Barratt et al. 2012), but also included those who had been living within the area for many years and were more familiar with the setting. After this formative stage, we conducted in-depth interviews with 50 young people living in the area, roughly evenly distributed by gender. Our recruitment approach involved approaching young people on the streets in the community and then adopting a snowballing approach, in which they would introduce the researchers to their friends. We followed up 30 of these same young people in a second individual interview approximately 6 months later. Although ideally our tapered sample would have been shaped by emerging analytical interests, given that several of the original sample had left the area and were no longer contactable, recruitment had instead to rely on availability. We invited those participants from the 30 interviewed, still resident in the area, to participatory workshops approximately 6 months later to discuss emerging findings and engage in co-design activities to develop an intervention model to address the concerns identified in the study. Thirteen participants attended. Four workshops were held: with eight young men and five young women.

Research ethics approvals were granted by all relevant institutional and national bodies. Participants were approached and invited to take part by the local research team and asked to provide written consent. Following Uganda National Council for Research and Technology guidance on Human Subjects Research (https://www.uncst.go.ug/guidelines-and-forms/), participants aged 16–17 living independently and providing for themselves financially were considered emancipated minors and able to give their own consent without requiring guardian approval.

We conducted an iterative thematic analysis of our data, discussing the data through weekly meetings during collection. This approach informed ongoing recruitment, sampling and revision of topic guides and formed the basis of analytical memos in which emerging themes were identified and explored. To expedite the data management process, we summarised audio-recorded data into detailed interview scripts in English using a mixture of reported speech and verbatim quotes. Pertinent linguistic phrases, such as idioms, were written verbatim and then translated into English with attention paid to capture their equivalent meaning. The completeness of the scripts was tested by transcribing verbatim some of the interviews and comparing them with draft scripts for detail. Requiring a high degree of training and skill, this is an approach increasingly adopted to facilitate timely analytical attention to emerging data, which can be disrupted by delays in transcription and translation (Bernays et al. 2018; Rutakumwa et al. 2019). Scripts were coded initially using an open-coding approach, then using a coding framework. Coded data were checked against themes identified in the team's ongoing analytical discussions. Emergent themes were corroborated between the analytical memos and the coding process and discussed by the team to ensure accuracy of representation. These were developed into the key findings.

19.3 Findings and Implications

The young people involved in this study lived in a trading town on the highway leading from Uganda to Tanzania and Rwanda or in the surrounding more rural areas in Kalungu District. The town has been a hub for the sale of produce from the rural areas, and from nearby fishing sites, for many years. Recently a rice farm and processing plant opened on the outskirts of the town, which employs several hundred young people as labourers.

19.3.1 What it Takes to 'Get by': Sex as a Currency

Young people's lives were characterised in many cases by exploitative employment situations, precarious living conditions and meagre incomes. Limited economic opportunities for these youth mean that transactional sex, where sex is used as a resource to be leveraged for material and social gain, has become increasingly normative (Bernays et al. 2020). Such sexual relationships tend to be transient in character, often concurrent and desired not only for their personal and relational pleasure, but also for their economic value. Within the context of these relationships, which are outside of explicitly commercial transactional sex, the acceptability of condom use is virtually nil; shaped by power, individual preference, and stigma associated with condoms. Jane (all names are pseudonyms) explains that should a man find a condom in a girl's house he will call her a 'Malaya' (prostitute). She goes on to describe the logic which disrupts the use of condoms for prevention.

> Generally, most young people do not want to abstain, but yet in not abstaining, they do not want to use these condoms they are giving out. In the majority of situations, you can ask him to use it and he says; 'Is a sweet eaten while in its cover?' That is what has caused illnesses among young people here. He or she thinks of what he or she is going to do that time without thinking of the consequences. (Jane, 22 years, IDI-1)

Engaging in unprotected sexual encounters, multiple relationships, and related substance use are described by young people as almost inevitable elements in what it means to be young: something that one must endure to 'get by' in the economic environment. Whilst acknowledging unprotected sex increased exposure to potential pregnancy, HIV and other sexually transmitted infections (STI) acquisition, these risks are 'traded-off' in favour of maximising immediate economic benefits.

It is very easy because if there is someone who has come having money, even if he is an old man these days us girls, we are not selective that that one is older than me. Whether he has given you how much, he does what he wants without you knowing about his status. We do not mind and there you also get infected because of the money you wanted. (Flavia, 17 years old, IDI-2).

It is surrendering oneself, tolerating whatever situation that comes her way in that relationship or whatever hardship she faces. You say whatever comes… when it fails then one gets into another relationship with someone else. (Jane, 22, and Edith, 21, workshop).

Effective HIV prevention, which in this context is to insist on condoms or pursue abstinence, 'costs' because it diminishes the value that can be gained from engaging in this pertinent economy, which is one of only a few available to young people. This extract from an interview summary with Betty illustrates the economic hardship she endured while she abstained, demonstrating that precious few real alternatives exist for the majority.

For the first two years Betty resisted taking up the option of sleeping with a man for financial support but relied singularly on her income as a waitress. This was insufficient to cover her basic needs and she either skipped meals or relied on her colleagues to share their food. Her colleagues encouraged her to adopt their approach and accept a man's proposals, so that she too could have more food to eat, buy herself cosmetics and get a phone. Both her colleagues and the patrons mocked her, asking: 'What are you waiting for? This is the way to survive.' Unable to find any alternatives to supplement her income, Betty now has a partner whom she sleeps with and he gives her money for items, previously beyond her means. (18, IDI-1).

Within a context characterised by risk, HIV is seen as just one of the many risks that they face. Other than financial hardship, young women voiced their desire to avoid unwanted pregnancy. Preventing the latter was their primary concern about unprotected sex, and if able to they used long acting contraception. However, the numbers that did were relatively low, with only two utilising the implant, and one the coil.

As a girl you do not want to get pregnant, at least you get HIV. It is because for HIV it is not seen that you are infected, but the pregnancy grows in front and there they will know that she got pregnant. (Sylvia, 23, IDI-2).

For these young women, accessing family planning and HIV testing services both carry some degree of social stigma. Integrating them into a broader delivery of combination sexual and reproductive health to go beyond a singular focus on HIV would have multiple advantages (Narasimhan et al. 2019). Services need to engage with the contextual drivers of risks to reduce the interconnected harms to which young people are exposed. We may increase the appeal of engaging in HIV prevention if we respond to the perceived risks of young people by targeting their priority concerns alongside HIV.

Table 19.1 Reported HIV testing behaviour of participants (at phase 2, n = 30)

	HIV test status
Females (n = 15)	13 tested for HIV within the last 6 months 2 tested for HIV more than 6 months ago 0 never tested for HIV
Males (n = 15)	6 tested for HIV within the last 6 months 3 tested for HIV more than 6 months ago 6 never tested for HIV

19.3.2   The 'Value' of HIV Testing a As Prevention Method

For young people who had recently migrated, who acknowledged that they might, at times, be at a heightened risk of acquiring HIV, negotiations around sex involve adopting prevention behaviour which did not diminish their opportunities to maximise the value of each sexual encounter or relationship. With condoms continuing to be an unappealing option and Pre-Exposure prophylaxis (PrEP) not widely available nor yet in considerable demand, many young people reported that they relied on HIV testing as their only HIV-prevention strategy (see Table 19.1).

Their engagement in HIV-testing was irregular, infrequent and often poorly timed. For example, young people described going for tests within a few days of having engaged in what they perceived to have been an acutely 'risky' sexual encounter ('The girl I had sex with looked ill'; 'I knew that she had a reputation of being with everyone'). This meant that the tests were commonly performed during the virus window period. Illustrative of this misunderstanding was that some young people berated the poor sensitivity of the locally available tests. Ahmed articulated a commonly held view:

> .....they (health workers) should ensure that they get machines (testing kits) that can detect the HIV virus immediately after you have contracted it because sometimes we do not have time to go back to the health facility again (23, workshop).

Testing was ordinarily done at the HIV clinic and given the continued social risks from the stigma associated with attending, young people were reticent to go often lest they be seen. Many participants described receiving a negative test result. While this was celebrated as a relief, their interpretation of the implications of these results illuminates a pivotal problem in the drive for people to get HIV-tested.

Testing has the advantage of operating as an entry point to facilitate young people's engagement in a combination of prevention options, such as access to condoms or, if available, PrEP, as well as nurses or counsellors to discuss monogamy and abstinence (Carlos et al. 2016; Starbird et al. 2016). The concerns surrounding sero-discordance within couples, which would threaten the protection of monogamy as a safe sex strategy, were not mentioned as being discussed. However, this relies on utilising the testing opportunity to enable discussion and provide relevant and targeted education. This was not a feature of the participants' experiences. Baker describes how informal payments were asked for to access explanatory counselling:

> ...when you reach there they tell you that the counsellor is not around and they ask you for money to give him/her a phone call [...]. He asks you for five thousand shillings, five hundred for beeping the health worker and four thousand five hundred his. And he asks you to wait for a few minutes for the health worker will be around (19, workshop).

Within the narrowing framework of the 95–95-95 global targets, it has been a national and regional trend for thinned resources to be increasingly prioritised towards linking those receiving a positive diagnosis into HIV treatment and care (Wong et al. 2019). Participants themselves observed that the local surge in testing drives had not been accompanied by increased access to HIV-counselling services, rather they reported reductions in the availability of counselling staff.

> I think counsellors should increase in number so that they come to the community and teach young people how they can protect themselves (about HIV). Right now, I see that the number of counsellors who used to come has reduced. When I was still young many counsellors used to come and mobilize young people and talk to them (Joshua, 21, IDI-1).

19.3.3   The 'Event' of Testing: Missed Opportunities for Primary Prevention

Testing is a part of a process (Church et al. 2017), yet considerations of the 'before' (what led someone to test) and the 'after' (what the consequences of the result are) which should be addressed in counselling around testing are increasingly been confined to those who receive a positive result. The policy of UTT creates health system pressures to move individuals through the HIV treatment cascade to achieve viral suppression as soon as possible (Witzel et al. 2017). This leaves little space to allow individuals the time they may need to come to terms with committing to a life on treatment (Mitiku et al. 2017; Kawuma et al. 2018; Horter et al. 2020).

Within our study for those who tested negative, the process was truncated into an event, with limited consideration of what provoked the decision to test, nor the after-effects of a negative result on risk exposure. Despite evident interest from the young people to receive pre and post-test counselling, only four (of 24) participants who received a negative test result reported being advised how to remain HIV-negative. Where advice was provided there was very little engagement with the contextual realities of young people's lives. Young people were advised to assume every person is HIV-positive and to use condoms if unable to abstain. The vast majority received nothing. In being shown the door upon receiving a negative result, critical opportunities are missed to respond to the reasons (and risks) that led these young people to get tested. Other studies have demonstrated a desire at a community level to have time for one-to-one discussions about testing options, implications and strategies to mitigate risk (Orne-Gliemann et al. 2016). This is a necessary component to augment the effectiveness of testing as a biomedical technology to encourage people to engage in and maximise the value of regular HIV testing, alongside ongoing investment in structural interventions which address broader gendered and economic configurations of risk (Malhotra et al. 2019).

Participants often entered the HIV testing facility with low HIV literacy, which explains their inappropriate timing. Critically though they left arguably with heightened risk, as they interpreted their test results as falsely reassuring about the limited risks of their behaviour.

> When you test HIV negative you do not go back for testing until you have had another woman because you are negative. You only go for testing after having sex with another woman and you are worried about this one having infected you with HIV (Ahmed, 23, workshop).

This approach to testing may potentially be an unintended consequence of self-testing too, where the linkage to prevention may be overshadowed by the narrow attention to those who need to be connected to care.

In settings of pressurised service delivery, such as resource-constrained areas, haste to embed testing within the treatment cascade risks rendering other essential prevention efforts perimetric. We are at risk of losing hard-won learning about combination prevention (Mannell et al. 2019). The push to meet ambitious targets funnel the care that is offered, which compromises the ability to meet the needs of uninfected young people. Current prevention efforts are failing if they do not engage with young people's concerns (Mulaudzi et al. 2018) and only then after their personal prevention strategies fail, and they have become HIV-positive.

19.3.4   The Moral Performance of Responsibility through Occasional Testing

Young people reported that they commonly relied on their own and their partner's test results, as a form of preventive sero-sorting to justify unprotected sex. Some men relied on their partners' HIV testing results, rather than their own, as their personal prevention strategy. Some attention was paid to recency of the test results; with evidence of negative test results within the last 12 months generally considered an adequate period.

> .... You also look at the date when the (HIV) test was done because you may bring a test slip of January and yet we are in December and there I can't trust you. At least you have to show me test results of the testing that was done around August or September (Samuel, 23, IDI-1).

Like a number of other participants, Samuel hinted at the fluidity of the evidential threshold required to satisfy his concerns, explaining that verbal confirmation would have been sufficient. He reported appraising the extent to which the prospective partner's body language indicated her confidence in the results. This was interpreted as a proxy assessment of her 'trustworthiness' and relatedly the authenticity of the test result.

Although the impact of an HIV test on expectations and engagement in prevention behaviours is complex, (Delavande and Kohler 2012) the configuration of this and the consequences of testing are shifting. The acceptability of HIV testing in part remains constrained by poor self-assessment of HIV risk (Corneli et al. 2014), however the shadow of stigma is changing shape as HIV testing among young people is increasingly infused with a moral tone in which it is framed as a 'responsible' act (Lambert et al. 2018) rather than singularly indicative of transgression. Engagement in occasional HIV testing thus constitutes a means to preserve the construction of being 'on the socially acceptable side' of HIV prevention, due to its linkage with an identity of 'responsibility' and positive self-image in the management of relative and occasional risk.

However, despite the commonalities that might be drawn elsewhere, for example in the UK, with PrEP as another strategy of 'responsibilised' HIV prevention, young people perceived there to be an important distinction between the two prevention technologies. The limited discussion that circulated around PrEP suggested that while testing may be perceived as a responsible approach to exercising preventive care, PrEP was perceived to align with ART as being an indicator of HIV. Young people wanted to distance themselves from both PrEP and ART, commensurate with emerging evidence from Kenya and Zimbabwe among the general population (Van der Elst et al. 2013; Gombe et al. 2020; Skovdal et al. this volume). Perceiving that the need to initiate either could be interpreted as a signal of having already 'fallen' and be a marker of individual culpability for engagement in undesirable behaviors.

19.4   Conclusion

The emphasis in global and national policy has been on combination prevention packages in sub-Saharan Africa for the past decade (Grabowski et al. 2017). However, there is a risk that if we observe the confluence of the funding emphasis, which privileges biomedical prevention technologies, and the inhibiting impact of the social landscape on young people's use of condoms, the principle of multiple prevention tools begins to disintegrate. The momentum towards investing in siloed prevention technologies, despite the compelling evidence for the need for integrated, combination prevention, has unintended consequences (Gilbertson et al. 2019). The young people's accounts demonstrate that an unintended consequence of the 'push' for HIV testing may be the justification of its replacement of other behavioural prevention strategies.

If, as in this case study, the uptake of widely available testing serves to justify not using condoms, which is a welcome pathway given that they are unappealing for sensual, social and economic reasons, then this becomes problematic. It is likely that the limited uptake of condoms or abstinence preceded the drive for HIV testing among youth, but its availability with limited counselling serves to erroneously justify infrequent testing as a singular, yet 'responsible', prevention strategy. This case study illustrates what impact such biomedical interventions may have if implemented as a priority and in isolation from the structural drivers of vulnerability: the social context of young people's lives.

References

Abdool Karim, S. S. (2019). HIV-1 epidemic control — Insights from test-and-treat trials. *New England Journal of Medicine, 381*(3), 286–288.

Abdool Karim, Q., Baxter, C., & Birx, D. (2017). Prevention of HIV in adolescent girls and young women: Key to an AIDS-free generation. *Journal of Acquired Immune Deficiency Syndromes, 75*(Suppl. 1), S17–S26.

Baisley, K. J., Seeley, J., Siedner, M. J., Koole, K., Matthews, P., Tanser, F., et al. (2019). Findings from home-based HIV testing and facilitated linkage after scale-up of test and treat in rural South Africa: Young people still missing. *HIV Medicine, 20*(10), 704–708.

Barratt, C., Mbonye, M., & Seeley, J. (2012). Between town and country: Shifting identity and migrant youth in Uganda. *The Journal of Modern African Studies, 50*(2), 201–223.

Bernays, S., Bukenya, D., Thompson, C., Ssembajja, F., & Seeley, J. (2018). Being an 'adolescent': The consequences of gendered risks for young people in rural Uganda. *Childhood, 25*(1), 19–33.

Bernays, S., Lanyon, C., Dlamini, V., Ngweny, N., & Seeley, J. (2020). Being young and on the move in South Africa: How 'waithood' exacerbates HIV risks and disrupts the success of current HIV prevention interventions. *Vulnerable Children and Youth Studies.* https://doi.org/10.1080/17450128.2020.1739359.

Bond, V., Hoddinott, G., Viljoen, L., Simuyaba, M., Musheke, M., & Seeley, J. (2016). Good health and moral responsibility: Key concepts underlying the interpretation of treatment as prevention in South Africa and Zambia before rolling out universal HIV testing and treatment. *AIDS Patient Care and STDs, 30*(9), 425–434.

Carlos, S., Nzakimuena, F., Reina, G., Lopez-del Burgo, C., Burgueño, E., Ndarabu, A., et al. (2016). Factors that lead to changes in sexual behaviours after a negative HIV test: Protocol for a prospective cohort study in Kinshasa. *BMC Public Health, 16*, 606.

Church, K., Machiyama, K., Todd, J., Njamwea, B., Mwangome, M., Hosegood, V., et al. (2017). Identifying gaps in HIV service delivery across the diagnosis-to-treatment cascade: Findings from health facility surveys in six sub-Saharan countries. *Journal of the International AIDS Society, 20*(1), 21188.

Corneli, A. L., McKenna, K., Headley, J., Ahmed, K., Odhiambo, J., Skhosana, J., et al. (2014). A descriptive analysis of perceptions of HIV risk and worry about acquiring HIV among FEM-prEP participants who seroconverted in Bondo, Kenya, and Pretoria, South Africa. *Journal of International AIDS Society, 17*(3 Suppl. 2), 19152.

Delavande, A., & Kohler, H. P. (2012). The impact of HIV testing on subjective expectations and risky behavior in Malawi. *Demography, 49*(3), 1011–1036.

Fox, K., Ferguson, J., Ajose, W., Singh, J., Marum, E., & Baggaley, R. (2013). *HIV and adolescents: Guidance for HIV testing and counselling and care for adolescents living with HIV: Annex 15: Adolescent consent to testing: A review of current policies and issues in sub-Saharan Africa.* Geneva: WHO.

Gilbertson, A., Ongili, B., Odongo, F. S., Hallfors, D. D., Rennie, S., Kwaro, D., et al. (2019). Voluntary medical male circumcision for HIV prevention among adolescents in Kenya: Unintended consequences of pursuing service-delivery targets. *PloS oOne, 14*(11), e0224548.

Gombe, M. M., Cakouros, B. E., Ncube, G., Zwangobani, N., Mareke, P., Mkwamba, A., et al. (2020). Key barriers and enablers associated with uptake and continuation of oral pre-exposure prophylaxis (PrEP) in the public sector in Zimbabwe: Qualitative perspectives of general population clients at high risk for HIV. *PLoS One, 15*(1), e0227632.

Gottert, A., Pulerwitz, J., Siu, G., Katahoire, A., Okal, J., Ayebare, F., et al. (2018). Male partners of young women in Uganda: Understanding their relationships and use of HIV testing. *PloS One, 13*(8), e0200920-e.

Govindasamy, D., Ferrand, R. A., Wilmore, S. M., Ford, N., Ahmed, S., & Afnan-Holmes, H. (2015). Uptake and yield of HIV testing and counselling among children and adolescents in subSaharan Africa: A systematic review. *Journal of the International AIDS Society, 18*(1), 20182.

Grabowski, M. K., Serwadda, D. M., Gray, R. H., Nakigozi, G., Kigozi, G., Kagaayi, J., et al. (2017). HIV prevention efforts and incidence of HIV in Uganda. *New England Journal of Medicine, 377*(22), 2154–2166.

Hargreaves, J. R., Delany-Moretlwe, S., Hallett, T. B., Johnson, S., Kapiga, S., Bhattacharjee, P., et al. (2016). The HIV prevention cascade: Integrating theories of epidemiological, behavioural, and social science into programme design and monitoring. *The Lancet HIV, 3*(7), e318–ee22.

Harichund, C., Kunene, P., Simelane, S., Abdool Karim, Q., & Moshabela, M. (2019). Repeat HIV testing practices in the era of HIV self-testing among adults in KwaZulu-Natal, South Africa. *PloS One, 14*(2), e0212343-e.

Havlir, D. V., Balzer, L. B., Charlebois, E. D., Clark, T. D., Kwarisiima, D., Ayieko, J., et al. (2019). HIV testing and treatment with the use of a community health approach in rural Africa. *New England Journal of Medicine, 381*(3), 219–229.

Havlir, D., Lockman, S., Ayles, H., Larmarange, J., Chamie, G., Gaolathe, T., et al. (2020). What do the universal test and treat trials tell us about the path to HIV epidemic control? *Journal of the International AIDS Society, 23*(2), e25455.

Hayes, R. J., Donnell, D., Floyd, S., Mandla, N., Bwalya, J., Sabapathy, K., et al. (2019). Effect of universal testing and treatment on HIV incidence – HPTN 071 (PopART). *New England Journal of Medicine, 381*(3), 207–218.

Horter, S., Seeley, J., Bernays, S., Kerschberger, B., Lukhele, N., & Wringe, A. (2020). Dissonance of choice: Biomedical and lived perspectives on HIV treatment-taking. *Medical Anthropology, 39*(8), 675–688. https://doi.org/10.1080/01459740.2020.1720981.

Iwuji, C. C., Orne-Gliemann, J., Larmarange, J., Balestre, E., Thiebaut, R., Tanser, F., et al. (2018). Universal test and treat and the HIV epidemic in rural South Africa: A phase 4, open-label, community cluster randomised trial. *The Lancet HIV, 5*(3), e116–ee25.

Kawuma, R., Seeley, J., Mupambireyi, Z., Cowan, F., & Bernays, S. (2018). REALITY trial team. "Treatment is not yet necessary": Delays in seeking access to HIV treatment in Uganda and Zimbabwe. *African Journal of AIDS Research, 17*(3), 217–225.

Lambert, R. F., Orrell, C., Bangsberg, D. R., & Haberer, J. E. (2018). Factors that motivated otherwise healthy HIV-positive young adults to access HIV testing and treatment in South Africa. *AIDS and Behavior, 22*, 733–741.

Malhotra, A., Amin, A., & Nanda, P. (2019). Catalyzing gender norm change for adolescent sexual and reproductive health: Investing in interventions for structural change. *Journal of Adolescent Health, 64*(4), S13–SS5.

Mannell, J., Willan, S., Shahmanesh, M., Seeley, J., Sherr, L., & Gibbs, A. (2019). Why interventions to prevent intimate partner violence and HIV have failed young women in southern Africa. *Journal of the International AIDS Society, 22*(8), e25380.

Mitiku, I., Addissie, A., & Molla, M. (2017). Perceptions and experiences of pregnant women about routine HIV testing and counselling in Ghimbi town, Ethiopia: A qualitative study. *BMC Research Notes, 10*(1), 101.

Mulaudzi, M., Dlamini, B. N., Coetzee, J., Sikkema, K., Gray, G., & Dietrich, J. J. (2018). Perceptions of counsellors and youth-serving professionals about sexual and reproductive health services for adolescents in Soweto, South Africa. *Reproductive Health, 15*(1), 21.

Nall, A., Chenneville, T., Rodriguez, L. M., & O'Brien, J. L. (2019). Factors affecting HIV testing among youth in Kenya. *International Journal of Environmental Research and Public Health, 16*(8), 1450.

Narasimhan, M., Yeh, P. T., Haberlen, S., Warren, C. E., & Kennedy, C. E. (2019). Integration of HIV testing services into family planning services: A systematic review. *Reproductive Health, 16*(1), 61.

Orne-Gliemann, J., Zuma, T., Chikovore, J., Gillespie, N., Grant, M., Iwuji, C., et al. (2016). Community perceptions of repeat HIV-testing: Experiences of the ANRS 12249 treatment as prevention trial in rural South Africa. *AIDS Care, 28*(Suppl. 3), 14–23.

Perkins, J. M., Nyakato, V. N., Kakuhikire, B., Mbabazi, P. K., Perkins, H. W., Tsai, A. C., et al. (2018). Actual versus perceived HIV testing norms, and personal HIV testing uptake: A cross-sectional, population-based study in rural Uganda. *AIDS and Behavior, 22*(2), 616–628.

Rutakumwa, R., Mugisha, J. O., Bernays, S., Kabunga, E., Tumwekwase, G., Mbonye, M., et al. (2019). Conducting in-depth interviews with and without voice recorders: A comparative analysis. *Qualitative Research, 20*(5), 565–581. https://doi.org/10.1177/1468794119884806.

Saul, J., Bachman, G., Allen, S., Toiv, N. F., Cooney, C., & Beamon, T. A. (2018). The DREAMS core package of interventions: A comprehensive approach to preventing HIV among adolescent girls and young women. *PLoS One, 13*(12), e0208167-e.

Seeley, J., Bond, V., Yang, B., Floyd, S., MacLeod, D., Viljoen, L., et al. (2019). Understanding the time needed to link to care and start ART in seven HPTN 071 (PopART) study communities in Zambia and South Africa. *AIDS and Behavior, 23*(4), 929–946.

Starbird, E., Norton, M., & Marcus, R. (2016). Investing in family planning: Key to achieving the sustainable development goals. *Global Health: Science and Practice, 4*(2), 191–210.

UNICEF. (2017). *Children and AIDS: Statistical update 2017.* https://data.unicef.org/wp-content/uploads/2017/11/HIVAIDS-Statistical-Update-2017.pdf Accessed 1 Mar 2020.

UNICEF. (2019). *Children, HIV and AIDS: Global and regional snapshots 2019.* https://data.unicef.org/resources/children-hiv-and-aids-global-and-regional-snapshots-2019/ Accessed 1 Mar 2020..

Van der Elst, E. M., Mbogua, J., Operario, D., Mutua, G., Kuo, C., Mugo, P., et al. (2013). High acceptability of HIV pre-exposure prophylaxis but challenges in adherence and use: Qualitative insights from a phase I trial of intermittent and daily PrEP in at-risk populations in Kenya. *AIDS and Behavior, 17*(6), 2162–2172.

WHO. (2016). *Consolidated guidelines on the use of antiretroviral drugs for treating and preventing HIV infection: recommendations for a public health approach. Report no. 9241549688.* Geneva: WHO.

Witzel, T. C., Lora, W., Lees, S., & Desmond, N. (2017). Uptake contexts and perceived impacts of HIV testing and counselling among adults in east and southern Africa: A meta-ethnographic review. *PLoS One, 12*(2), e0170588.

Wong, V., Jenkins, E., Ford, N., & Ingold, H. (2019). To thine own test be true: HIV self-testing and the global reach for the undiagnosed. *Journal of the International AIDS Society, 22*(Suppl. 1), e25256.

Open Access This chapter is licensed under the terms of the Creative Commons Attribution 4.0 International License (http://creativecommons.org/licenses/by/4.0/), which permits use, sharing, adaptation, distribution and reproduction in any medium or format, as long as you give appropriate credit to the original author(s) and the source, provide a link to the Creative Commons license and indicate if changes were made.

The images or other third party material in this chapter are included in the chapter's Creative Commons license, unless indicated otherwise in a credit line to the material. If material is not included in the chapter's Creative Commons license and your intended use is not permitted by statutory regulation or exceeds the permitted use, you will need to obtain permission directly from the copyright holder.

Chapter 20
Entangled Bodies in a PrEP Demonstration Project

Lisa Lazarus, Robert Lorway, and Sushena Reza-Paul

20.1 A Community-led PrEP Demonstration Project in South India

> After I took [PrEP], my life has turned out good. [Before] I would have body pain, I would get white discharge always, eyes would burn, always. I would have pain, my stomach was bloated. After I started taking tablets, my stomach got reduced. I would get leg pain if I walk a bit, now after I started taking these tablets, I don't have any pain. I was not sleeping well. I would always get irritation. I would have a lot of pain when urinating. I felt that I am not going to live. I started feeling good after I started taking these tablets. [In the past] I have gone to so many doctors, eaten so many tablets, visited so many temples. After taking these tablets, I have not gone to any hospitals, I have not gone to any temples; now after I started taking these tablets I don't have any problems. (Aahna, participant, Mandya)

Following the celebration of high-efficacy levels in pre-exposure prophylaxis (PrEP) clinical trials, multilateral funders such as the United States Agency for International Development (USAID) and the Bill & Melinda Gates Foundation launched multi-country demonstration projects to assess the 'real-world' effectiveness of PrEP when rolled out as part of a routine programme (Reza-Paul et al. 2019a). Although less scientifically stringent than a randomised control trial, lacking a control group for instance, PrEP demonstration projects nevertheless are conducted under technically-regulated conditions based on rigid measures that track retention, adherence, risk behaviours, and clinical biomarkers. These data on PrEP effectiveness certainly hold

L. Lazarus (✉) · R. Lorway
Institute for Global Public Health, Rady Faculty of Health Sciences, University of Manitoba, Winnipeg, Canada
e-mail: Lisa.Lazarus@umanitoba.ca

S. Reza-Paul
Institute for Global Public Health, Rady Faculty of Health Sciences, University of Manitoba, Winnipeg, Canada

Ashodaya Samithi, Mysore, India

© Springer Nature Switzerland AG 2021
S. Bernays et al. (eds.), *Remaking HIV Prevention in the 21st Century*, Social Aspects of HIV 5, https://doi.org/10.1007/978-3-030-69819-5_20

importance for programme planning and help to inform how new interventions can be incorporated within existing health systems; however, this knowledge, which treats 'the body' in universalistic terms, fails to account for the divergent ways in which people experience their bodies across societies and in relation to pharmaceutical consumption, biomedical experimentation, and public health programmes (Das 2001; Ecks 2005; Bharadwaj 2007). As medical anthropologists have long shown, 'the body' is enmeshed in webs of socio-cultural and political signification (Scheper-Hughes and Lock 1987; Yates-Doerr 2017a), thereby resisting portrayals that reduce the body to its biochemical and physiological functioning, as though isolatable from sociality and lived experience.

Based on the findings from an extensive ethnographic study of a PrEP demonstration project conducted in South India among female sex workers, we analyse a constellation of narratives in which participants claim PrEP as a kind of 'cure all' for a range of physical ailments and afflictions, including stomach and abdominal pain, white discharge, fatigue and weakness, poor appetite, skin and eye irritations, and so on. Many claimed that taking the medication created an improved overall sense of wellness. Through the lens of 'local biologies' in global health (Lock 1994; Lock and Kaufert 2001; Brotherton and Nguyen 2013), it becomes clear how participation in a transnationally-mediated project has compelled these women to cultivate a particular relationship with their bodies, one that has led them to more intensely reflect on and track various bodily changes pertaining to wellness and illness. In many ways, these women came to view the demonstration project as their own opportunity to test and 'discover' PrEP. Indeed, unexpected health subjectivities emerge around the taking of PrEP, wherein 'the body' becomes a highly reactive and connective site that entangles the life histories of global health science, sex workers' collective engagements in health promotion, and individualistic regimes of care. Following on assertions made by Lock and Nguyen (2010), we draw on the PrEP demonstration project to illustrate how biological and social life come to be mutually constructed, and how the women in our study, based on their understanding of research, make sense of their own bodily responses to PrEP in experimental terms.

20.2 'Local Biologies' and the Importance of Situatedness

Margaret Lock (1994) introduced the term 'local biologies' to account for her findings that symptoms related to menopause differed dramatically among women in Japan, Canada, and the USA. The concept of local biologies refers to 'the way in which the embodied experience of physical sensations, including those of well-being, health, and illness, is in part informed by the material body, itself contingent on evolutionary, environmental, social and individual variables' (Lock 1994 in Niewöhner and Lock 2018, p. 684). This 'embodiment' is informed by localised meanings and experiences, connecting material and social processes while pointing toward the importance of 'situatedness', where human and environmental entanglements impact health and illness (Niewöhner and Lock 2018). Emily Yates-Doerr

(2017b), who examines how scientific experts in Guatemala problematise the assumed boundaries between nature and culture in their characterisations of childhood growth and development, stresses the importance of 'situatedness' as an 'attempt to strengthen [local biologies] by tethering it [to] an ethnographic sensitivity for treating concepts and objects alike as mobile, empirically situated, not-quite-ever-things' (p. 382). In other words, rather than asking the overly rehearsed question of 'what is nature versus culture?', Yates-Doerr instead points toward the materiality of the body in its relational *doings*—how biological notions of the body circulate and attach to expert discourses, techniques of measurement and forms of care in particular localities (also see Lazarus 2019).

Employing the concept of local biologies to better understand patterns of untreated HIV and the rapid onset of AIDS in Papua New Guinea, Leslie Butt (2013) and her team interviewed indigenous persons living with HIV and health care workers. Her findings found linkages between stigma and barriers to treatment that bring to light the interrelatedness of biological processes (i.e., the rapid onset of AIDS) and local social and institutional conditions (such as, the fear of stigma and gaps in appropriate care). According to Butt, through the lens of local biologies we can go further than other studies of the social context of health by viewing the impact of biomedical knowledge on health outcomes. Furthermore, subjective experiences are portrayed as inexorably intertwined with biological patterns and the physiological effects of health services. In our study, we explored how participants as 'lay persons' draw upon biomedical knowledge to interpret forms of bodily health and illness, such that their technical understandings become 'part of their repertoires of experience, including embodied experience' (Nunes 2012, p. 67). More specifically, we illuminate how participants redeploy technical knowledge in and through their bodily journeys with PrEP, in ways that allow them to participate in embodied forms of 'scientific discovery', which tend to often go unnoticed and unreported by clinical researchers and programme implementers running the demonstration project.

20.3 Ashodaya Samithi

A three-to-four-hour drive southwest from the Bangalore airport is the nearby city of Mysore, known as the 'City of Palaces' for its rich history and architecture. Located at the foot of the Chamundi Hills, about 150 kilometers from Bangalore, Mysore shares a spill-over from the IT sector that is reflected in a rapidly expanding urban context, which increasingly reflects Bangalore's cosmopolitan culture (Sudhira et al. 2007). Famous for its temples and palaces, silk sarees, sandalwood oil and soaps, and coffee, Mysore draws a steady flow of national and international tourists (Mudde 2017). Mysore is also known for its festivals, such as the annual Dasara festival, a 10-day event celebrating the victory of good over evil that takes place in September or October and culminates in a procession attended by ministers of the state, who gather to watch the enactment of various traditions through dance, music, and floats (Srinivas 2001). While considered a mid-size city, Mysore is considerably calmer than Bangalore. Mandya, located between these two rapidly urbanising cities, has a distinctive working-class urban culture that is tied to the sugarcane manufacturing sector (Rotti 2017). Compared with Mysore, people are more tightly interconnected through patrilineal kinship networks that can be traced to the surrounding villages and talukas (sub-districts).

In 2004, the Gates Foundation's Avahan Initiative began to fund an HIV prevention programme in Mysore, in the state of Karnataka. Avahan sought to address the HIV epidemic in six high prevalence states across India, including Karnataka (Ramakrishnan and Alexander 2006; Rao 2010). In 2006, Ashodaya Samithi, which translates to Dawn of Hope, was registered as a community-based organisation. To ensure that the organisation remained by and for the community of sex workers, members of the organisation democratically elected a board of governance, made up of male, female, and hijra (transgender or 'third gender')[1] sex workers who elected to work in solidarity. Since its inception, Ashodaya operated as an inclusive space, where people of all gender identities came together to form a unified 'community'. Based on a philosophy of building community capacity, sex workers were paired with project managers, who were mostly trained social workers, to shadow and learn their roles, with the expectation of taking over the operations of the organisation. As an early activity, a community clinic was opened, with sex workers playing a major role in designing the clinic and hiring medical staff. Within the first year, nearly 75% of Ashodaya members had accessed clinic services (Dixon et al. 2012). At the end of its first year, Ashodaya opened a project office in the neighbouring city of Mandya that similarly included a drop-in centre space for sex workers, and its own clinic space so that women would no longer have to travel the hour distance to be seen by the physician in Mysore, who would instead come to them.

Ashodaya has continued to grow over the years, with organisational activities expanded to include outreach to community, sex work and health-related advocacy at the district, state, and national levels, social and economic empowerment through the establishment of a cooperative bank, addressing sexual and gender-based violence through community responses, the provision of non-discriminatory clinical services (including sexual and reproductive health services), and community-based research (Reza-Paul et al. 2008, 2012, 2016, 2019b). Ashodaya's governance structure remains grounded in democratic processes, with community needs at the forefront of its agenda. The Board of Directors ensures that Ashodaya remains driven by the priorities of the communities of sex workers it serves. Ashodaya's current membership base is estimated to include around 8000 sex workers across the state of Karnataka.

Between March 2016 and November 2016, 647 women were enrolled into a PrEP demonstration project in Mysore and Mandya. The project was funded by the Bill &

---

[1]We avoid the term transgender women because many hijras today see themselves as distinct from men or women; a distinction that is reinforced by relatively newer state government regulations that allow hijras to claim a separate identity on voter and ration identification cards as 'transgender'.

Melinda Gates Foundation and implemented in partnership with the University of Manitoba. Women were provided PrEP free of cost for the 16-month project, and followed up for quarterly clinical screenings and questionnaires, along with community-led support throughout the duration of the project. At project end, 640 of the women had completed their follow up. The findings presented in this chapter are based on fieldwork conducted as part of the first author's PhD research, which took place between January 2015 and April 2018 and included six trips to the Ashodaya offices (in January 2015; June and September/October 2016; April and November/December 2017; and April 2018). In particular, we focus on a set of interview transcripts conducted with thirty-six women taking PrEP towards the end of the demonstration project in November/December 2017. While analysis initially focused on the community-based project processes, here we focus on a set of narratives that emerged surrounding PrEP and the body. Our interpretation of these data is based on over 15 years of fieldwork and collaboration on community-based projects with the organisation. This long-standing role as the allies and technical partners of Ashodaya afforded us an intimate positionality from which to closely interact with and directly learn from our interlocutors throughout the project. Ashodaya's own reputation as a trusted community-led organisation further played an important role in facilitating the roll-out of the larger PrEP study, as we further explore in the next section.

20.4   Entangled Bodies

To make sense of a curious set of participant narratives that emerged during interviews, we appeal to the concept of 'local biologies', as we elaborate above, to understand the effects on the body described by participants in a community-led PrEP demonstration project. In the next sections, we highlight the numerous physical benefits that women ascribe to PrEP, followed by their experimental engagement with PrEP as a new prevention technology and with health services, thereby revealing transformed ways of experiencing the body. Finally, we ground these findings in the history of Ashodaya collectivisation, and community health activism and promotion.

20.4.1   PrEP as a 'Cure all'

Ashodaya community outreach workers began to enrol women into the demonstration project in March 2016. As part of enrolment, all participants had to first undergo, free of charge, extensive medical screenings, including testing for pregnancy, HIV, syphilis, Hepatitis B, and kidney and liver function. This took place in a health facility with which Ashodaya had cultivated rapport in order to facilitate the testing process and rapidly receive results. From its infancy, engagement in the project involved an increased attention on the body and health. As women initiated taking PrEP, experiences with side effects, including nausea, vomiting, and dizziness, were initially reported within the first few weeks of participation, as described by Jayita.

> Experiences means...when I started taking the tablets I felt dizzy and also vomited a few times. Then I called the office and told them. They advised me to continue to take it and that it will stop. So I continued taking it and after a few days it stopped. Daily at 10 in the morning I would punctually take it. Before [taking PrEP], I had white discharge and severe pains in the lower abdomen, but after I started taking the tablets all that disappeared and I am taking it and I feel fine now. (Jayita, participant, Mysore).

As part of their enrolment in the project, participants were closely followed by the clinical team who quickly addressed these initial complaints, with the Ashodaya physician providing treatment for nausea and white discharge. Bodies soon adjusted to daily intake of the new pill, with the reassurance of Ashodaya staff and community leaders who were the first to try PrEP.

> No. they would tell me. When we give them tablets, we will ask them about what happened to them, some people would complain about giddiness, vomiting, diarrhea, etc. What happens when we take tablets is that, now when the medicine goes in through injection when we have fever, the fever comes out, similarly, when the good things from tablet goes into our body, whatever is bad inside will come out, this is what I would tell them. I would tell them that this tablet is good for our body and life and so take them regularly. (Kyra, participant, Mysore).

As a community-led project, support for side effects from community outreach workers and the clinic doctor, alongside other social adjustments to pill-taking led to continued adherence (see for example, Lazarus 2019). Interestingly, as women continued taking PrEP, their experiences shifted dramatically from initial side effects and discomfort, to describing PrEP as healing a number of different ailments. As expressed by Kyra in the above quotation, PrEP was seen as pushing out the 'bad inside'. The women that we spoke with shared a number of different health concerns cured by PrEP, from pains, vaginal discharge and bleeding, to increased energy and appetite. Aahna also describes how PrEP began to have positive effects on her body, sleep, and appetite.

> ... Before taking tablets [PrEP], I would not eat properly, now after taking tablets, I eat nicely in the morning, afternoon, and night, I sleep well. I had no proper sleep for so many years. Now after I started taking these tablets, I sleep well, eat well, and then I used to get heartburn every day. If I take this much of tea, I would not eat any food the whole day. Then after that, after I started coming to Ashodaya, after I started taking tablets, only then I became healthy. I don't have any problem except for a bit of throat irritation. Otherwise I am healthy and happy. (Aahna, participant, Mandya).

Participation and engagement in biomedical research directs focus on one's bodily health, making up the body as its own experimental site. Participants enrolled in the study engaged in self-surveillance as a way of exploring and discovering PrEP for themselves. The experimental nature of PrEP as a new intervention compelled a focus on the body, with women tracking and monitoring their own experiences. While women understood that PrEP was rolled out as a new HIV prevention option, it soon came to be viewed as providing other health benefits. Direct bodily experiences with PrEP led women to uncover and draw association with other benefits of PrEP that go beyond the therapeutic goal of the tablet. As Maanika (Mysore) put it, 'There must be some medicine in it, it is for our good, only, [that] they have made it madam'. Similarly, Padma, Sadhana, Vaanya, and Kaashi all list a number of different diseases and ailments they felt were improved by taking PrEP.

> After taking the tablet, HIV, blood cancer, uterine cancer, white discharge warts are all under control now. (Padma, participant, Mysore).

> There is no white discharge, no foul smell during menstruation. I feel my uterus is clean because of this tablet. Everything is clear and clean. I feel good now. (Sadhana, participant, Mandya).

> Pains stopped, there was no back pain, burning sensation also stopped, I would get burning sensation in the urinating area and the area where I have sex, I used to get burning sensation also. Now there is no such problems. So I got a lot of trust in the tablet. This tablet is providing us nutrition, so I started trusting this tablet more. (Vaanya, participant, Mandya)

> It could be white discharge, or excessive bleeding or warts or any such things, we need not worry about them because of this tablet [name of interviewer]. I haven't got any of these things from the time I have started taking this tablet. I don't have any burning sensation when I pass urine or any such thing from the time I started this tablet. (Kaashi, participant, Mysore)

In the above quotations, women express 'feeling good' and 'not needing to worry'. Extending beyond the physical, PrEP's benefits also were linked to an overall sense of wellness and improvement in mental health. Many women, such as Lata and Vaanya, described an increase in appetite, with PrEP as having a 'food component'.

> My friend and I speak about it and say it is good that we are taking this tablet. Before that we both were scared we may get some infection. We are happy now that we are taking the tablet. We feel safe and we don't have that fear anymore. Now we are eating well and I have put on weight. Earlier I could not eat properly and I was thin. From the time I started taking the tablet I am eating well and have added weight and am able to do my work well. I was also weak then, now I am fine. (Lata, participant, Mysore)

> If you see the food we are eating now, it has no nutrition factors in it. Whatever we eat we don't get enough nutrition to our body. But this tablet is very powerful. If it is giving so much of benefit, we can imagine how much of food component is there in the tablet. So we like to take PrEP tablet. (Vaanya, participant, Mandya)

Along with an increased appetite and the 'nutrition' provided by PrEP, women also described having increased energy, allowing them to work more. Aahna tells of how she used to find it difficult to walk due to leg pain and would feel tired after meeting with a client. Since starting PrEP, she feels able to work more. Nandini echoes this sentiment, sharing how PrEP allows her to see more clients and earn more money.

> Advantage is, now if I go somewhere or walk a bit, I would feel tired and get leg pain. I have come back by doing only one party, I would feel tired after doing one party. Now after taking these tablets, I do 3 or 4 party. Earlier I would feel tired with one person, I would feel weak when the condoms would break, when they brought me here and got my checkup done in Mysore, after that they gave me tablets, they told me to come every month for checkup, they gave me tablets, after that I became healthy. Now after I started taking these tablets, I feel

that I am capable of maintaining 3–4 people [clients]. Otherwise I did not have the capacity to do more than one person. So I want to take tablets. I come here to the office and take the tablets. Even if I go out for work, I come here to take the tablets. (Aahna, participant, Mysore).

After starting the tablet I feel like taking more clients. Earlier if I take one or two clients I would get bodily pains, burning sensation down there and pain in the lower abdomen and would feel like stopping after two clients. Now after starting the tablet I feel like taking more clients and earn more money. (Nandini, participant, Mysore).

Women described feeling more energetic and confident during sex with intimate partners as well as with clients, linked to the HIV prevention benefits of PrEP and highlighting the psychological benefits and peace of mind they felt while taking PrEP.

I am a sex worker and if I drink and go with a client and during sex if the condom breaks I used to have a fear that I may get infected. Now that I am taking the tablet I don't have that fear and this tablet has given me that confidence. Now I can look after my children, I can educate my son and I have that confidence now. This is a big help for me. (Radhika, participant, Mandya).

I had a fear of getting HIV, how long I would take care of my children, now since they have provided these tablets, I don't have any fear. They call us here, once in three months they get me here for test, I will not have any fear if the test is done, and they come home and give tablets. (Anu, participant, Mysore).

As described in the above quotation by Anu, this peace of mind and confidence is also linked to increased interactions with the health care system. The unexpected benefits explored in this section need to be understood within the context of PrEP being rolled out by a well-established and trusted community-led sexual health organisation. While introducing PrEP as a new HIV prevention option, the endorsement of PrEP by Ashodaya leaders led to beliefs by the community that PrEP must be 'good for us'. Outreach workers known to participants were responsible for delivering PrEP and providing ongoing adherence support, stressing the benefits of continued adherence and dispelling any concerns or doubts, with messaging reinforced by Ashodaya's clinical team. Further entanglements with health systems are explored in the next section.

20.5 Experimental Entanglements: Screenings and Follow Ups

Embedded in the study were increased health screenings. These included quarterly screenings for HIV, sexually transmitted infections (STIs), syphilis, pregnancy, creatinine and a bi-annual cervical cancer screening, the results of which were fed back to the participants, allowing them to assume an active role in monitoring and surveying their own health, alongside formal project tracking. Although these screenings were linked to monitoring PrEP safety and side effects related to potential changes in condom use, they additionally increased participants' interactions with health systems (including the Ashodaya community clinic) and opportunities to process their health. Improved health, energy, and overall well-being became deeply entangled with the experimental process, in other words, connecting participants embodied experiences with PrEP to the routine screening and testing practices of the demonstration project. Lata describes in detail her interactions with health screenings as part of her involvement in the project.

> They conducted a meeting here in the office and told us about PrEP. Then they took us to a private hospital and got our blood, urine, stools tested. And our kidneys and scanning everything was done. They said it normally costs more than Rs. 5000/– [approx. $67USD] but we will get it done for you and they did it. Our heart and kidneys they got scanned and then they told this tablet is good for you and from that day I started taking the tablet. (Lata, participant, Mysore).

As Lata states, this type of full body screening would normally be inaccessible to most of the women participating in the study because of the high cost of testing. She goes on to explain that stigma and discrimination often faced by sex workers acts as an additional barrier to accessing care (Dixon et al. 2012; Lazarus et al. 2012a, b; Chevrier et al. 2016).

> Yes, the office took the responsibility for it. They said it is expensive and then once in two months we need to go for tests again. If we go out we cannot openly tell our problems even to a lady doctor. We may have some problems but we cannot openly tell them the symptoms, so they have their own clinic in the office and a doctor and they get us examined here itself. If there is anything wrong with us they will give the medicines. They also encourage us to talk openly about the problems, pains and symptoms.

Through PrEP participation, women gained access to usually unavailable health services and were provided with repeated opportunities to 'talk openly about the problems, pains and symptoms' in a safe and supportive space. Furthermore, Kareena shares how undergoing the screening process also led to *receiving treatment* for any diagnosed health issues.

> They do a health checkup. They test for STIs. There could be white discharge, or warts, or pain in lower abdomen, and they treat us for it. So we come here once in three months for a health checkup. If there is anything else then they refer us to the big hospital [government hospital]. If there are any warts they give an injection and tablets and we have to take it for three weeks. After that they will do another health checkup to see if we have been cured or not. Then if we are fine then they tell us we are cured. (Kareena, participant, Mysore).

In addition to testing and treatment, women were also provided with the opportunity to collect copies of their test results and make sense of them with the support of the clinic team. Increasing health contact in the context of the project created opportunity for women to become engaged patients, discussing, interrogating, and processing test results with Ashodaya clinic staff.

> I felt scared then because they [the clinical team] will do blood tests and the apprehension is we have had sex without condom at one time, so would we have got HIV, or STIs, or syphilis or herpes or gonorrhoea…there would be a lot of fear in the mind. When they show the reports and then explain it then we don't feel it [fear] anymore. Now whenever they call we will gladly come and get blood tests done and even if they don't call we will get ICTC [HIV testing at an Integrated Counselling and Testing Centre] and RPR [rapid plasma regain

syphilis test] done. Then we will insist on the reports. It will take about three days and we can't spend and come from the village often. So after a week we would come and collect reports. Another thing is we can't go to any other hospital we have to come here for examination because we feel whether we get fever or anything else only the doctor in Ashodaya Samithi should treat us. (Preeti, participant, Mysore).

Through the process of participation in the PrEP project, women were provided with ongoing opportunities to engage with their bodies through access to normally inaccessible testing and health screenings, treatment for diagnosed health concerns, and sharing and processing test results. The clinical screening required at enrolment, along with the quarterly follow up testing provided women with the opportunity to continually interrogate and understand their health in ways that went beyond simply taking a daily pill. In this way, women became active participants in monitoring and responding to their health.

20.6 Understanding Place in Scaling Up PrEP

The women that we spoke with shared complicated narratives of how they embodied their experience as biomedical research participants. As similarly described by Butt (2013) in her research, our participants express how 'the drugs they were given were central to their stories' (p. 189). As Butt goes on to articulate, 'in addition to constructed meanings around medications, the material presence of the drugs them-selves—running the gamut from aspirin to painkillers, from vitamin C to tubercu-losis medication—also reinforce the client's sense that he or she is doing something about his or her problem, trying to mediate the structural and material problems with the quality of care on offer' (p. 189). Whether the women enrolled in the PrEP project experienced PrEP as a sort of 'cure all' for various physical ailments, found 'peace of mind' and energy stemming from its prophylaxis qualities, or engaged more widely with their health and health systems as 'experimental subjects' (see for example, Petryna 2009), we see in these participant narratives how biomedical technologies get taken up in non-universalistic terms in differing contexts. Our analysis adds to the rich body of work by medical anthropologists who have shown how 'the body' is experienced through socio-cultural and political milieus (Scheper-Hughes and Lock 1987; Yates-Doerr 2017a), particularly where rich histories of collectivisation and community health activism exist, such as is the case with Ashodaya. Attention to 'entangled bodies', as we call them, points to important limitations of biomedical knowledge employed in global efforts to scale-up PrEP. Instead, special attention to local context sheds important light on how these new technologies are utilised and understood. Our findings illustrate how participation in this project has intensified a relationship with their bodies, where 'the body' becomes a highly reactive site that entangles HIV research, sex workers' engagements in health promotion, and regimes of self-care. In order to more fully understand how biomedical interventions and technologies are understood, they must be further interrogated beyond biomedical markers to appreciate how they are embodied within particular local contexts. Engaging with local biologies, as we have done here, can provide important insights for the design and implementation of biomedical interventions, and for understanding how PrEP is experienced by communities.

References

Bharadwaj, A. (2007). Biosociality and biocrossings: Encounters with assisted conception and embryonic stem cells in India. In S. Gibbon & C. Novas (Eds.), *Biosocialities, genetics and the social sciences* (pp. 108–126). New York: Routledge.

Brotherton, P. S., & Nguyen, V. K. (2013). Revisiting local biology in the era of global health. *Medical Anthropology, 32*(4), 287–290.

Butt, L. (2013). Local biologies and HIV/AIDS in highlands Papua, Indonesia. *Culture, Medicine, and Psychiatry, 37*(1), 179–194.

Chevrier, C., Khan, S., Reza-Paul, S., & Lorway, R. (2016). 'No one was there to care for us': Ashodaya Samithi's community-led care and support for people living with HIV in Mysore, India. *Global Public Health, 11*(4), 423–436.

Das, V. (2001). *Stigma, contagion, defect: Issues in the anthropology of public health. Stigma and Global Health:* Developing a Research Agenda, 5–7.

Dixon, V., Reza-Paul, S., D'Souza, F. M., O'Neil, J., O'Brien, N., & Lorway, R. (2012). Increasing access and ownership of clinical services at an HIV prevention project for sex workers in Mysore, India. *Global Public Health, 7*(7), 779–791.

Ecks, S. (2005). Pharmaceutical citizenship: Antidepressant marketing and the promise of demarginalization in India. *Anthropology & Medicine, 12*(3), 239–254.

Lazarus, L. (2019). *In search of success: The politics of care and responsibility in a PrEP demonstration project among sex workers in India* (doctoral thesis). University of Manitoba.

Lazarus, L., Deering, K. N., Nabess, R., Gibson, K., Tyndall, M. W., & Shannon, K. (2012a). Occupational stigma as a primary barrier to health care for street-based sex workers in Canada. *Culture, Health & Sexuality, 14*(2), 139–150.

Lazarus, L., Reza-Paul, S., Pasha, A., Jairam, S., Hafeez Ur Rahman, S., O'Neil, J., & Lorway, R. (2012b). Exploring the role of community-based peer support in improving access to care and antiretroviral treatment for sex workers in Mysore, India. *Journal of HIV/AIDS & Social Services, 11*(2), 152–168.

Lock, M. M. (1994). *Encounters with aging: Mythologies of menopause in Japan and North America.* Berkeley and Los Angeles: University of California Press.

Lock, M., & Kaufert, P. (2001). Menopause, local biologies, and cultures of aging. *American Journal of Human Biology, 13*(4), 494–504.

Lock, M., & Nguyen, V. K. (2010). *An anthropology of biomedicine.* Oxford: John Wiley & Sons.

Mudde, R. (2017, March). Mysore- of history and places. *Karnataka.* Retrieved May 5, 2020, from https://www.karnataka.com/mysore/about-mysore/.

Niewöhner, J., & Lock, M. (2018). Situating local biologies: Anthropological perspectives on environment/human entanglements. *BioSocieties, 13*(4), 681–697.

Nunes, J. A. (2012). "I have become a microscope for my own body": Local biologies and the embodiment of biomedical knowledge. *Antropologia Portuguesa, 29*, 65–74.

Petryna, A. (2009). *When experiments travel: Clinical trials and the global search for human subjects.* Princeton: Princeton University Press.

Ramakrishnan, A., & Alexander, A. (2006). Practicing theory: Management in HIV intervention. *Harvard International Review, 28*(2), 58.

Rao, P. J. (2010). Avahan: The transition to a publicly funded programme as a next stage. *Sexually Transmitted Infections, 86*, i7–i8.

Reza-Paul, S., Beattie, T., Syed, H. U. R., Venukumar, K. T., Venugopal, M. S., Fathima, M. P., et al. (2008). Declines in risk behaviour and sexually transmitted infection prevalence following a community-led HIV preventive intervention among female sex workers in Mysore, India. *AIDS, 22*, S91–S100.

Reza-Paul, S., Lorway, R., O'Brien, N., Lazarus, L., Jain, J., Bhagya, M., et al. (2012). Sex worker-led structural interventions in India: A case study on addressing violence in HIV prevention through the Ashodaya Samithi collective in Mysore. *The Indian Journal of Medical Research, 135*(1), 98.

Reza-Paul, S., Lazarus, L., Doshi, M., Rahman, S. H. U., Ramaiah, M., Maiya, R., et al. (2016). Prioritizing risk in preparation for a demonstration project: a mixed methods feasibility study of oral Pre-Exposure Prophylaxis (PREP) among female sex workers in South India. *PloS One, 11* (11), e0166889.

Reza-Paul, S., Lazarus, L., Jana, S., Ray, P., Mugo, N., Ngure, K., et al. (2019a). Community inclusion in PrEP demonstration projects: Lessons for scaling up. *Gates Open Research, 3*, 1504.

Reza-Paul, S., Lazarus, L., Maiya, R., Venukumar, K. T., Lakshmi, B., Roy, A., et al. (2019b). Delivering community-led integrated HIV and sexual and reproductive health services for sex workers: A mixed methods evaluation of the DIFFER study in Mysore, South India. *PLoS One, 14*(6), e0218654.

Rotti, J. (2017, Sept). Mandya- of sugar and rivers. *Karnataka*. Retrieved May 5, 2020, from https://www.karnataka.com/mandya/about-mandya/.

Scheper-Hughes, N., & Lock, M. M. (1987). The mindful body: A prolegomenon to future work in medical anthropology. *Medical Anthropology Quarterly, 1*(1), 6–41.

Srinivas, S. (2001). *Landscapes of urban memory: The sacred in India's silicon valley*. Minneapolis: University of Minnesota Press.

Sudhira, H. S., Ramachandra, T. V., & Subrahmanya, M. B. (2007). Bangalore. *Cities, 24*(5), 379–390.

Yates-Doerr, E. (2017a). Counting bodies? On future engagements with science studies in medical anthropology. *Anthropology & Medicine, 24*(2), 142–158.

Yates-Doerr, E. (2017b). Where is the local? Partial biologies, ethnographic sitings. *HAU: Journal of Ethnographic Theory, 7*(2), 377–401.

Chapter 21
An Unfinished History: A Story of Ongoing Events and Mutating HIV Problems

Marsha Rosengarten

21.1   An Unfinished History: A Story of Ongoing Events and Mutating HIV Problems

In an interview by one of his colleagues at the 2019 International AIDS Conference, Director of the US National Institute of Allergy & Infectious Diseases, Anthony Fauci stated: 'now we have the tools [antiretroviral drugs], if we implement them properly, aggressively, to the extent that we can, we can *theoretically turn off the dynamics of the epidemic*.' (my emphasis).[1] Referring to the Joint United Nations Programme on HIV/AIDS (UNAIDS)/World Health Organization (WHO) '90-90-90' goals—that by 2020, 90% of all people living with HIV will know their HIV status; 90% of all people with diagnosed HIV infection will receive sustained antiretroviral therapy; and 90% of all people receiving antiretroviral therapy will have viral suppression—he stressed that the biomedical prevention technology, PrEP (HIV Pre-Exposure Prophylaxis), should be included in regimes to redress the problem of HIV incidence. He also stated that PrEP should become available not only as a daily pill but additionally in the form of a long term acting injectable or implant suitable for women. The proposal to refashion PrEP was made with reference to the failure of a recent PrEP pill behavioural randomised control trial (RCT) conducted with women called SMART (Sequential Multiple Assignment Randomised Trial). As we shall see, this RCT was preceded by other PrEP RCTs that also failed to find relevance for women.

---

[1] The interview is titled 'Dr. Fauci Discusses Ending the HIV Epidemic from the 2019 IAS Conference on HIV Science'. It was was conducted by Anne Rancourt and is available online at https://www.niaid.nih.gov/news-events/ias-2019-fauci-discussion [accessed November 2019]

M. Rosengarten (✉)
Goldsmiths, University of London, London, UK
e-mail: M.Rosengarten@gold.ac.uk

© Springer Nature Switzerland AG 2021   289
S. Bernays et al. (eds.), *Remaking HIV Prevention in the 21st Century*, Social Aspects of HIV 5, https://doi.org/10.1007/978-3-030-69819-5_21

Without disputing the affordances of PrEP, in either pill or long-term acting form or, indeed, the concreteness of HIV, what I want to dramatise in this chapter is how the relevancies of HIV prevention regimes have become folded into a particular scientific logic and why this should concern us. By reflecting on the thinking that has come to prevail with regard to women and HIV and, doing so, by working back through an albeit brief outline genealogy of the development of PrEP, I suggest that the WHO/UNAIDS goals and, no less, Fauci's optimism for a future end to the dynamics of the epidemic is founded on a misplaced conception of what is at stake. Drawing on a conception of problems provided by a branch of process philosophy that has earned the term 'event-thinking' (Fraser 2009), I propose that if biomedicine is to be responsive to the relevancies of those affected by HIV, a different conception of what is assumed of the 'dynamics of the epidemic' may be warranted.

21.2   The 'Essence' of the Problem for Biomedicine

As I discuss later, underpinning the premise for 90-90-90 goals and proposals about PrEP, is the idea that problems arise from a *deficit* in what is assumed to be the normal course of events (Schillmeier 2017), namely, a deficit in social conduct or in the functioning of the body as a consequence of disease. This is not surprising, it is the commonplace conception of the problem of HIV. Nor is the idea surprising that a solution, devised in terms of pinpointing and fixing the deficit, could make HIV disappear. The means for devising a solution is sought through knowledge-making and, as mentioned with regard to the SMART trial, the most lauded method is an RCT. It provides the data for evidence-based medicine (EBM) and also, increasingly so, for evidence-informed health policymaking (EIHP). The former mode for EBM is premised on a problem pre-identified as a deficit in the biology of the human body, namely a lack of capacity to ward of HIV infection. And it is in response to this that RCTs have shown antiretroviral drugs to be highly efficacious. The latter mode for EIHP is premised on a problem pre-identified as a deficit in the sociality of human subjects, namely a lack in individual or community conduct for preventing the biological body becoming exposed to what it cannot ward off either for acquiring or transmitting infection. This distinction between two orders of reality—the biological and the social—orchestrates much of the field of HIV intervention.

While this distinction has been important to cultivating approaches for the prevention of HIV infection prior to the introduction of biomedical technologies and, specifically, prior to antiretroviral drugs for treatment and, more lately PrEP, when adopted as if self-evident rather than a useful but limited construction, it serves to elide the relationship between a complex nexus of situated factors (see for example, Kippax and Stephenson 2012, p. 789; Race 2012). Here, I suggest that the distinction and its presupposition that the problem of HIV can be assigned first and foremost to a deficit or lack in either the body or the social subject, goes to the heart of the claim by social scientists that the epidemic has become 'biomedicalised' (Kippax and Race 2003; Kippax and Stephenson 2012; Young et al. 2016). While there is some debate on what is meant by the term 'biomedicalised' (Flowers and Davis 2013), there is no doubt that the achievement of efficacious antiretroviral drugs as a solution to the biological problem of HIV has given those in the natural sciences an increasingly more authoritative role in determinations for thwarting or assuaging the effects of HIV. Determinations that extend to both sides of the distinction.

If we leave aside for now different styles of critical engagement with the mode of the RCT (see for example, Kippax and Van de Ven 1998; Michael and Rosengarten 2013; Savransky and Rosengarten 2016), it could be argued that the SMART trial and, subsequently, Fauci's proposal for refashioning PrEP show an appreciation for a long-standing neglect of women's HIV needs (see for example, Sheth et al. 2016). One of the most concerning epidemiological findings of the epidemic is that girls and women make up more than half of the 37.9 million people living with HIV (UNAIDS 2019). The SMART trial was designed to compare the efficacy of different kinds of dosing adherence support for women in order to address difficulties previously identified as a problem of lack, a deficit, in reference to dosing with the PrEP pill. The trial recruited 400 women who at the outset consented to participate. It randomised consenting participants to brief counselling and either WhatsApp groups or weekly two-way SMS messages to facilitate daily dosing with PrEP. At 3 months into the trial there was 80% adherence but by 12 months, despite the different modes of support, only 9% were found to be continuing with PrEP (Celum et al. 2019). This finding has provided the reasoning for a refashioned PrEP (as an implant or injectable) as the new solution.

However, what we shall see in the genealogy to follow gives cause for questioning the premise for refashioning of PrEP and more, broadly, the presumption that biotechnologies serve as a solution to 'end' the dynamic of HIV. Without refuting the importance of antiretroviral drugs for preventing HIV infection from becoming AIDS, they have not made the problem of HIV disappear but, rather, they have developed it in new ways. For instance, they have been shown to have contributed to an alteration in risk assessments and hence prevention practices (Flowers 2001; Blumenthal and Haubrich 2014; Holt and Murphy 2017) and have introduced new issues to clinical practice (Newman et al. 2019; Nicholls and Rosengarten 2019). When it comes to women, a complex nexus of situated factors suggestive of women's HIV needs (Fleck 2013; Valencia-Garcia et al. 2017) have become developed into a problem *of* the women. Indeed if, as Mariam Motamedi Fraser (Fraser 2009, p. 76) states, 'the best . . . a solution can do is to do develop a problem', the solution of PrEP and also biomedical technologies for treatment have contributed to a shifting dynamic of new concerns or 'problems.'

21.3   A Genealogy of the Inheritances of 'Research Events'

The impetus for the SMART trial completed in 2019 was drawn from the findings of two of the largest PrEP trials with women, Fem-PrEP and VOICE, conducted between 2009 and 2012 (van der Straten et al. 2012). Together they enrolled 'over 5000 young single women' in Kenya, South Africa, Tanzania, Uganda, and Zimbabwe. FEM-PrEP (N = 2120) and VOICE (N = 5029). Areas with very high rates of HIV incidence in the epidemiological category of young women. However, both trials were deemed to have failed in demonstrating PrEP's efficacy. The same number of women in the treatment groups became infected as those in the placebo groups. To understand how their failure was wholly unexpected by the HIV biomedical prevention field, and notwithstanding the iPrEX trial that found PrEP highly efficacious in the epidemiological categories of gay men, men who have sex with men and transgender women (N = 2499) (Grant et al. 2010), it is necessary to put the two trials in the context of another large trial called the Partners PrEP trial in Kenya and Uganda. This trial found PrEP to be highly efficacious in women who made up half the number enrolled (N = 5000) (Baeten et al. 2012), as did a smaller study with heterosexual women and men in Botswana (N = 1219) (Thigpen et al. 2012).[2]

It would be an understatement to say that the 'failure' of both the Fem-PrEP and VOICE trials was baffling to the trialists. But since the trial protocols were based on what has come to be accepted as 'the gold standard' RCT mode and were entirely in keeping with what has been established as bioethical principles, no fault was thought to reside in the research practice or, indeed, its aims. That is to say, no questions were raised of the pre-determined assumption that PrEP, if found efficacious, is a solution to the HIV prevention needs of women. With this view consolidated and further scientific evidence based on follow up analysis of drug levels in the women's blood collected during the trial (Koenig et al. 2013), we can see how a problem for women was rendered a problem of the women: although the women reported that were adhering to daily dosing, they had not only failed to take the drug, they had lied about doing so.

In 2013, a summary of Fem-PrEP was provided by Gus Cairns at AIDSMap. It was titled 'Magical thinking? FEM-PrEP trial may have failed because participants used testing as prevention.' Noting that retention in the study was high, 82% of participants continued to attend monthly visits throughout its duration, Cairns reported on a follow up interview-based study with some of the female participants. The study concluded that many of the women remained for the monthly HIV tests provided by the trial but, in the words of Cairns: 'used the test, and participating in the trial itself, as a way of getting reassurance that they did *not* have HIV.' Cairns

---

[2]There are a host of reasons that might be offered to explain why women did adhere to using PrEP in these two trials and not the others. For instance, knowing that a sexual partner is HIV positive was likely to be significant in the Partners PrEP trial. However, the smaller Botswana trial did not involve serodiscordant couples. Arguably, the most plausible is that the situated nature of the trials affected the outcome (see Rosengarten and Savransky 2018).

added: 'The trial itself, in the *minds of the women*, became the prevention method offered' [my emphasis] (Cairns n.d.). There are of course many explanations that could be offered for the finding of the qualitative study. Elsewhere, I have discussed the Fem-PrEP women's 'lack of dosing adherence' as a mode of recalcitrance (Rosengarten 2017). Although the women gave the answer that they perceived scientists wanted, as often happens with human research subjects (Stengers 2011), their actions suggested that what was *relevant to them* was different from the scientists' requirement. Here, I suggest, by neglecting this difference—and what might be considered a shifting multi-factorial terrain—a problem of the women themselves was able to take hold in the imaginaries of those invested in a biomedical solution and, as we have seen, apparent in the design of the SMART trial and, arguably, in the proposal for a refashioned PrEP.[3]

If we go further back in the biomedical record of the first planned PrEP RCTs in 2004/2005, we can see another unexpected outcome for science but, also, how bioethics became established in a manner that enabled FEM-PrEP, VOICE and SMART to hold fast to the view that the research itself was beyond question. Two of these earlier trials were specifically targeted at female sex workers in Cameroon and Cambodia. A third trial, with people who inject drugs, was in Thailand. All three drew intense opposition from the research participants who were supported by civil society organisations for sex workers and people who inject drugs. The opposition was clear in denouncing the research for the manner in which it exploited the health and economic conditions of the targeted research participants (Women's Network for Unity 2004; Jintarkanon et al. 2005). For a complex set of reasons following the opposition, the Cameroon and Cambodian trials with female sex workers were eventually cancelled (see Michael and Rosengarten, 2013). The Thai trial continued, although not without contention, most of which concerned the fact that the trial did not provide clean needles and syringes known to prevent HIV transmission. The trialists were not permitted by US politics to do so but justified the implementation of the trial without these on the basis that they could be purchased in Thai pharmacies. The trial participants, often with limited financial means, stated that visiting a pharmacy for obtaining these crucial prevention aids put them at high risk of incarceration because drug use was outlawed in Thailand (Michael and Rosengarten 2013). However, what I want to pursue here is how the opposition to the trials was taken up as a serious concern for the viability of future HIV RCTs.

Two separate international consultations by WHO/UNAIDS (2006) and the International AIDS Society (IAS 2005) were designed to study the controversies, taking into account longstanding issues pertaining to 'off-shore' RCT that often mean findings serve to benefit others in considerably more advantageous socio-economic locations. The goals of both consultations were captured in the IAS report:

---

[3]I have purposely resisted speculating on what might comprise this multi-factorial terrain. First, because I do not want to attempt to speak for the women. Second, consistent with what I later propose of possibles, I do not want to impose a conventional and, no doubt, frequently pragmatically helpful disciplinary distinction of a social and a biological realm. As Whitehead remarks: 'No one ever says, here I am and I have brought my body with me' (Whitehead 1938/1968, p. 114).

'to develop guidance on processes for reaching agreements on the design, conduct and oversight of HIV prevention trials in developing countries'; and 'to build consensus on emerging issues in HIV prevention research and, hopefully, to develop norms and standards that can be used in this research' (IAS 2005, p. 14). The consultations provided a series of recommendations to ensure the regulatory conditions approach would be met in the future. This included the provision of treatment and care as well as prevention interventions for research participants; ensuring they possessed an otherwise lacking research literacy; and inclusion of consensual community representatives in the planning of trials (see Michael and Rosengarten 2013, p. 40). As the IAS goals indicate, the focus was on retaining and shoring up the future of RCTs. While 'research literacy' and 'community inclusion' were nominated concerns, they were rendered as necessary to the pre-decided importance of future RCTs taking place without opposition that could put future biomedical research in jeopardy. What was to be provided in return was the instituting of bioethical parameters to guarantee levels of health care for research participants. Thus, despite what might be said of the attempt to appreciate the needs of research participants, the two consultations consolidated not only the authority of science in determining the problem but introduced an approach that would foreclose on discord. In effect, they took what was voiced in the opposition as politico-ethical concerns and rendered them as considerably narrower bioethical concerns. The contrast I am drawing here between the ethical and the bioethical pertains to whether we see ethics as immanent to a situation or dependent on an overlay of regulatory procedures addressing biomedical issues. To put this another way, insofar as bioethical rules and norms are presupposed to protect research participants, bioethics shares the same world view as science on what matters.

With the benefit of hindsight, the additional bioethical regulatory provisions worked or, more accurately, they worked for science. There have been no similar overt protests displayed against RCTs. Indeed, I shall go as far as to suggest that it inoculated SMART, FEM PREP and VOICE from any questions pertaining to the pre-determined problem for which evidence was sought to validate PrEP as a solution. And what I have suggested above of the recalcitrance of the women in the Fem-PrEP trial was simply understood as deception or, as Cairns suggests in reference to a qualitative study on their behaviour, due to a deficit in their logic.

I will finish this genealogy with a 'before' to PrEP and the achievement of antiretroviral drugs that now serve as the basis for U=U (Undetectable virus = Untransmittable) in the UNAIDS/WHO '90-90-90' goals. In the late 1980s, members of the women's health field linked with others to forge the Global Campaign for Microbicides (GCM n.d.; Forbes 2013). The aim was to secure the development of 'barrier/contraceptive methods and virucides that could be woman-controlled and used 'without detection by their sexual partners'. As the feminist epidemiologist, Zena Stein stressed, evidence that condoms were efficacious for preventing HIV was irrelevant if a woman was unable to persuade her partner to use them (Stein 1990, p. 2). While we might applaud the efforts of this early feminist movement to enlist science, what we have seen above is a series of selected inheritances that have led to a reformulation of the problem. Although microbicides could be argued to have been superseded by PrEP, as either a pill or a long term injectable or implant, the orientation to women's needs arising from their relationship with a sexual partner has shifted to a focus on the women's individual capacity or lack thereof to conform to a biomedical expectation. Put simply, we might say that the feminist goal to find ways of meeting a need has been transformed to become less open to what this might demand. This does not preclude the possibility that PrEP might be more preferable than a vaginal microbicide. But ingesting a drug is, in conventional speak, 'socially' and 'biomedically' different from using a topical intervention.

In some key respects, the early feminist efforts parallels those of gay activism to enlist science in dealing with the problem of HIV. But both have evolved in a manner that can now be viewed as a highly biomedicalised approach to the epidemic. The distinction between the biological and social has been developed on the premise that the essence of the problem resides in an order of biological substances for which biomedicine has a solution but at risk from a lack in social conduct. In sum, the reality of HIV as a viral object that threatens life has grown in stature and, with it, a concern for biomedical advance in place of what makes the threat a relevant concern for the sociality of life.

21.4 Possibles in the Becoming of a History without 'End'

In the remainder of this chapter, I want to reflect on the biomedically posed problem that renders the social as both external yet central to its achievement of '*turning off the dynamics of HIV*'. This conception of the problem has been arrived at through a series of elements selectively inherited in a manner that matches what has been achieved by scientific advance. That is to say, we have arrived at a situation where what was initially sought from science to deal with a problem understood to be posed by a virus, has developed or, perhaps more aptly, mutated to match a radically reduced conception of what is at stake in treatment and prevention. As Kippax and Stephenson (2012, p. 789) see this in reference to prevention, biomedical solutions have become privileged but, in being so, they fail 'to realize that all HIV prevention interventions must engage with the everyday lives of people and be integrated into their social relations and social practices'. While some might argue that the proposal to refashion PrEP to provide a semi-permanent drug delivery without requiring dosing, not unlike the instituting of bioethical principles to shore up the viability of RCTs, is an important advance by science, it does not address the question of what may or may not make it meaningful for a heterogeneous category of persons. Persons whose individual circumstances may differ, including in relation to sex and to HIV. Instead HIV prevention and, arguably, much to do with what biomedicine understands as PrEP's efficacy, has become a fixed concern that is universally applied to an epidemiological category homogeneous in its risk of HIV.

In what follows I shall draw on a series of event thinkers, asking: what might enable an appreciation of the divergent realities that can be deduced in the relation between biomedicine and those for whom it presumes to act and, more so, decide for? Relatedly, I ask: what might enable a more relevant and, thus, ethico-practicable response in place of what has been formulated as a sustained deficit or absence in those affected?

To do so, I begin with a summary account of Alfred North Whitehead's radical revision of the notion of an event (1920/1964, pp. 106–110). While there are numerous elements from which we may make sense of the significance of an event, we inevitably select only a few and, with them, presume that the event is an independent happening. To be so, however, an event must be composed of stable sequential elements that can be viewed in the same way by all. Yet, as Whitehead points out, it is not beyond our awareness that what we perceive is a partial aspect of the multiple dynamic relations of objects and relations; and, also that its discernment is achieved in relation to other events (1920/1964, p. 10). If we pause here to consider the event of HIV infection, it is not beyond awareness that there is more than what we make of it and that others may perceive it differently. It is also not beyond our awareness that its happening is 'positive' in the sense that it makes a difference. Hence, counter to the view that what is at stake is a deficit or lack that presupposes an absence, this making of difference suggests that, on the contrary, there must first be a presence for its occurrence. To put this another way, any claim of a deficit is arrived at by way of a comparison between different 'things' and not *no* things. This leads me to a further aspect of Whitehead's account of events. The activity of the objects that constitute an event, what he terms 'adventures', 'determine the subsequent events to which they will pass on the objects situated in them' (Whitehead 1920/1964, p. 109). That is to say, elements are inherited into the making of a new event as we have seen with what has been made of the findings of research. Moreover, as I have argued, they have become inoculated from challenge by the inheritance of a correlative notion of bioethics determinant of their unquestioned legitimacy.

It is this making of findings and what has been made of them in the design of new research events that brings me to the notion of *problems*. As Giles Deleuze states, although events may be understood as problematising they are not, he says, in themselves, problematic. That is to say, they do not define what is *formulated from them* as a problem (Deleuze 1990, p. 54). Counter to the commonplace assumption that leads us to think 'problems are given ready-made, and they disappear in the responses or the solution' (Deleuze 1994, p. 158), we have a role in their formulation and, hence, in the required response. In the words of Martin Savransky, problems 'demand to be inherited, but they do not dictate the terms by which their heirs might inherit them' (Savransky 2018, p. 218). For Savransky this means that problems remain 'open' for what can be cultivated as a response to an event.

When reflecting on Steven Epstein's (1998) history of the HIV epidemic in the United States, Savransky describes a radically different conception of the dynamic to that of Fauci's. In Savransky's words: 'modes of togetherness involving viruses, medical specialisms, novel modes of gay activist socialities, antiretroviral drugs …

and prevention became together as provisional, evolving cases of solution to the problem posed by the event of HIV/AIDS'. With reference to my own work on the generative work of intervention, Savransky adds that in their inheritance: 'these solutions have never ceased to mutate' (Savransky 2018, p. 222; see also Rosengarten 2009). Arguably, the most topical example at the present time is the mutation of the initial normalisation of condoms to prevent HIV. While their use was promoted in relation to the problematic posed by AIDS, they have become a benchmark for many of the debates that now circulate on the 'whys' and 'where-fores' for PrEP. Nonetheless, these debates also suggest that condom use signifies differently in the context of biomedical interventions (see Blumenthal and Haubrich 2014; Auerbach and Hoppe 2015; Cáceres et al. 2015; Race 2016; Rosengarten and Murphy 2019).

However, it is the 'openness' of problems raised by Savransky that I want to pursue in order that we might arrive at a different kind of problem to that formulated by biomedicine. Here I turn to Isabelle Stengers description of the response to what she terms the 'AIDS event' in France, prior to the advent of antiretroviral treatments. Although similar in manner Savransky's conception of modes of togetherness, it adopts a more 'human-centred' approach to give emphasis to how a choice was made, in Stenger's words: 'of not yielding to the urgency of the strictly medical problem, of resisting demagogic and security-seeking temptations'. Instead, as she puts this, it involved a choice *'to pose the problem [HIV] clearly'* (Stengers and Ralet 1997, p. 216.7). The account does not detail the immense difficulties faced in making this choice, nor does it mention the inventiveness of cultivating the use of condoms as a protective barrier method *for* sex, in contrast to a public health insistence on abstinence (Kippax and Race 2003; Rosengarten and Murphy 2019). Nevertheless, it dramatises the importance of a *formulation* of the HIV problem that is *relevant* to those who live the response to it. To put this another way, the problem of HIV was not taken as if self-evident as now seems so for a prevalent biomedical authority.

In a recent article, Dean Murphy and I have suggested that this early phase of the epidemic can be regarded as the cultivation of a pragmatic response to the problem of HIV. Pragmatic in the sense that foremost in the response was a concern that it should be relevant to *living with* the given reality or the prospect of such a reality of a communicable infection and, moreover, without presuming to know in advance what would become (Rosengarten and Murphy 2019). By working with what was relevant to those affected by the event of AIDS, this early response to what otherwise seemed as a 'given' problem was effectively altered (Kippax and Race 2003; Kippax and Stephenson 2012).

If we now revisit the 'failure' of Fem-PrEP with the above arguments in mind, we can say that it was achieved by a selective process drawn from elements or charac-teristics known to comprise the trial protocol. For instance, bioethical requirements of consent forms, diagnostic technologies, research participants and so on. Elements that were assembled on the premise of a problem of a deficit in the body's capacity to ward off HIV and for which PrEP was decided as if the solution. Contrary to what I have offered of an earlier pre-antiretroviral phase of the epidemic, this was not a problem posed by modes of togetherness to which the women contributed, and according to what was relevant to them. Rather, it was and continues to be a problem formulated and matched *to* the gains achieved by pharmaceutical interventions. To put this another way, the problem of 'failure' for which the women were able to be held responsible was a formulation based on isolating a 'certain chunk' in the transitory life of multiple relations and objects that made the trial an event. And, as part of that 'chunk', the women were able be regarded as no more than a stable object of scrutiny. Bearing in mind what I have covered in this chapter and without presuming to know what might have become, we might nonetheless consider what other possibles might have emerged with an appreciation for what the women provided. *Not a deficit in the course of the event but a difference as the event.* That is, a difference achieved, as Savransky above might say, through the modes of togetherness involved in the trial. Thus, in contrast to the authoritative determinations of biomedicine of events and what has become of them.

To refer again to the recent SMART trial, despite additional support provided by the trial that did not achieve the difference anticipated, the problem remains for biomedicine and global health as resolutely tied to a deficit. Hence, the problem has not disappeared but has been developed to require a more insistent mode of PrEP, that is, a mode intended to bypass whatever the women's reasons were for not dosing and to the exclusion of what might, instead, be considered a complex nexus of factors. This does not exclude the possibility that PrEP in the form of long-term implants or injectables may have significant relevance for some women. Nor does it exclude that if so, HIV incidence would be reduced. But let us recall Fauci's suggestion that biomedical technologies need to be implemented 'properly, aggressively'. In light of the complex dynamics that have reduced the problem of HIV to a deficit in the women, we might wonder about what this will demand of their diverse and evolving realities as well as those of others for whom biomedicine decides.

Here it may be helpful to consider what Fraser, cited earlier, says of her discipline of sociology with its particular reliance on concepts such as structures, capitalism, and power to bring about change: these, she says, are 'abstractions that make sociology relevant to itself' (Fraser 2009, p. 76). I suggest that the same may be said of scientific concepts of bodies and viruses regarded as the essential stuff but also abstractions, in this case from the concreteness of HIV. As such they make science relevant to itself and, as I have sought to stress, have enabled it to increasingly extend its purview. While Fraser is not suggesting that we reject the perceptions of sociologists, nor do I suggest that we reject the perceptions of science. Rather, by treating events as the difference that is felt or registered between a 'before' and an 'after'—and not as if discernible according to an objective determination of time and space—we can appreciate, as Stengers (2000, p. 66) proposes, what a scientist perceives of an event while, also, appreciating that they do not have a privileged knowledge of what the difference made signifies.

21.5   Conclusion

Insofar as some might wish to believe that at last the feminist goal is to be achieved with long-term PrEP injectables or implants and that, the dynamic of the epidemic will be turned off, what I have endeavoured to suggest is that to see the epidemic in this way is to agree to what science has decided as relevant. To be sure, some *factors* in the dynamic may well become 'turned off'. We have already seen this to a significant degree with the introduction of antiretroviral drugs and the prevention of AIDS. But this has not made absent the inheritances of problems for which lay individuals and communities are held responsible and from which science is absolved. On the contrary, it has shored up a privileged scientific view of reality afforded by the licence provided by a conception of *bio*ethics, that is, a set of transcendental principles added in a manner that inoculates from challenge what science pre-determines as relevant.[4]

While HIV infection could well serve as the exemplar of the negative outcome of an event, that is, as creating a lack in the body's capacity to endure, it is nonetheless a happening involving not first and foremost an absence of elements but the very presence of elements to create the happening. It is the achievement of a felt experience, as are the solutions posed to the problems formulated from it. They are felt for the difference they make, a difference that impregnates the becoming of future events. Unwanted but real. If they weren't real we wouldn't be members of a field mobilised by matters of concern that I have argued are open to formulation. It is this that leads me to conclude that we have before us an unfinished history where events do not cease but, instead, remain generative due to the problematics they pose. A history where, to be sure, there is no guarantee of what will become, only the guarantee that a new difference will become of what has passed. And of which only some factors will acquire realisation in this difference. How they acquire realisation will depend on what will be taken up from prior events and by whom and/or what, including humans, viruses, research methods, publications and numerous other factors that may not be discerned. To put this another way, by assuming that problems are the bare fact of an event and due to a deficit or lack, we neglect its possibles. It is this that makes me hesitate about the promise of 'turning off the dynamics of the event' and doing so, as Fauci states, 'aggressively'. A promise that, for now, relies on first and foremost correcting a deficit. In sum, as if what matters is an absence in what makes HIV a matter of concern rather than, as I have sought to suggest here, according to what is relevant to those presupposed as central to the concern.

---

[4]For process thinkers, ethics can be more constructively appreciated as immanent to the value created by the dynamics of its situated happening (see for example: Savransky 2014; Sehgal 2018).

References

Auerbach, J. D., & Hoppe, T. A. (2015). Beyond "getting drugs into bodies": Social science perspectives on pre-exposure prophylaxis for HIV. *Journal of the International AIDS Society, 18*(4, Suppl 3), 19983.

Baeten, J. M., Donnell, D., Ndase, P., Mugo, N. R., Campbell, J. D., Wangisi, J., et al. (2012). Antiretroviral prophylaxis for HIV prevention in heterosexual men and women. *New England Journal of Medicine, 367*(5), 399–410.

Blumenthal, J., & Haubrich, R. (2014). Risk compensation in PrEP: An old debate emerges yet again. *The Virtual Mentor, 16*(11), 909–915.

Cáceres, C. F., Goicochea, P., Sow, P.-S., Mayer, K. H., & Godfrey-Faussett, P. (2015). The promises and challenges of pre-exposure prophylaxis as part of the emerging paradigm of combination HIV prevention. *Journal of the International AIDS Society, 18*(4 (Suppl 3)), 19949.

Cairns, G. (n.d.). *Magical thinking? FEM-PrEP trial may have failed because Participants used testing as prevention.* Aidsmap.Com. Retrieved January 9, 2020, from https://www.aidsmap.com/news/jul-2013/magical-thinking-fem-prep-trial-may-have-failed-because-participants-used-testing.

Celum, C., Mgodi, N., Bekker, L., Hosek, S., Anderson, P., & Dye, B., et al. (2019) PrEP use in young African women in HPTN 082 effect of drug Level Feedback. *Slide Presentation 23.* Retrieved April 12, 2020, from http://www.natap.org/2019/IAS/2019CelumIAS_082primaryfindings_FINAL.pdf.

Deleuze, G. (1990). *The logic of sense,* C.V. Boundas (Ed.) (M. Lester & C. Stivale, Trans.). (Reprint ed.). New York: Columbia University Press.

Deleuze, G. (1994). *Difference and repetition* (P. Patton, Trans.). New York: Columbia University Press.

Epstein, S. (1998). *Impure science: AIDS, activism and the politics of knowledge* (New ed.). Berkeley: University of California Press.

Fleck, F. (2013). The new Women's health agenda. World Health Organization. *Bulletin of the World Health Organization, 91*(9), 628–629.

Flowers, P. (2001). Gay men and HIV/AIDS risk management. *Health: An Interdisciplinary Journal for the Social Study of Health, Illness and Medicine, 5*(1), 50–75.

Flowers, P., & Davis, M. D. M. (2013). Understanding the biopsychosocial aspects of HIV disclosure among HIV-positive gay men in Scotland. *Journal of Health Psychology, 18*(5), 711–724.

Forbes, A. (2013). Mobilizing women at the grassroots to shape health policy: A case study of the global campaign for Microbicides. *Reproductive Health Matters, 21*(42), 174–183.

Fraser, M. (2009). Facts, ethics and event. In C. Bruun Jensen & K. Rodje (Eds.), *Deleuzian intersections in science, technology and anthropology* (pp. 57–82). New York: Berghahn Books.

Global Campaign for Microbicides (GCM). (n.d.). Retrieved December 20, 2019, from http://www.global-campaign.org/about.htm.

Grant, R. M., Lama, J. R., Anderson, P. L., McMahan, V., Liu, A. Y., Vargas, L., et al. (2010). Preexposure chemoprophylaxis for HIV prevention in men who have sex with men. *New England Journal of Medicine, 363*(27), 2587–2599.

Holt, M., & Murphy, D. (2017). Prevention optimism related to HIV pre-exposure prophylaxis: Shifting the focus from individual to community-level risk compensation. *American Journal of Public Health, 107*(10), 1568–1571.

IAS (International AIDS Society). (2005). *Building collaboration to advance HIV prevention: Global consultation on tenofovir pre- exposure prophylaxis research.* Retrieved July 1, 2012, from https://library.iasociety.org/MediaView.aspx?media_id=3391.

Jintarkanon, S., Napapiew, S., Tiendudom, N., Suwannawong, P., & Wilson, D. (2005). Unethical clinical trials in Thailand: A community response. *Lancet, 365*(9471), 1617–1618.

Kippax, S., & Race, K. (2003). Sustaining safe practice: Twenty years on. *Social Science & Medicine, 57*(1), 1–12.

Kippax, S., & Stephenson, N. (2012). Beyond the distinction between biomedical and social dimensions of HIV prevention through the Lens of a social public health. *American Journal of Public Health, 102*(5), 789–799.

Kippax, S., & Van de Ven, P. (1998). An epidemic of orthodoxy? Design and methodology in the evaluation of the effectiveness of HIV health promotion. *Critical Public Health, 8*(4), 371–386.

Koenig, L. J., Lyles, C., & Smith, D. K. (2013). Adherence to antiretroviral medications for HIV pre-exposure prophylaxis. *American Journal of Preventive Medicine, 44*(1), S91–S98.

Michael, M., & Rosengarten, M. (2013). *Innovation and biomedicine: Ethics, evidence and expectation in HIV*. Basingstoke: Palgrave Macmillan.

Newman, C., Hughes, S., Persson, A., Truong, H.-H. M., & Holt, M. (2019). Promoting 'equitable access' to PrEP in Australia: Taking account of stakeholder perspectives. *AIDS and Behavior, 23*(7), 1846–1857.

Nicholls, E., & Rosengarten, M. (2019). PrEP (HIV pre-exposure prophylaxis) and its possibilities for clinical practice. *Sexualities*. https://doi.org/10.1177/1363460719886556.

Race, K. (2012). Framing responsibility: HIV, biomedical prevention, and the performativity of the law. *Journal of Bioethical Inquiry, 9*(3), 327–338.

Race, K. (2016). Reluctant objects: Sexual pleasure as a problem for HIV biomedical prevention. *GLQ: A Journal of Lesbian and Gay Studies, 22*(1), 1–31.

Rosengarten, M. (2009). *HIV interventions: Biomedicine and the traffic between information and flesh. In vivo*. Seattle: University of Washington Press.

Rosengarten, M. (2017). Pluralities of action, a lure for speculative thought. In A. Wilkie, M. Savransky, & M. Rosengarten (Eds.), *Speculative research: The lure of possible futures* (pp. 71–83). Abingdon: Routledge.

Rosengarten, M., & Murphy, D. (2019). A wager on the future: A practicable response to HIV pre-exposure prophylaxis (PrEP) and the stubborn fact of process. *Social Theory & Health, 18*, 1–15. https://doi.org/10.1057/s41285-019-00115-y.

Rosengarten, M., & Savransky, M. (2018). A careful biomedicine? Generalization and abstraction in RCTs. *Critical Public Health, 29*(2), 181–191.

Savransky, M. (2014). *The adventure of relevance: An ethics of social inquiry*. London: Palgrave Macmillan.

Savransky, M. (2018). The social and its problems: On the problematic of sociology. In N. Marres, M. Guggenheim, & A. Wilkie (Eds.), *Inventing the social* (pp. 212–233). Manchester: Mattering Press.

Savransky, M., & Rosengarten, M. (2016). What is nature capable of? Evidence, ontology and speculative medical humanities. *Medical Humanities, 42*, 166–172.

Schillmeier, M. (2017). *Eventful bodies*. Oxfordshire and New York: Routledge.

Sehgal, M. (2018). Aesthetic concerns, philosophical fabulations: The importance of a "new aesthetic paradigm.". *SubStance, 47*(1), 112–129.

Sheth, A. N., Rolle, C. P., & Gandhi, M. (2016). HIV pre-exposure prophylaxis for women. *Journal of Virus Eradication, 2*(3), 149–155.

Stein, Z. A. (1990). HIV prevention: The need for methods women can use. *American Journal of Public Health, 80*(4), 460–462.

Stengers, I. (2000). *The invention of modern science* (D. W. Smith, Trans). Minneapolis: University of Minnesota Press.

Stengers, I. (2011). Sciences were never "Good.". *Common Knowledge, 17*(1), 82–86.

Stengers, I., & Ralet, O. (1997). Drugs: Ethical choice or moral consensus. In I. Stengers (Ed.), *Power and invention: Situating science (Paul Bains, P. Trans.)* (pp. 215–232). Minneapolis and London: University of Minnesota Press.

Thigpen, M. C., Kebaabetswe, P. M., Paxton, L. A., Smith, D. K., Rose, C. E., Segolodi, T. M., et al. (2012). Antiretroviral Preexposure prophylaxis for heterosexual HIV transmission in Botswana. *New England Journal of Medicine, 367*(5), 423–434.

UNAIDS. (2019). *19.6 million girls and women living with HIV*. Retrieved November 5, 2019, from https://www.unaids.org/en/resources/infographics/girls-and-women-living-with-HIV.

Valencia-Garcia, D., Rao, D., Strick, L., & Simoni, J. M. (2017). Women's experiences with HIV-related stigma from health care providers in Lima, Peru: "I would rather die than go back for care". *Health Care for Women International, 38*(2), 144–158.

van der Straten, A., Van Damme, L., Haberer, J. E., & Bangsberg, D. R. (2012). Unraveling the divergent results of pre-exposure prophylaxis trials for HIV prevention. *AIDS, 26*(7), F13–F19.

Whitehead, A. N. (1920/1964). *The concept of nature* (Reprint ed.). Cambridge: Cambridge University Press.

Whitehead, A. N. (1938/1968). *Modes of thought. 1st free press paperback*. New York: Fireside.

WHO/UNAIDS. (2006). Creating effective partnerships for HIV prevention trials: Report of a UNAIDS consultation, Geneva 20–21 June 2005. *AIDS, 20*(6), W1–W11.

Women's Network for Unity, Cambodia. (2004, June 15). *Protests drug trial recruitment tactics*. Public statement released by WNU Secretariat.

Young, I., Flowers, P., & McDaid, L. (2016). Can a pill prevent HIV? Negotiating the Biomedicalisation of HIV prevention. *Sociology of Health & Illness, 38*(3), 411–425.